THE CRAFT BEER
COOKBOOK & PARING GUIDE

© 2025 Chef Charles Michael Landutsch
All rights reserved.

No part of this publication may be reproduced, stored in a retrieval system, or transmitted in any form or by any means—electronic, mechanical, photocopying, recording, or otherwise—without prior written permission of the publisher, except for brief quotations in reviews or critical articles.

ISBN: 978-0-9825925-5-7
Library of Congress Control Number: 978-0-9825925-5-7

Published by
Chef Media and Publishing Group
Phillips, WI, USA

Wisconsin Edition

This book is intended for informational and entertainment purposes only. Recipes and cooking techniques should be followed with care and attention to safety. The author and publisher assume no responsibility for accidents, injuries, or damages resulting from the use or misuse of the information contained herein. Always follow proper food-handling practices, verify internal cooking temperatures from reliable sources, and consume alcoholic beverages responsibly.

Artificial intelligence tools were used during the development of this book for tasks including brainstorming, organization, and text editing. The author exercised full editorial control over the final content, and all recipes were personally developed and tested. AI systems do not guarantee accuracy, and readers should verify critical information such as food safety practices, cooking temperatures, and health-related considerations through authoritative sources. The author and publisher assume no liability for reliance on AI-assisted content.

Printed in the United States of America.

Website: www.CraftBeerCookbook.com

*Dedicated to all the bartenders
who have tolerated my shenanigans,
as I've drank across the World who I probably
didn't tip enough to not tell on me.*

Foreword

There's magic that happens when the right beer meets the right bite. It is not just about flavor—it is about harmony. A smoky porter that deepens the richness of braised short ribs. A crisp Pilsner that cuts through the heat of spicy wings. A citrusy IPA that lifts the zest of grilled shrimp. These are not just pairings—they are conversations between glass and plate.

This cookbook is a tribute to that dialogue. It is for the cooks who see beer not just as a beverage, but as an ingredient. For the brewers who dream of their creations being sipped alongside something unforgettable. And for the flavor chasers who know that the best meals are the ones that linger—on the tongue, in the memory, and in the stories we tell.

Inside, you will find recipes that celebrate the diversity of craft beer—from bold Stouts to funky Saisons—and the foods that bring them to life. Each dish complements, contrasts, or elevates the beer with which it is paired. Whether you are hosting a backyard barbecue, plating up comfort food classics, or experimenting with something new, this book is your guide to building unforgettable pairings.
So, pour a pint, fire up the grill, and let your taste buds lead the way. When beer and food come together with intention, every meal becomes a celebration.

Cheers to flavor. Cheers to craft. Cheers to you.

Contents

Beer Pairing 101 10
    Hop Flavor 11
    Bitters Flavor 12
    Malt Flavor 13
    Yeast Flavors 14
    Adjuncts and Additions 15
    Water Flavors 16
    Brewing Process 17
    Color 18

How to Taste and Evaluate Beer 19
    The Evaluation Process 20
    Craft Beer Evaluation Checklist 22
    Style/Flavor Reference 23

Cooking with Beer: Enhancing Flavors and Techniques 24
    Cooking with Beer: Style-by-Style Usage Chart 25
    Beer Favorite Recipes to Google 26
    Craft Beer & Food Pairing 27
    Beer Style Guide to this Book 28
    Beer Categories & Beer Style 29
    Outstanding Beer Pairing 30

Ale Beers 24
    Introduction to Pale Ales 26
    Pale Ale 27
    Beer Can Chicken 28
    American Pale Ale 29
    Pan Fried Pork Chops 30
    Bitter (ESB) 31
    Chicken Fried Chicken Recipe 32
    Imperial Pale Ale 33
    Bacon Smash Burger 34
    English Pale Ale 35
    Spiced Pork Chops with Apple Chutney 36
    Belgian Golden Strong Ale 37
    BBQ Brisket Nachos 38
    Belgian Pale Ale 39

- Cedar Planked Salmon ... 40
- Dubbel ... 41
- Braised Beef Short Ribs ... 42
- Saison | Farmhouse Ale ... 43
- Crock-Pot Dr. Pepper Shredded Beef ... 44
- Blonde Ale ... 45
- Shrimp Tacos with Mango Salsa ... 46
- Tripel ... 47
- Santa Fe Pork Medallions with Peach Salsa ... 48
- Quadrupel ... 49
- Grilled Leg of Lamb With Garlic and Lemon ... 50

IPA's ... 52
- American IPA ... 53
- Fish Tacos ... 54
- East Coast IPA ... 55
- The Best Ever Cheeseburger ... 56
- West Coast IPA ... 57
- Cioppino (Fisherman's Stew) ... 58
- Triple IPA ... 59
- Crispy Smoked Pork Belly Recipe ... 60
- Black IPA ... 61
- Slow Cooker Short Ribs ... 62
- Belgian IPA ... 63
- Roast Chicken with Rosemary and Lemon ... 64
- Sessions IPA ... 65
- Grilled Chicken Thighs ... 66
- Double IPA ... 67
- Grilled Ham and Cheese Sandwich ... 68

Sour Ales ... 69
- Wild ... 70
- Ceviche ... 71
- Lambic ... 72
- Smoked Chicken Wrap ... 73
- Beliner Weisse ... 74
- Bratwurst Stewed with Sauerkraut ... 75
- Flanders ... 76
- Smoked Ribeye ... 77

Wheat Beer 78
    Wheat Ales 79
    Shrimp Po' Boy 80
    Hefeweizen 81
    Chicken Satay with Peanut Sauce 82
    Gose 83
    Smoked Skirt Steak 84
    Dunkel 85
    Beef Rouladen 86
    Witbiers 87
    Vietnamese Pork Banh Mi Sandwiches 88

Brown Ales 89
    American Brown 90
    Smoked Brisket 91
    English Brown 92
    Pulled Pork Sandwich with Apple Slaw 93

Porters 94
    Baltic (English) 95
    Smoked Ham and Grilled Cheese 96
    Robust (American) 97
    Cowboy Sliders 98

Stouts 99
    Dry Stout 100
    Pepper Stout Beef 101
    Sweet (Chocolate) Stout 102
    Pulled Pork Mac and Cheese 103
    Oatmeal Stout 104
    Sticky Ribs 105
    Imperial Stout 106
    KC Burnt Ends 107
    Foreign Stout 108
    Crockpot Bourbon BBQ Meatballs 109
    Milkshake Stout 110
    Jamaican Jerk Chicken 111
    American Stout 112
    Smoked Baby Back Ribs 113

Lagers Beers 114

- Pale Lagers 116
  - Pale Lager 117
  - Chicken in White Wine Sauce 118
  - Light Lager 119
  - Green Chile Stew 120
  - Euro Pale Lager 121
  - Carolina Pulled-Pork Sandwiches 122
  - Pilsner 123
  - Crispy Beer Batter Fish 124
  - Czech Pilsner 125
  - Pork Cabbage Rolls 126
  - German Pilsner 127
  - Carne Asada Street Tacos 128
  - American Lager 129
  - Grilled Chicken Caesar Salad 130
  - Dortmunder 131
  - Smoked Pork Tenderloin 132
  - California Common- Steam Beer 133
  - Santa Maria Grilled Tri-Tip Beef 134
- Dark Lagers 135
  - Dark Lager 136
  - Savory Smoked Sausage and Potatoes 137
  - Helles 138
  - Chicken Sausage and Vegetable Foil Packet Dinner 139
  - German Pilsner 140
  - Flat Iron Steak 141
  - Munich\Dunkel 142
  - Caramelized Pork Ribs 143
  - Schwarzbier 144
  - Taco Chicken Enchiladas 145
- Ambers Beers 146
  - Amber Ales 148
  - Amber Ale 149
  - Blackened Salmon 150
  - Irish Red Ales 151
  - Sausage Mushroom Pizza 152
  - Amber Lager 153

Beer Braised Chicken with Carrots and Red Potatoes	154
Rauchbier (Smoked Lager)	155
BBQ Dry Rub Ribs	156
Marzen (Lager)	157
Bourbon Brown Sugar Smoked Pork Loin	158
Vienna	159
Smoked Sirloin Steak	160
Bocks	161
German Bock	162
German Pot Roast in the Slow Cooker (Sauerbraten)	163
Maibock/Helles Bock	164
Sausage & Pepper Flatbread Pizza	165
Doppelbock	166
Smoked Bologna and Pimiento Cheese Sandwich	167
Eisbock	168
Stout Beer Chili Recipe	169
Specialty Beers	170
Barleywines Ales	172
Rancher's Texas Chili Recipe (Chili con Carne)	173
English Ale	174
London Broil	175
American Ale	176
Oven Fried Nashville Hot Chicken	177
Strong Ales	178
Chicken in Ale Sauce	179
Scotch Ale	180
Brown Sugar Glazed Pork Chops	181
Christmas Ale	182
Baked Ham with Pineapple and Brown Sugar Glaze	183
Weizen	184
Garlic Grilled Shrimp Skewers	185
Altbier	186
Hot Smoked Salmon	187
Cream Ale	188
Hot Honey Butter Grilled Chicken	189
Wheat Wine	190
Penne Arrabiata with Smoked Sausage	191

- Kolsch 192
- Reuben Sandwich 193
- Fruit/Herb/Spice Lagers 194
- Slow-Cooker Carnitas Tacos 195
- Seasonal Lagers 196
- Honey Dijon Mustard Pork Loin 197
- Weiss Lagers 198
- Dry Rub Smoked Chicken Wings 199
- Cider Beers 200
- Crisp Cider-Braised Pork Belly 201

Beer Style Comparison Chart 202
BBQ Style and Beer Varietal Recommendations 203
Plan a Party 205
Recipe Index 206
Wisconsin Brewery Directory 210
Wisconsin Microbrewery Directory 211
Wisconsin Taphouse Directory 212
Wisconsin Brewpub Directory 213

Beer Pairing 101

Definition of Tastes in Beer

When describing the taste of beer, there are a few general definitions to help you understand how the flavors in beer are typically described:

- **Hops:** Many times, people use "hoppiness" to describe how bitter a beer tastes, but not all hoppy beers are bitter. The taste of a hoppy beer depends on when the hops are added in the brewing process. The earlier the hops are added, the more bitter the beer. Hops themselves have a versatile flavor and aroma that can enhance flowery and fruity flavors in the beer.
- **Bitter:** Bitterness is a distinct flavor profile found in many types of beer, although the amount of bitterness varies between the styles of beer. Many breweries rate how bitter a beer is with an IBU number. IBU stands for International Bitterness Units, and the higher the IBU, the stronger the bitterness.
- **Malt:** Malt comes from the barley grain, and it is usually roasted before it is added to the brew. Roasting barley gives the beer a nutty flavor and a toasty aroma. Plus, during the roasting process, the sugars in the barley caramelize, bringing out a slightly sweet, caramel taste.
- **Yeast is the unsung hero of craft beer**—a microscopic powerhouse that not only creates alcohol and carbonation but also defines the beer's personality. Its influence stretches from the brewing process to the dining table, making it essential for both beer making and food pairing.
- **Water is the silent architect of craft beer**—often overlooked, yet essential. It makes up 90–95% of a beer's composition and plays a pivotal role in shaping flavor, texture, and even how well a beer pairs with food.
- **The brewing process is the heartbeat of craft beer**—it transforms raw ingredients into a flavorful, aromatic, and textured beverage. Every step, from mashing to fermentation, influences not only the beer's final taste, but also how well it pairs with food.
- **Adjuncts and additions are the creative spark in craft beer**—they are what allow brewers to break the mold, push boundaries, and infuse their beers with unexpected flavors. From honey and spices to fruit and coffee, these ingredients transform beer into a culinary experience and open exciting food pairing possibilities.
- **Dark:** While it may seem more like a description of the color, dark can also describe how a beer tastes. Dark beers are made with malt grain that is roasted until it reaches a dark color. Dark beers typically roasted longer than malty beers, giving them a richer and heavier taste. The malt's nutty, caramel flavor turns to darker notes of chocolate and coffee with a longer roast time.
- **Light:** Light beer is usually known for having a clean and crisp taste that is refreshing. Typically, light beers do not have a strong flavor and are not very bitter or hoppy. Most light beers also have a low alcohol content.

Notes on Alcohol by Volume (ABV) & Flavor
Lower ABV (3.5–4.5%): Crisp, refreshing, ideal for long sessions.
Mid-range ABV (4.5–6.5%): Balanced hop-malt profile, classic pale ale territory.
Higher ABV (6.5%+): More intense hop character, fuller body, sometimes bordering on IPA territory.

Hop Flavor

Hop flavors are a cornerstone of craft beer—not just in brewing, but in how beer interacts with food. Their aromatic complexity and bitterness shape the beer's identity and open exciting possibilities for culinary pairing.

Importance of Hop Flavors in Craft Beer Making

- **Flavor & Aroma Profile:** Hops contribute citrus, pine, floral, herbal, tropical, and earthy notes. These flavors define styles like IPAs, pale ales, and Saisons.
- **Bitterness & Balance:** Hops counteract the sweetness of malt, creating a balanced beer. The timing of hop additions—early for bitterness, late or dry-hopped for aroma—affects the final taste.
- **Brewer's Creative Tool:** Craft brewers blend hops varieties to create signature profiles. For example, combining Citra (tropical) with Mosaic (berry and herbal) can yield a juicy, layered IPA.
- **Preservation & Stability:** Historically, hops were used to preserve beer. Their antimicrobial properties still help extend shelf life today.

Hop Flavors and Food Pairing

Hop-forward beers like IPAs and pale ales can elevate food pairings through **contrast, complement, and intensity** matching:

Contrast Pairings
- **Spicy Foods:** Bitterness from hops cools heat. IPAs pair beautifully with Indian curries, buffalo wings, or Mexican dishes.
- **Rich Meats:** Hoppy bitterness cuts through fatty textures—think grilled sausages or pork belly.

Complement Pairings
- **Citrus Hops + Citrus Dishes:** Cascade or Amarillo hops echo lemon or orange zest in seafood or salads.
- **Herbal Hops + Herb-Infused Foods:** Pair herbal hops with rosemary chicken or thyme-roasted vegetables.

Intensity Matching
- **Bold Beers with Bold Flavors:** Double IPAs or West Coast IPAs match well with sharp cheeses, charred meats, or umami-rich dishes.
- **Light Hoppy Beers with Delicate Foods:** Session IPAs or hoppy pilsners go well with grilled shrimp, sushi, or goat cheese.

Quick Pairing Guide using Hops Flavor

Beer Style	Malt Flavor Notes	Ideal Food Pairings
West Coast IPA	Pine, resin, citrus	BBQ ribs, blue cheese, spicy tacos
NEIPA (Hazy IPA)	Tropical, juicy	Thai curry, mango salsa, grilled chicken
Pale Ale	Floral, earthy	Burgers, roasted veggies, cheddar
Saison	Spicy, fruity	Soft cheese, seafood, vinaigrette salads

Pairing craft beer with food is like composing music—hops are the melody that can harmonize or play counterpoint to the dish.

Bitters Flavor

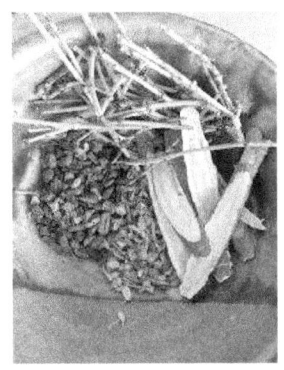

Bitterness is the backbone of many craft beers - defining a flavor that shapes the drinking experience and opens bold possibilities for food pairing. Far from being just a sharp taste, bitterness adds depth, balance, and complexity.

Importance of Bitter Flavors in Craft Beer Making

As a balance against sweetness, bitterness from hops (especially alpha acids) counteracts the natural sweetness of malt, creating a harmonious flavor profile. Without it, beer would taste cloying or flat.

- **Style Definition:** Bitter flavors are essential to iconic styles like IPAs, pale ales, ESBs (Extra Special Bitters), and even some stouts. The level of bitterness—measured in IBUs (International Bitterness Units) - helps distinguish these styles.
- **Ingredient Expression:** Bittering hops added early in the boil release alpha acids that define the beer's bitterness. Later additions (flavor and aroma hops) contribute complexity without overwhelming bitterness.
- **Palate Cleansing:** Bitterness acts as a natural palate cleanser, making bitter beers ideal for pairing with rich, fatty, or spicy foods.
- **Cultural & Historical Role:** Historically, bitterness helped preserve beer during long voyages (like the birth of IPAs). Today, it is a hallmark of craft brewing creativity.

Bitter Flavors and Food Pairing

Bitterness in beer can **cut, contrast, or complement** flavors in food, depending on how it's used:

Cut Through Richness
- **Fatty Meats**: Bitter beers slice through the richness of pork belly, duck confit, or burgers.
- **Creamy Dishes**: Try a bitter pale ale with mac & cheese or Alfredo pasta to refresh the palate.

Contrast Spicy Heat
- **Spicy Cuisine**: Bitterness cools the burning of chili peppers. IPAs pair well with Indian curries, Thai stir-fries, or buffalo wings.

Complement Savory & Umami
- **Sharp Cheeses**: Blue cheese, aged cheddar, or Gouda match the intensity of bitter beers.
- **Grilled Veggies & Roasts**: Bitterness enhances caramelized flavors in roasted mushrooms, Brussels sprouts, or steak.

Quick Pairing Guide using Bitters Flavor

Beer Style	Bitterness Level	Flavor Notes	Best Food Pairings
West Coast IPA	High (60–100+ IBU)	Pine, citrus, resin	BBQ ribs, spicy tacos, sharp cheddar
ESB (Extra Special Bitter)	Medium (30–50 IBU)	Toasty, earthy, balanced	Meat pies, bangers & mash, aged cheese
Pale Ale	Moderate (30–45 IBU)	Floral, citrus, herbal	Burgers, grilled chicken, nachos
Barleywine	High but balanced	Boozy, bittersweet	Stilton cheese, roasted lamb, chocolate cake

Bitterness isn't just a flavor—it's a tool for contrast, a bridge between ingredients, and a signature of craft beer artistry.

Malt Flavor

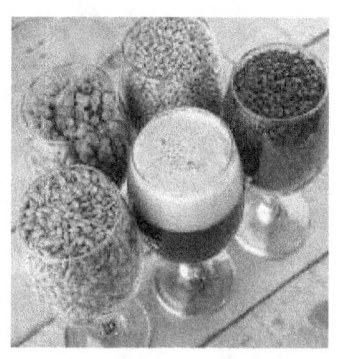

Malt flavors are the heart and soul of craft beer—they provide the body, sweetness, and depth that define a beer's character. While hops often steal the spotlight, malt is the unsung hero that makes beer rich, complex, and incredibly food-friendly.

Importance of Malt Flavors in Craft Beer Making
- **Fermentable Sugars** Malted grains (usually barley) supply the sugars that yeast converts into alcohol. Without malt, there is no fermentation—and no beer.
- **Flavor Foundation** Malt contributes flavors ranging from light and bready to dark and roasted.
- **Pilsner Malt**: Crisp, grainy, clean; **Munich Malt**: Toasted, biscuit-like; **Crystal/Caramel Malt**: Sweet, caramel, toffee; **Chocolate/Roasted Malt**: Coffee, cocoa, burnt sugar.
- **Style Identity:** Malt-forward styles like stouts, porters, brown ales, and bocks rely heavily on malt character. Even hop-forward beers need malt to provide balance.

Malt Flavors and Food Pairing
Malt flavors are incredibly versatile in food pairing because they offer **sweetness, toastiness, and umami-like dept**h that can complement or contrast a wide range of dishes.

Contrasting Pairings
- **Aged cheeses:** Gouda, Manchego, or Gruyère contrast malt's sweetness with umami and salt.
- **Cured meats:** Prosciutto or salami offer salty richness that highlights malt's depth.
- **Roasted nuts and olives:** Their earthy bitterness balances malt's sweetness.

Complementary Pairings
- **Roasted Meats**: A porter or brown ale with roasted malt pairs beautifully with brisket, ribs, or grilled mushrooms.
- **Caramelized Dishes**: Amber ales and bocks echo the sweetness of caramelized onions, roasted root vegetables, or glazed ham.

Intensity Matching
- **Low-intensity malts** (e.g., Pilsner, Pale Ale malt): Pair with subtle hops, light fruits (pear, apple), or mild cheeses. Ideal for clean, crisp beers or light desserts.
- **Medium-intensity malts** (e.g., Munich, Crystal 40°L): Match with richer flavors like caramelized onions, roasted poultry, or aged cheddar. Great for amber ales or malt-forward lagers.
- **High-intensity malts** (e.g., Chocolate malt, Black Patent): Balance with bold ingredients: espresso, dark chocolate, smoked meats. Use sparingly to avoid overpowering bitterness.

Quick Pairing Guide using Malt Flavor

Beer Style	Malt Flavor Notes	Ideal Food Pairings
Amber Ale	Toasty, caramel	Grilled chicken, roasted veggies, cheddar
Brown Ale	Nutty, chocolaty	BBQ pork, mushroom risotto, pecan pie
Stout	Roasted coffee, cocoa	Oysters, chocolate cake, blue cheese
Bock	Rich, sweet, toasted	Sausages, pretzels, aged Gouda
Scotch Ale	Deep caramel, smoky malt	Lamb stew, smoked meats, toffee desserts

Malt is more than just a brewing ingredient—it is a culinary bridge that connects beer to food in warm, flavorful harmony.

Yeast Flavors

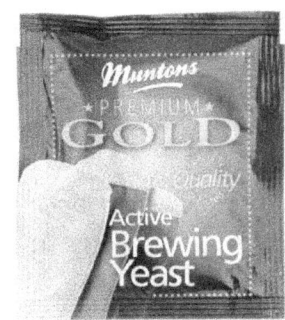

Yeast is the unsung hero of craft beer—a microscopic powerhouse that not only creates alcohol and carbonation but also defines the beer's personality. Its influence stretches from the brewing process to the dining table, making it essential for both beer making and food pairing.

Importance of Yeast in Craft Beer Making

- **Fermentation Engine:** Yeast consumes sugars from malt and converts them into alcohol and carbon dioxide. Without yeast, beer would be a sweet, flat liquid—not the bubbly.
- **Flavor Creator:** Yeast produces esters (fruity notes like banana, pear) and phenols (spicy notes like clove, pepper). Different strains yield dramatically different profiles: Ale yeast (Saccharomyces cerevisiae): Fruity, complex; Lager yeast (Saccharomyces Pastorious): clean, crisp; Wild yeast (Brettanomyces): Funky, sour, earthy.
- **Style Definition**: Yeast is the defining ingredient in styles like: Hefeweizen: Banana and clove from ale yeast, Saison: Peppery, earthy from farmhouse strains, Sour ales: Tart and funky from wild yeast.
- **Aroma & Mouthfeel:** Yeast affects carbonation levels, which influence texture and aroma release. Some yeasts leave residual sugars or proteins that enhance body and creaminess.

Yeast-Driven Flavors and Food Pairing

Yeast contributes **fruity, spicy, funky, or tart notes** that can elevate food pairings through contrast or harmony.

Complement: Match yeast flavors with similar notes in food:
- Hefeweizen (banana/clove) + banana bread or spiced pork
- Belgian Tripel (pear, spice) + pear tart or creamy brie
- Saison (peppery, citrus) + herbed chicken or citrus salad

Contrast: Use opposing flavors to create tension and balance:
- Funky Brett beer + sweet, glazed pork or pineapple salsa
- Sour ale + fatty cheese (triple cream brie) or rich duck confit
- Spicy phenols + cooling dishes like yogurt-based sauces or mild cheeses

Enhance: Highlight and amplify flavors through synergy:
- Estery yeast + fruit-forward dishes (stone fruit tart, citrus ceviche)
- Phenolic yeast + smoked meats or aged cheeses
- Clean lager yeast + delicate seafood or sushi

Quick Pairing Guide by Yeast-Driven Beer Style

Beer Style	Yeast Flavor Profile	Ideal Food Pairings
Hefeweizen	Banana, clove	Soft cheeses, grilled chicken, fruit salad
Saison	Peppery, earthy	Lamb, charcuterie, roasted root vegetables
Belgian Dubbel	Raisin, fig, spice	Braised beef, aged Gouda, bread pudding
Sour Ale	Tart, funky	Duck, blue cheese, berry compote
Lager	Clean, crisp	Sushi, pretzels, grilled fish

Yeast isn't just a fermenter—it's a flavor architect.

Adjuncts and Additions

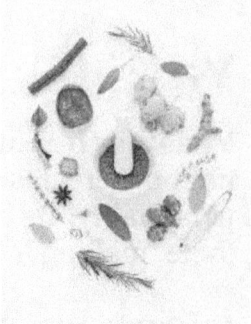

Adjuncts and additions are the creative spark in craft beer—they're what allow brewers to break the mold, push boundaries, and infuse their beers with unexpected flavors. From honey and spices to fruit and coffee, these ingredients transform beer into a culinary experience and open exciting food pairing possibilities.

Importance of Adjuncts & Additions in Craft Beer Making

1. **Flavor Innovation**
   - Adjuncts like oats, rice, corn, and rye modify texture and taste.
   - Additions such as fruit, spices, herbs, chocolate, coffee, and even chili peppers introduce bold, unique flavors.
   - Brewers use these to create seasonal beers, experimental styles, and signature brews.
2. **Style Expansion**
   - Adjuncts help define modern styles like:
   - Milk Stout: Uses lactose for sweetness and creaminess.
   - Fruit IPA: Adds mango, grapefruit, or passionfruit for juicy complexity.
   - Pumpkin Ale: Incorporates pumpkin and spices for autumnal warmth.
3. **Mouthfeel & Body**
   - Oats and wheat add smoothness and haze (common in NEIPAs).
   - Sugar, like honey or maple syrup, lightens the body while boosting alcohol.
4. **Visual & Aromatic Appeal**
   - Additions can enhance color (e.g., hibiscus for pink hues) and aroma (e.g., vanilla, cinnamon, citrus zest).

Adjuncts & Additions to Food Pairing

These ingredients make beer more versatile at the table, allowing for flavor matching, contrast, and thematic pairings:

Fruit Additions: Pair with salads, goat cheese, grilled chicken, berry desserts
Spices & Herbs: Pair with Indian cuisine, Moroccan dishes, roasted meats
Chocolate & Coffee: Pair with BBQ, mole sauce, chocolate cake, tiramisu
Sweeteners (Honey, Maple, Lactose): Pair with glazed ham, roasted nuts, creamy desserts

Pairing Guide by Adjunct Type

Adjunct/Additions	Flavor Profile	Ideal Food Pairings
Fruit (e.g., mango, cherry)	Juicy, tart, sweet	Grilled chicken, fruit tarts, soft cheeses
Spices (e.g., cinnamon, clove)	Warm, aromatic	Roasted meats, curries, gingerbread
Coffee & Chocolate	Roasty, bittersweet	BBQ, mole, chocolate desserts
Honey & Maple Syrup	Sweet, floral, earthy	Glazed pork, nuts, creamy cheeses
Oats & Wheat	Smooth, creamy	Sushi, creamy pasta, seafood

Adjuncts and additions are the brewer's spice rack—they turn beer into a canvas for culinary creativity.

Water Flavors

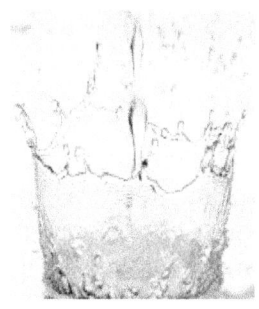

Water is the silent architect of craft beer—often overlooked, yet essential. It makes up 90–95% of a beer's composition and plays a pivotal role in shaping flavor, texture, and even how well a beer pairs with food.

Importance of Water in Craft Beer Making

1. Mineral Content Shapes Flavor: Water isn't just H2O—it contains minerals like calcium, magnesium, sulfate, and bicarbonate. These minerals influence:
- **Hop expression**: Sulfates enhance bitterness and crispness (ideal for IPAs).
- **Malt smoothness**: Chlorides round out sweetness and mouthfeel (great for stouts and ambers).
- **Fermentation health**: Calcium stabilizes enzymes and yeast activity.

2. Regional Water Profiles Define Styles: Famous beer styles emerged from local water chemistry:
- **Burton-upon-Trent (UK)**: High sulfate water → dry, hoppy pale ales
- **Pilsen (Czech Republic)**: Soft water → delicate, smooth lagers
- **Dublin (Ireland)**: Hard water → rich, roasted stouts

3. pH and Brewing Efficiency: Water pH affects mash efficiency and flavor extraction. Ideal pH (~5.2–5.6) ensures proper enzyme activity during mashing and a clean fermentation.

4. Water Treatment = Flavor Control: Modern brewers often adjust water profiles to match desired styles. Reverse osmosis water allows full customization of mineral content.

Water's Role in Food Pairing

Water affects **mouthfeel, bitterness, and sweetness**, which influences how beer interacts with food.

Pairing Examples Based on Water Profile

- **West Coast IPA (high sulfate)** Crisp, bitter → pairs with spicy tacos, sharp cheddar, grilled meats
- **New England IPA (high chloride)** Juicy, soft → pairs with sushi, creamy pasta, mango salsa
- **Stout (hard water, roasted malt)** Rich, smooth → pairs with oysters, chocolate cake, smoked brisket

Quick Pairing Guide Mineral Balance & Impact

Mineral	Flavor Effect	Pairing Benefit
Sulfate	Enhances bitterness	Cuts through fatty foods like BBQ or cheese
Chloride	Boosts malt sweetness	Complement desserts, roasted meats
Bicarbonate	Buffers acidity	Balances sour or spicy dishes

Water may be invisible in the glass, but it's foundational to flavor and pairing success. It's the canvas on which hops, malt, and yeast paint their masterpiece.

Brewing Process

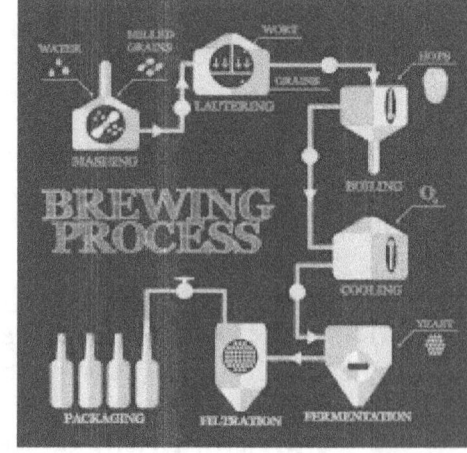

The brewing process is the heartbeat of craft beer—it transforms raw ingredients into a flavorful, aromatic, and textured beverage. Every step, from mashing to fermentation, influences not only the beer's final taste, but also how well it pairs with food.

Importance of the Brewing Process in Craft Beer Making

1. **Mashing**
   - Convert the starch in malt into fermentable sugars.
   - **Impact**: Determines sweetness, body, and alcohol potential.
   - **Pairing Tip**: Fuller-bodied beers from higher mash temperatures pair well with rich foods like stews or creamy pasta.
2. **Boiling**
   - Adds hops for bitterness, flavor, and aroma.
   - **Impact**: Controls bitterness and sterilizes the wort.
   - **Pairing Tip**: Bitter beers (like IPAs) cut through spicy or fatty dishes.
3. **Fermentation**
   - Yeast converts sugars into alcohol and CO_2.
   - **Impact**: Defines flavor profile—fruity, spicy, clean, funky.
   - **Pairing Tip**: Yeast-driven beers (like Saisons or hefeweizens) pair beautifully with herb-roasted meats or tangy cheeses.
4. **Conditioning & Aging**
   - Refines flavors, smooths harsh notes, and develops complexity.
   - **Impact**: Adds especially in barrel-aged or sour beers.
   - **Pairing Tip**: Aged beers match well with bold flavors like smoked meats or chocolate desserts.
5. **Carbonation**
   - Adds effervescence and affects mouthfeel.
   - **Impact**: Enhances aroma and refreshes the palate.
   - **Pairing Tip**: Highly carbonated beers cleanse the palate between bites—ideal for fried foods or creamy sauces.

Brewing Process & Food Pairing: Why It Matters

Brewing Step	Flavor Influence	Food Pairing Benefit
Mashing	Sweetness, body	Matches richness in meats or sauces
Boiling	Bitterness, hop aroma	Cuts through spice, fat, or strong cheeses
Fermentation	Yeast character	Complement herbs, fruits, and savory dishes
Aging	Complexity, smoothness	Pairs with bold flavors and desserts
Carbonation	Texture, refreshment	Cleanses the palate, enhances fried or creamy food

Craft beer isn't just brewed—it's crafted, and every step in the process is a flavor decision.

Color

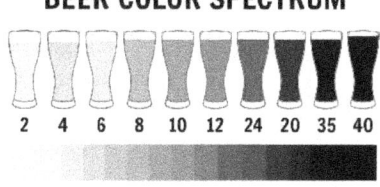

Color in craft beer is more than visual appeal—it's a window into the beer's soul. It hints at the ingredients, brewing process, and even the flavor profile you're about to experience. Here's how color plays a key role:

What Beer Color Indicates
1. Malt Type & Roasting Level: The primary driver of beer color is malt. Lightly kilned malts produce pale beers, while roasted malts yield darker hues. For example:
- **Pale gold**: Pilsner or pale ale malts.
- **Amber to copper**: Caramel or Munich malts.
- **Brown to black**: Chocolate, roasted barley, or black patent malts.

2. Flavor Expectations: Color often correlates with flavor intensity:
- **Light-colored beers** (SRM 2–6): Crisp, clean, subtle—think lagers, blond ales
- **Amber to copper beers** (SRM 7–15): Toasty, caramel, nutty—like amber ales or bocks
- **Dark beers** (SRM 16+): Roasty, chocolatey, coffee-like—stouts, porters, Schwarzbiers

3. Brewing Process: Longer boil times and Maillard reactions (browning of sugars and amino acids) deepen color and add complexity. Caramelization during malt roasting also darkens the beer and introduces sweet, burnt sugar notes.

4. Style Identification: Color helps quickly identify beer styles:
- Pale yellow: Pilsner, Kölsch
- Deep amber: Red ale, Vienna lager
- Dark brown to black: Porter, stout, imperial brown ale

<u>**Color & Food Pairing:**</u>
Color can guide food pairing by hinting at flavor intensity:
- **Light beers**: Pair with seafood, salads, soft cheeses
- **Amber beers**: Great with grilled meats, roasted veggies, aged cheeses
- **Dark beers**: Match with BBQ, chocolate desserts, rich stews
- So, the next time you raise a glass, take a moment to admire the hue—it's telling you a story about what's inside

Measuring Beer Color: SRM Scale

SRM Value	Color Description	Common Styles
2–5	Pale straw to gold	Pilsner, Blonde Ale, Kölsch
6–10	Amber to copper	Pale Ale, Vienna Lager
11–20	Deep amber to brown	Brown Ale, Bock, ESB
21+	Dark brown to black	Porter, Stout, Schwarzbier

SRM (Standard Reference Method) is the most common scale used in the U.S. to measure beer color scientifically.

How to Taste and Evaluate Beer

Beer tasting, much like wine tasting, is a sensory experience built on sight, aroma, flavor, and mouthfeel. Both traditions share the same goal: to understand, appreciate, and evaluate the beverage through its ingredients, craftsmanship, and balance. Yet the way beer expresses aroma, taste, and texture often makes the experience even more layered, more diverse, and sometimes more surprising than wine.

While wine begins with a single ingredient—grapes—beer is shaped by four core elements that each contribute differently to your senses:
- Malt brings sweetness, breadiness, roast, caramel, and color.
- Hops add bitterness, aroma, and flavors like citrus, pine, floral, or herbal notes.
- Yeast creates fruity esters, spicy phenols, dryness, or clean fermentation character.
- Water affects body, softness, minerality, and overall balance.

This combination makes beer tasting fundamentally more varied than wine tasting. Where wine's spectrum is wide but grape-driven, beer's spectrum is almost unlimited because changing even one ingredient can completely transform aroma, flavor, color, or mouthfeel.

Similarities Between Beer Tasting & Wine Tasting

1. Both Use Sequential Sensory Evaluation: Wine tasters move from appearance → aroma → taste → finish.
Beer follows the same structure, giving tasters a familiar rhythm.

2. Both Rely on a "Flavor Memory": To judge complexity and quality, tasters refer to a library of scents and flavors—fruits, spices, flowers, breads, chocolates, herbs, woods, acidity levels, and more.

3. Both Seek Balance: A well-made wine balances fruit, acidity, tannin, and alcohol. A well-made beer balances sweetness, bitterness, acidity, carbonation, malt, and hops.

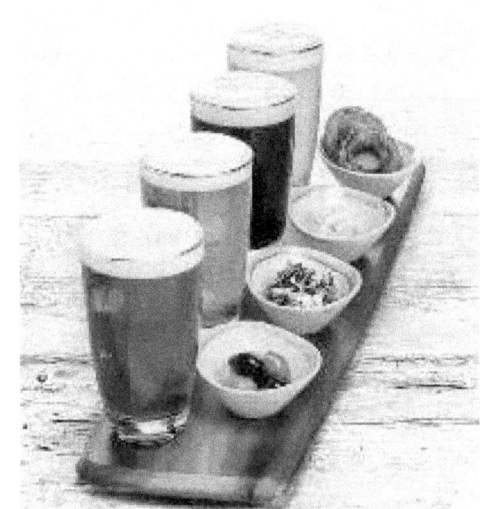

4. Both Highlight Craftsmanship: Every step in brewing—like fermentation temperature, hop additions, and malt selection—mirrors the decisions winemakers make with grape selection, oak aging, or fermentation choices.

Key Differences Between Beer Tasting & Wine Tasting

1. Beer Has Far More Aroma & Flavor Variety. Wine expresses grape varietals; beer expresses grains, hops, yeast strains, adjuncts, and brewing techniques.

A beer tasting can swing from:
- bright citrus (IPAs)
- deep chocolate roast (stouts)
- funky farmhouse spice (saisons)
- sour fruit acidity (sours)
- clean crisp grain (lagers)

Wine rarely covers this many flavor families.

2. Carbonation Plays a Major Role. Wine has bubbles sometimes; beer has them always.
Carbonation impacts:
- Aroma release
- Mouthfeel
- Perceived bitterness
- How a beer "cuts" through food

This is why beer often excels with rich, fatty, or spicy foods.

3. Beer Has More "Moving Parts" to Evaluate. Wine evaluation focuses heavily on aroma and texture. Beer evaluation requires analyzing:
- sweetness
- bitterness
- acidity
- roast
- hop character
- carbonation
- aftertaste
- mouthfeel
- malt complexity
- and overall balance of these features

This is what makes beer tasting more dynamic and interactive.

Beer tasting is not about being a critic—it's about training your palate, recognizing the craftsmanship behind each pint, and appreciating beer as one of the world's most diverse and expressive beverages.

The Evaluation Process

When tasting beer like a professional, every sip begins long before the beer touches your lips. A complete evaluation uses three core components—Appearance, Swirl & Smell, and Taste. Each one reveals different clues about the beer's ingredient quality, brewing technique, freshness, and style accuracy.

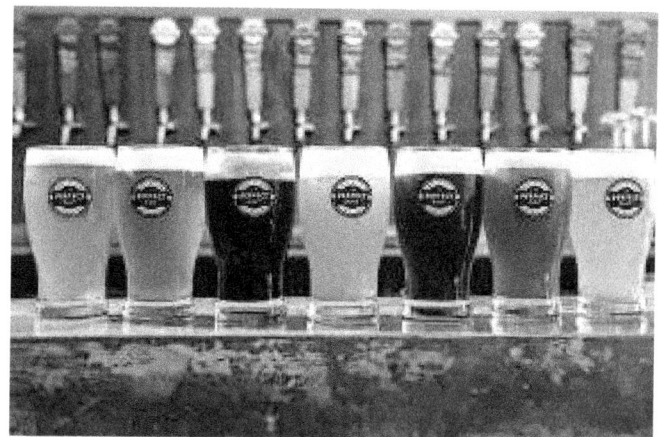

Just as wine sommeliers visually inspect wine, swirl it to unlock aromatics, and then taste for balance and finish, beer tasting follows a similar—but more dynamic—process. Beer's malt, hops, yeast, carbonation, and brewing methods create a wider range of aromas and textures than wine, making these three steps essential for understanding the full character of any beer.

These three components work together to give you complete sensory experience:
- **Appearance.** Your first impression of a beer comes from how it looks in the glass. Color, clarity, foam, and carbonation all speak to freshness, brewing precision, and style authenticity. Appearance sets the expectations for what the beer should smell and taste like.
- **Swirl & Smell.** A gentle swirl releases the beer's aroma—its most important sensory signal. Much of what we "taste" actually comes from smell. Malt, hops, fermentation notes, esters, phenols, and off-aromas all reveal themselves here. This step prepares your palate and frames your expectations for the first sip.
- **Taste.** Flavor is where everything comes together: sweetness, bitterness, acidity, malt complexity, hop character, carbonation, balance, and the lasting aftertaste. Taste confirms or contradicts what the appearance and aroma suggested, offering the full picture of the beer's quality and craftsmanship.

Lets explore each component further:

1. APPEARANCE

The first evaluation happens before the glass touches your lips. Beer appearance tells you a lot about style accuracy, freshness, and brewing technique. *What to Look For*
- Color – Straw, gold, amber, copper, brown, black.
- Clarity – Brilliant, clear, hazy, cloudy, opaque.
- Head Formation – Height, stability, and texture of foam.
- Lacing – Patterns of foam left on the glass. Indicates protein content and carbonation level.
- Carbonation Activity – Slow bubbles, lively streams, or CO_2 bursting at the top.

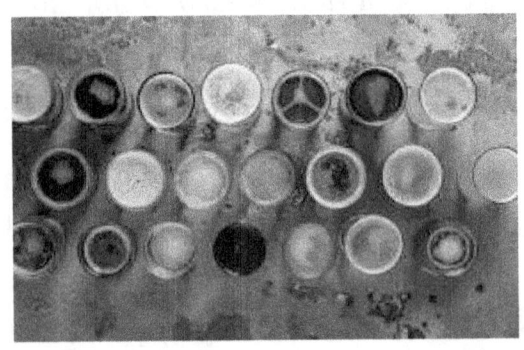

Appearance Evaluation Questions
- Does the beer match the expected style color?
- Is the head thick and lasting, or does it disappear quickly?
- Is the clarity appropriate for the style (e.g., hazy IPA vs. lager)?
- ABC, IBU, Description...What might you expect?

2. SWIRL & SMELL (AROMA)

Swirling releases volatile aromatics—the soul of the beer. *How to Swirl:* Give the glass a gentle rotation. This wakes up aromas without over-foaming. *Aroma Components*
- Malt Aromas – Bread, biscuit, caramel, toffee, chocolate, coffee.
- Hop Aromas – Citrus, pine, resin, tropical fruit, floral, earthy, spicy.
- Yeast Aromas – Banana, clove, pepper, fruity esters, funky phenols (Belgian, saisons).
- Fermentation/Process – Alcohol notes, smoke, oak, sourness.

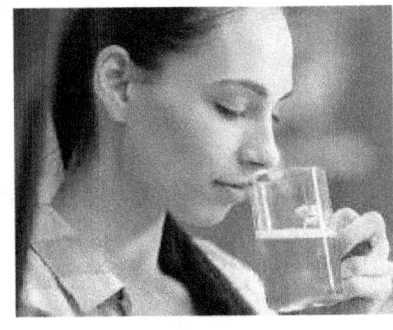

3. Taste

Flavor is where everything comes together: sweetness, bitterness, acidity, malt complexity, hop character, carbonation, balance, and the lasting aftertaste. Taste confirms or contradicts what the appearance and aroma suggested, offering the full picture of the beer's quality and craftsmanship.

Core Sensory Attributes to Evaluate

Key Attribute What to Consider? Acidity Lactic, citric, vinegar-like? Sharp or soft?

Sweetness	Malt-driven sugar perception. Light, moderate, high?
Bitterness	Hop-derived? Sharp, lingering, resinous?
Mouthfeel	Light, creamy, slick, astringent, full-bodied?
Aftertaste	Clean, lingering, bitter, sweet, dry, fruity?

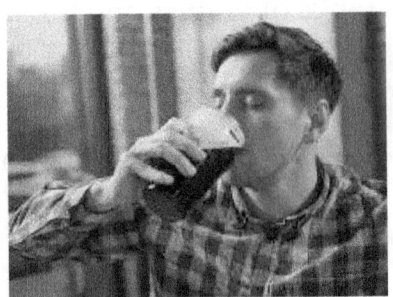

Why These Three Steps Matter

Evaluating beer through Appearance, Smell, and Taste helps you:
- Understand how ingredients and brewing techniques express themselves
- Identify what distinguishes one style from another
- Recognize quality, balance, and brewing flaws
- Describe beer more confidently
- Pair beer with food more effectively

Together, these components create a structured, reliable way to enjoy beer at a deeper level—whether you're a brewer, a taster, or simply a craft beer enthusiast.

Craft Beer Evaluation Checklist

Beer Name: _____   Style: _____
Brewery: _____ ABV: _____ IBU: _____
Date: _____

1 APPEARANCE

Color: ☐ Straw ☐ Gold ☐ Amber ☐ Brown ☐ Black ☐ Other: _____ **Clarity:** ☐ Brilliant ☐ Clear ☐ Slight Haze ☐ Hazy ☐ Murky **Carbonation (Visual):** ☐ Low ☐ Medium ☐ High **Head (Foam):** **Color:** ☐ White ☐ Off-white ☐ Tan **Retention:** ☐ Excellent ☐ Good ☐ Average ☐ Poor **Texture:** ☐ Creamy ☐ Frothy ☐ Fizzy ☐ Thin	**Appearance Notes:**

2 SWIRL & SMELL (AROMA)

Intensity: ☐ Low ☐ Medium ☐ Strong ☐ Very Strong **Aroma Characteristics:** ☐ Malty ☐ Bready ☐ Caramel ☐ Toasty ☐ Hoppy – Citrus ☐ Pine ☐ Floral ☐ Earthy ☐ Fruity – Esters ☐ Tropical ☐ Stone Fruit ☐ Spicy ☐ Yeasty ☐ Funky ☐ Sour/Tart ☐ Alcohol ☐ Off-aroma: _____ **Balance (Malt vs Hop):** ☐ Malt-forward ☐ Balanced ☐ Hop-forward **Aroma Quality:** ☐ Clean ☐ Complex ☐ Muted ☐ Off	**Swirl & Smell Notes:**

3 TASTE (FLAVOR & MOUTHFEEL)

Bitterness: ☐ Low ☐ Medium ☐ High ☐ Intense **Flavor Notes:** ☐ Malt – Bread / Toast / Roast / Caramel ☐ Hop – Citrus / Pine / Floral / Spicy / Herbal ☐ Fruit – Tropical / Berry / Stone Fruit ☐ Yeast – Phenolic / Spicy / Funky ☐ Other – Chocolate / Coffee / Smoke / Spice / Sour **Mouthfeel:** ☐ Light ☐ Medium ☐ Full ☐ Creamy ☐ Smooth ☐ Sharp ☐ Astringent ☐ Carbonation: ☐ Low ☐ Medium ☐ High **Aftertaste / Finish:** ☐ Clean ☐ Lingering ☐ Bitter ☐ Sweet ☐ Dry **Sweetness:** ☐ Dry ☐ Semi-Dry ☐ Medium ☐ Sweet	**Taste Notes:**

4 OVERALL IMPRESSION

Balance: ☐ Excellent ☐ Good ☐ Acceptable ☐ Needs Work **Drinkability:** ☐ High ☐ Medium ☐ Low **Flaws Present?** ☐ None ☐ Oxidation ☐ Diacetyl (buttery) ☐ Acetaldehyde (green apple) ☐ Phenolic (band-aid) ☐ Astringent	**Overall Notes:**

Final Score (0–50): _____

Style/Flavor Reference

Style	Flavor
Pale Ales	hoppy, citrusy, floral, lightly malty
IPAs	bitter, piney, citrus, tropical fruit
Sours	tart, fruity, acidic, sometimes funky
Wheats	light, bready, citrus, banana, clove
Browns	nutty, toasty, caramel, mild chocolate
Porters	roasty, coffee, chocolate, caramel
Stouts	roasty, coffee, cocoa, creamy, bitter
Pale Lagers	light, crisp, bready, slightly floral or gr
Dark Lagers	toasty, caramel, nutty, mild roast
Amber Ales	malty, caramel, toasty, ligntly hoppy
Amber Lagers	toasty, caramel, biscuity, lightly sweet
Specialty Ales	varies – can include spicy, fruity, herbal, or experimental flavors
Specialty Lager	varies – can include roasted, herbal smoked, or fruit-infused tones

Cooking with Beer: Enhancing Flavors and Techniques

In the culinary arts world, the incorporation of beer into cooking is a refined technique that can significantly elevate the complexity, depth, and richness of various dishes. Beer is not simply a liquid ingredient; it is a complex amalgamation of malt sugars, hop-derived bitterness, yeast-produced esters, carbonation, and sometimes acidity or smoky elements. Each component contributes uniquely to the overall flavor profile of a dish. When used with precision and understanding, beer can transform ordinary recipes into extraordinary culinary experiences, making it an invaluable resource for students, aspiring chefs, and seasoned cooks alike.

Understanding the interaction between beer and heat is crucial for mastering its application in cooking. The ingredients within beer respond predictably under heat, leading to specific flavor developments:

- **Malt sugars** undergo caramelization when simmered, producing notes of caramel, toffee, and toasted flavors, especially in styles such as amber ales, brown ales, porters, and stouts.
- **Hop bitterness** intensifies during reduction, requiring careful selection of hop-forward beers like IPAs and pale ales for sauces and glazes.
- **Yeast esters and phenols** soften with heat, imparting subtle complexity suitable for chicken dishes, braises, and bread baking.
- **Carbonation** acts as a natural tenderizer, lightening batters, tempura, and fry coatings, resulting in a crisp texture without excessive heaviness.

Choosing the appropriate beer for a specific dish can greatly enhance the final flavor profile. For example:

- Simmering sausages or bratwurst in a German lager adds a malty sweetness and depth of flavor.
- Finishing barbecue sauces with hoppy IPAs introduces a bright, bitter contrast that balances smoky richness.
- Baking bread with stout provides a rich, roasted flavor that complements hearty dishes.
- Marinating beef in Belgian Dubbel infuses the meat with fruity and spicy notes, enhancing tenderness and aroma.

Each beer style offers distinct characteristics that can complement various ingredients and culinary applications:

- **Stouts**: Known for deep chocolate and coffee notes, ideal for stews, gravies, and desserts.
- **Belgian Ales**: Fruity and spicy flavors suitable for roasted poultry and creamy sauces.
- **Lagers**: Light and crisp, perfect for seafood, chicken, and light appetizers.
- **Sours and Goses**: Bright acidity, excellent for marinades, ceviches, and dressings, providing a refreshing alternative to traditional citrus or vinegar-based flavors.

Ultimately, beer is a versatile ingredient that celebrates craftsmanship and creativity in the kitchen. Its ability to add character, aroma, and flavor transforms everyday recipes into memorable dishes. Whether used as a marinade, cooking liquid, or flavor enhancer, beer bridges brewing and culinary arts, offering endless possibilities for those eager to explore new flavors and techniques in their culinary journey.

Cooking with Beer: Style-by-Style Usage Chart

Beer Style	Best Uses in Cooking	Flavor Contributions	Notes / Tips
Pilsner / Pale Lager	Steaming seafood, light batters, chicken marinades, braising vegetables	Crisp, clean, lightly bready	Great for light dishes that need subtle flavor; enhances tempura and fish fry batters.
Helles / Kölsch	Chicken dishes, soups, light sauces, bread dough	Soft malt, gentle sweetness	Adds body without bitterness; ideal for delicate glazes.
Wheat Beer (Hefeweizen, Witbier)	Salad dressings, seafood, chicken, desserts	Citrus, banana, clove, soft malt	Perfect for marinades and fruity desserts. Avoid in long reductions to prevent overpowering spice notes.
Pale Ale	BBQ sauces, chili, marinades, roasted vegetables	Citrus, herbal, mild bitterness	Adds brightness and depth; bitterness intensifies when reduced—use carefully.
IPA	Spicy foods, glazes, bold BBQ sauces	Citrus, pine, strong hop bitterness	Works well for cutting through heat and fat. Avoid heavy reductions (can turn harsh).
Amber Ale	Burger mixes, stews, braises, chili, caramelized dishes	Toasty, caramel, malty sweetness	Excellent general-purpose cooking beer; adds warmth and color.
Irish Red Ale	Shepherd's pie, roasted meats, glazes, stews	Caramel, biscuit, light roast	Great for rich sauces and reductions; balances savory flavors.
Brown Ale	Gravies, roasted chicken, pork dishes, marinades	Nutty, toasty, caramel	Versatile for savory dishes; excellent base for pan sauces.
Porter	Chili, BBQ brisket, braised beef, chocolate desserts	Coffee, chocolate, roast	Adds rich depth to meat dishes; superb for brownies and cakes.
Stout (Dry, Sweet, Oatmeal)	Stews, braises, BBQ sauces, desserts	Chocolate, coffee, dark roast, creaminess	Great in baked goods, beef stews, and smoked meats. Sweet stouts excel in desserts.
Belgian Dubbel	Ham glazes, pork roasts, braises, sweet-savory sauces	Dark fruit, toffee, spice	High complexity; ideal for holiday dishes or rich sauces.
Belgian Tripel	Seafood, chicken, creamy sauces	Fruity esters, spice, soft warming alcohol	Use sparingly in reductions; adds gourmet flavor to white sauces.
Saison / Farmhouse Ale	Herb sauces, chicken, seafood, pickling	Peppery, fruity, dry	Enhances herbal or citrusy dishes; excellent for pickling or poaching.
Sour Ales (Gose, Berliner Weisse, Fruited Sours)	Ceviche, vinaigrettes, marinades, fatty meats	Bright acidity, fruitiness	Cuts through rich dishes beautifully; adds tang like vinegar or citrus.
Smoked Beer (Rauchbier)	BBQ marinades, beans, braised pork, baked beans	Smoky, savory, malty	Adds smoke complexity without a smoker. Use lightly—strong flavor.
Bock / Doppelbock	Pork roasts, braised meats, hearty stews	Rich malt, caramel, dark fruit	Great for winter dishes and heavy braises; adds velvety body.

Beer Style	Best Uses in Cooking	Flavor Contributions	Notes / Tips
Barrel-Aged Beers	Sauces, reductions, desserts	Oak, vanilla, bourbon, tannin	Use sparingly—intense flavors. Excellent for dessert sauces or bourbon-style glazes.

Beer Favorite Recipes to Google

COMMON BEER-BASED MARINADES

For Beef & Pork
- Stout & Molasses Marinade
- Porter & Soy-Garlic Marinade
- Amber Ale BBQ Marinade
- Brown Ale Steak Marinade
- IPA Citrus-Herb Marinade
- Doppelbock Mustard-Pepper Marinade
- Belgian Dubbel Maple Marinade

For Chicken
- Wheat Beer Citrus Marinade
- Pilsner-Lime Garlic Marinade
- Saison Herb Marinade
- Kölsch Honey-Garlic Marinade

For Seafood
- Lager–Lemon Dill Marinade
- Witbier Orange-Coriander Marinade
- Gose Lime-Chili Marinade (excellent for shrimp)

COMMON BEER BRAISES

Beef & Pork
- Stout Braised Short Ribs
- Porter Braised Beef Chuck Roast
- Brown Ale Braised Bratwurst with Onions
- Doppelbock Braised Pork Shoulder
- Dubbel Braised Ham Shanks

Chicken Dishes
- Belgian Ale Braised Chicken Thighs
- Amber Ale Beer Can Chicken
- Wheat Beer Braised Chicken with Citrus & Herbs
- Saison Braised Chicken & Vegetables

Seafood
- Lager Braised Mussels
- Ale-Braised Fish Stew
- Gose-Braised Shrimp with Chili & Lime

Vegetarian Braises
- Amber Ale Braised Root Vegetables
- Porter Braised Mushrooms
- Saison Braised Cabbage

COMMON BEER GLAZES

Sweet & Savory
- Stout Chocolate Glaze
- Honey-IPA Glaze for Chicken or Wings
- Brown Ale Maple Glaze for Pork
- Dubbel Brown Sugar Glaze for Ham
- Amber Ale Mustard Glaze
- Tripel Citrus Glaze for Seafood
- Porter Balsamic Glaze

Dessert Glazes
- Chocolate Stout Donut Glaze
- Fruited Sour Berry Dessert Glaze
- Caramel-Stout Sticky Bun Glaze

COMMON BEER-BASED SAUCES

Savory Sauces
- Stout Peppercorn Cream Sauce
- Amber Ale Caramelized Onion Sauce
- Porter Mushroom Pan Sauce
- IPA Beer Cheese Sauce
- Brown Ale Gravy
- Belgian Tripel Butter Sauce (great on seafood)
- Bock Beer Demi-Glace Reduction

BBQ & Chili Sauces
- IPA Spicy Beer BBQ Sauce
- Porter Sweet Molasses BBQ Sauce
- Rauchbier Smoky BBQ Sauce
- Amber Ale Chili Base
- Stout Beer Chili Sauce

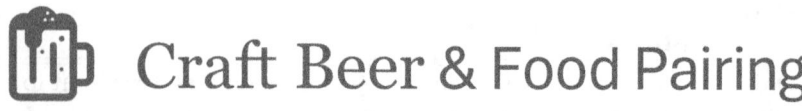
Craft Beer & Food Pairing

Pairing Information
Field Notes:
Beer Name / Style:

Food Dish:
Tasting Date:
Evaluator:

PAIRING PRINCIPLE SCORES (0–10 each)

Pairing Category	What to Evaluate	Score (0–10)	Notes
Complement	Do the beer and food share similar flavors?		
	Do malt, sweetness, spice, or roast enhance the dish?		
Contrast	Do differences (sweet vs spicy, bitter vs sweet) create balance or excitement?		
	Does the contrast work?		
Cut	Does carbonation, bitterness, acidity, or dryness "cut through" richness, fat, heat, or sweetness?		
	Subtotal:	___ / 50	

FLAVOR ALIGNMENT SCORES (0–10 each)

Attribute	What to Consider	Score (0–10)	Notes
Sweetness Alignment	Do sweetness levels clash or harmonize?		
Acidity Alignment	Does acidity brighten or overwhelm the dish?		
Bitterness Alignment	Does bitterness enhance or fight with flavors?		
Mouthfeel Match	Body, carbonation, creaminess, density—do they align with the dish?		
Aftertaste Alignment	Does the finish work with the lingering flavors of the food		
	Subtotal:	___ / 50	

OVERALL IMPRESSION

Category	Score (0–10)	Notes
Overall Pairing Success Would You Serve This Pairing Again? (0–10)		
Total Score		(Out of 110):

TOTAL PAIRING SCORE

Rating Level	Score Range	*Optional Add-On: Quick Pairing Summary Box*	Notes: (Complement / Contrast / Cut / Mouthfeel, etc.)
World-Class Pairing	95–110	Best Attribute	
Excellent	80–94	Weakest Attribute	
Good	65–79	Why Pairing Works?	
Average	50–64	What Would Improve It?	
Needs Work	Below 50		

Beer Style Guide to this Book

There are over 100+ distinct styles of beer (over 73 different ales, over 25 different lagers, Ambers, and a handful of hybrid styles) but to confuse the classification process, there are even more ways to group and/or sub-categorize beer. For example, you could group beers by flavor, by color, by bitterness, by ingredients, by region/country, by alcohol percentage, and so on. In this book, we cover four primary categories of beer: Ales, Lagers, Ambers and Specialty beers, broken into fourteen styles of beer and broken into about forty sub-styles of beer. Technically, Ambers & Specialty beers are brewed in an Ale or Lager style, but their taste profile can be so different they have their own categories.

1. **Pale ales** : Steak, barbecue, and Mexican food
2. **IPA ales:** Barbecue with rub or light sauce
3. **Sours:** Fatty cuts of beef BBQ, vinegar-based sauces, brisket, sausages, and hot links
4. **Wheat beer**: Spicy food and fruity desserts
5. **Brown ales**: Sausage, sushi, fish
6. **Porters**: Seafood, coffee-flavored desserts, game meats
7. **Stouts**: Chocolate desserts, shellfish, Mexican food
8. **Pale lagers**: Spicy food, burgers, salads
9. **Dark lagers**: Pizza, burgers, hearty stews
10. **Bocks**: Cajun food; jerk chicken; beef; sausage; seared foods
11. **Amber ales**: Spicy and smoked foods, such as chili, BBQ ribs, grilled chicken, and beef
12. **Amber lagers**: Tomato reduction sauces, foods flavored with basil and oregano
13. **Specialty Ales**: Strong cheeses or rich, sweet chocolate and caramel desserts
14. **Specialty Lagers**: Char-grilled and seared meats or hearty, spicy Mexican dishes

Pairing to Individual Styles and Sub-Styles of Beer

1. Crisp beers like Pilsners, Kolsch & Hoppy Lagers can cut through the fat of the meat.
2. Richer, maltier beers, like Brown Ales, Porters, and Smoked Beer, can add nicely to the decadence of meat.
3. Hoppy and malty beers, Black IPA & Barley Beers offer sweetness complementing the meat, while the bitterness cuts through the savoriness of the meat.
4. Dry, roasty and boozy beers, like Stouts, Porters, and Ales, can offset the fat and umami nicely.
5. Dark ales — Brown, Amber, and Black with not too much hoppiness — work best with leaner cuts.
6. Malty beers with caramel and dark fruit notes, like Tripels, Doppel, and Dunkelweizen are great for pulling out the best flavors of the meat and sauce.
7. For dry-rubbed ribs and less saucy meats, use sweet beers, like Witbiers or Hefeweizens, that will not overpower the delicate pork flavors.
8. Versatile beers like Rauchbier and Strong Pale Ales work well with sauced and dry-rubbed ribs, pork, or beef.
9. Brighter beers like Pale Ales, Dry-Hopped Lagers, and Saisons work well with citrus, herbal marinades of fish or chicken.
10. Heavy-sauced chicken develops caramel-sweet skin and pairs well with a Helles Lager.
11. Crisp, bitter beers like Kolsch or IPAs help cool down your tongue with spicier meats, even jerk chicken.
12. Light beers like German and Czech Pilsners go great with vegetables mild in flavor.
13. More acidic light beers like Gose or Berliner Weisse go well with coleslaws and potato salads.
14. Pair beers like Pale Ales or Saisons with toppings like cheese or ketchup for veggie burgers.

Beer Categories & Beer Style

Ale: Ale is a type of beer brewed using a warm fermentation method, resulting in a sweet, full-bodied, and fruity taste.	**Pale Ales:** Run the gamut from light and refreshing to heavy and unpalatable; they are known for their trademark bitterness
	IPAs: India Pale Ale is a hoppy beer style known for its strong flavors and aromas, originating from England, changing the craft beer scene.
	Sours: With yogurt-like tartness, sours can be soured in many ways, from introducing certain yeast strains to leaving the beer exposed and letting nature have at it.
	Wheats: Wheat beers can be light or medium-bodied and are very versatile when it comes to adding other flavors or ingredients.
	Browns: Dark ales are dark and nutty and usually medium-bodied without too much hop flavor.
	Porters: Porters originated in the UK, and are identified by their dark color, a light roastiness, and a hint of molasses-like sweetness.
	Stouts: Stout is dark, heavy, and roasted. Guinness is the most famous. Stout can be made in a variety of ways with several added ingredients.
Lagers: Lagers are light in body and crisper than ales, but there are exceptions. The taste is usually clean, and they are better served very cold.	**Pale Lagers:** The pale lager is a modern style of beer. Light in color and body, pale lagers are slightly hoppy and well carbonated.
	Dark Lagers: Darker than pale lagers, dark lagers are usually lightly hopped and, despite the color, not very heavy.
	Bocks: Bocks are brown to deep black with a medium-heavy body and a flavorful maltiness, with little hop character.
Ambers: Ambers can be easily identified by their color, which can run from amber to deep red. Amber beers can be ales, like Irish Reds lagers or smoked beers.	**Amber Ales:** - are characterized by a medium mouthfeel and colors that range from amber to a deep reddish-gold. These beers have strong flavors of malt, and there are notes of sweet caramel that complement the roasted malt taste. Many amber ales have a dry and crisp finish.
	Amber Lagers: are a medium-bodied lager with a toasty or caramel-like malt character. Hop bitterness can range from exceptionally low to medium-high. Brewers may use decoction mash and dry hopping to achieve advanced flavors. Brewed and conditioned at low temperatures.
Specialty: Some beer fails to fall into a category altogether. These can include strong ales, like barleywines, seasonal beers, and fruit or spiced beers.	**Ales:** Any specialty beer that does not fit other specialty beer styles would be appropriately considered here. Examples can include sahti, steinbier, white IPA, session IPA and more.
	Specialty Lagers: Are unique, creative interpretations of traditional lager styles. Brewed at cool fermentation temperatures, they maintain a clean, crisp profile while showcasing distinct ingredients or techniques—such as smoked malts, added spices, fruit infusions, or barrel aging.

Outstanding Beer Pairing

Pale Ales & IPAs
- American Pale Ale + Cheeseburger with sharp cheddar
- English Pale Ale + Roast beef sandwich
- West Coast IPA + Spicy Thai curry
- New England IPA + Mango salsa fish
- Session IPA + Fried pickles
- Double IPA + Korean BBQ ribs
- IPA + Jalapeno poppers
- Hazy IPA + Coconut shrimp
- Black IPA + Grilled lamb chops
- Pale Ale + Chicken tikka masala

Belgian & Sour Styles
- Saison + Herb-roasted chicken
- Belgian Tripel + Lobster with butter
- Belgian Blonde + Ham and Gruyère sandwich
- Lambic (Framboise) + Dark chocolate tart
- Gose + Ceviche
- Kriek + Duck breast with cherry glaze
- Gueuze + Charcuterie board
- Belgian Strong Dark + Beef bourguignon
- Saison + Goat cheese crostini
- Sour Ale + Watermelon feta salad

Wheat Beers (Hefeweizen, Witbier)
- Hefeweizen + Grilled shrimp skewers
- Belgian Witbier + Orange-glazed chicken
- American Wheat + Summer salad with goat cheese
- Dunkelweizen + Banana bread
- Kristallweizen + Lemon pepper chicken
- Witbier + Mussels in white wine sauce
- Hefeweizen + Apple strudel
- Wheat Beer + Avocado toast
- Belgian White + Chicken satay
- Dunkelweizen + Sweet potato fries

Brown Ales
- English Brown Ale + Bangers and mash
- American Brown Ale + Grilled portobello mushrooms
- Nut Brown Ale + Aged Gouda
- Belgian Dubbel + Braised short ribs
- Brown Ale + Maple-glazed bacon
- Brown Ale + Roasted root vegetables
- Nut Brown + Chicken mole
- Dubbel + Beef stew
- Brown Ale + Pecan-crusted salmon
- English Brown + Sticky toffee pudding

Porters & Stouts
- Dry Stout + Oysters on the half shell
- Milk Stout + Chocolate lava cake
- Imperial Stout + Blue cheese
- Coffee Porter + Tiramisu
- Baltic Porter + Smoked brisket
- Oatmeal Stout + Chili con carne
- Chocolate Stout + Black Forest cake
- Stout + Espresso-rubbed steak
- Porter + BBQ ribs
- Imperial Stout + Dark chocolate truffles

Light Lagers & Pilsners
- Pilsner + Bratwurst with mustard
- American Lager + Buffalo wings
- Helles Lager + Pretzel with beer cheese
- Mexican Lager + Fish tacos with lime crema
- Japanese Rice Lager + Sushi rolls
- Czech Pilsner + Fried calamari
- Italian Pilsner + Prosciutto and melon
- Light Lager + Grilled corn on the cob
- Rice Lager + Tempura vegetables
- Pilsner + Crab cakes

Amber & Red Ales
- Amber Ale + BBQ pulled pork
- Irish Red Ale + Shepherd's pie
- Vienna Lager + Chicken enchiladas
- American Red Ale + Pepperoni pizza
- Altbier + Roasted duck
- Red Ale + Meatloaf with gravy
- Amber Ale + Sweet potato casserole
- Vienna Lager + Cuban sandwich
- Irish Red + Corned beef and cabbage
- Altbier + Mushroom risotto

Strong & Barrel-Aged Styles
- Barleywine + Stilton cheese
- Belgian Quadrupel + Fig and prosciutto flatbread
- Bourbon Barrel-Aged Stout + Pecan pie
- Doppelbock + Roasted pork loin
- Eisbock + Dark chocolate truffles
- Barrel-Aged IPA + Grilled ribeye
- Scotch Ale + Smoked salmon
- Old Ale + Beef Wellington
- Strong Ale + Lamb shanks
- Barrel-Aged Saison + Duck confit

Fruity & Specialty Styles
- Fruit Beer + Strawberry spinach salad
- Pumpkin Ale + Roasted turkey with stuffing
- Honey Ale + Cornbread and chili
- Spiced Ale + Moroccan lamb stew
- Coconut Porter + Pineapple upside-down cake
- Ginger Beer + Teriyaki chicken
- Cherry Ale + Chocolate mousse
- Vanilla Cream Ale + Bread pudding
- Coffee Cream Ale + Breakfast sandwich
- Blueberry Wheat + Lemon bars

Ale Beers

Ale is one of the oldest and most diverse categories of beer, known for its rich flavors, aromatic profiles, and top-fermentation brewing style. Unlike lagers, which ferment at cooler temperatures with bottom-fermenting yeast, ales use top-fermenting yeast and ferment at warmer temperatures, resulting in a wide range of bold and complex flavors.

Origins & History
- Ancient Egyptians consumed ale daily for nutrition and refreshment. It was so vital that Cleopatra VII faced backlash for taxing it.
- Arthur Guinness began brewing ales in Dublin in the mid-1700s before switching to porters and stouts by 1799.
- In the late 20th century, the craft beer movement reignited interest in traditional ale styles like IPAs, stouts, and Belgian ales.

Key Characteristics
Fermentation: Top-fermented: Ale yeast rises to the top during fermentation.
Maturation: Most ales mature in 1 to 3 weeks, though stronger styles may take longer.
Taste: Fruity esters, Spicy phenols, Bold and complex: Often richer than lagers.
ABV Range: Typically, 4.5% to 9% depending on style.

Common Ale Styles

Style	Flavor Notes	Color Range	ABV Range
Pale Ale	Hoppy, citrus, pine	Pale amber	4.5–6.2%
India Pale Ale	Intense hops, tropical fruits	Golden to copper	5.5–7.5%
Brown Ale	Nutty, caramel, chocolate	Brown	4.2–6.0%
Porter	Roasty, coffee, dark chocolate	Dark brown	4.5–6.5%
Stout	Rich, creamy, espresso	Jet black	5.0–8.0%
Belgian Ale	Spicy, fruity, complex	Golden to amber	6.0–9.5%

Food Pairings
Pale Ale: Grilled chicken or fish, Spicy tacos, Sharp cheddar cheese, Fried foods (e.g., fish and chips)
India Pale Ale (IPA): Spicy curries, Buffalo wings, Blue cheese, Barbecue ribs
Brown Ale: Roasted pork or duck, Mushroom dishes, Gouda or Swiss cheese, Toasted nuts, Breads
Porter: Smoked meats, Grilled steak, Chocolate desserts, Aged cheeses
Stout: Oysters, Beef stew, Chocolate cake or brownies, Stilton or Roquefort cheese,
Belgian Ale: Roast chicken with herbs, Brie or Camembert cheese, Fruit tarts, Spiced sausages

BEER PAIRINGS

PALE ALE	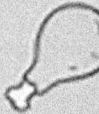 GRILLED CHICKEN	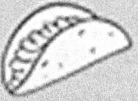 FISH TACOS	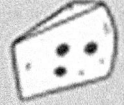 CHEODAR
INDIA PALE ALE	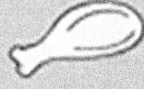 SPICY WINGS	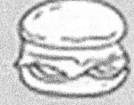 PULLED PORK	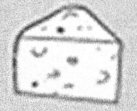 BLUE CHEESE
SOUR ALE	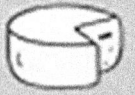 GOAT CHEESE	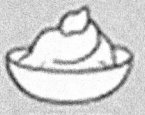 FRUIT DESSERTS	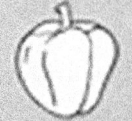 VEGETABLES
WHEAT BEER	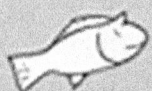 SEAFOOD	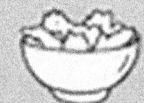 BRATWURST	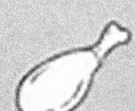 LEMON CHICKEN
BROWN ALE	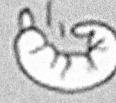 SMOKED SAUSAGE	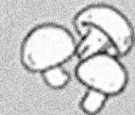 MUSHROOMS	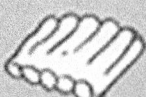 RIBS
PORTER	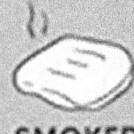 SMOKED BRISKET	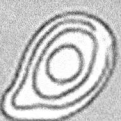 MOLE	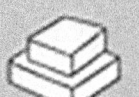 CHOCOLATE
STOUT	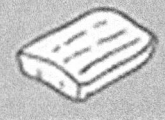 BABY BACK RIBS	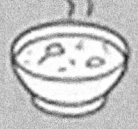 CHILI	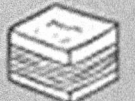 TIRAMISU

Introduction to Pale Ales

What Is a Pale Ale?
Pale Ale is a golden to amber-colored beer brewed with pale malt and ale yeast. It's known for its balanced flavor—malt sweetness meets hop bitterness—and moderate alcohol content, typically ranging from 4.5% to 6.5% ABV. Pale ales are the backbone of modern craft brewing, offering a wide spectrum of flavors from earthy and herbal to citrusy and tropical.

Flavor Profile Breakdown

Characteristic	Typical Range
Color	Golden to copper (4–16 SRM)
Bitterness	Moderate (20–50 IBU)
ABV	4.5% – 6.5%
Aroma	Citrus, pine, floral, earthy, fruity (varies by style)

Pale Ale Styles by Region

English Pale Ale
- Substyles: Bitter, Best Bitter, Extra Special Bitter (ESB)
- Flavor: Malty, earthy, floral hops
- Examples: Fuller's ESB, Bass Pale Ale

American Pale Ale (APA)
- Flavor: Bold hops—citrus, pine, resin—with a clean malt backbone
- Examples: Sierra Nevada Pale Ale, Dale's Pale Ale

Belgian Pale Ale
- Flavor: Fruity esters, spicy yeast, subtle hops
- Examples: Orval, De Koninck

Other Variants
- Australian Pale Ale: Tropical hops, light malt
- Hazy Pale Ale: Juicy, low bitterness, soft mouthfeel
- Session Pale Ale: Lower ABV, crisp and refreshing

Food Pairing Tips
- Grilled meat: The bitterness cuts through fat, while malt complements char.
- Spicy dishes: Hops amplify spice while malt soothes heat.
- Cheese: Try with cheddar, Gouda, or blue cheese for contrast.

Awesome Food Pairings

Pale Ale Style	Best Pairings
English Pale Ale	Roast chicken, shepherd's pie, cheddar
American Pale Ale	Burgers, tacos, spicy wings
Belgian Pale Ale	Mussels, charcuterie, creamy cheeses
Hazy Pale Ale	Sushi, Thai curry, grilled pineapple
Session Pale Ale	Fish and chips, salads, light pasta

Pale Ale

These are on the lighter end when it comes to heaviness, but the citrusy, floral blend of flavors will still hold up to the pork with enough malt and pair very well. Hops bitterness contrasts with spicy, heat-charred, smoky, or aromatic flavors, such as those in Stilton and blue cheese. These pair nicely with Texas-style BBQ. Pale ales and IPAs are great when paired with pork, poultry, veggie burgers, and even red meats.

Pale Ale: Key Characteristics		Notable American Pale Ales:
Attribute	**Description**	Fulton Pils
ABV	Typically, 4.4%–5.4%, offering moderate strength	Bass Pale Ale
IBU (Bitterness)	Ranges from 30–50, with noticeable hop bite but not overwhelming	Mirror Pond Pale Ale
Color	Deep gold to light brown or copper	Zombie Dust
Body	Medium-bodied, with a clean finish	Pale 31
Carbonation	Higher than English styles—crisp and refreshing	Anchor Liberty Ale
Flavor Profile	Balanced between citrusy/floral American hops and light malt sweetness	
Aroma	Bright hop-forward notes—think grapefruit, pine, or tropical fruit	
Finish	Smooth, slightly dry, with a lingering hop bitterness	

Taste: Malty | Hoppy | Refreshing Carbonation
Food Pairings: Cheese | Salmon | Grilled Meats | Mildly Spicy Dishes

Food Pairing Guide for Pale Ale
Pale ales are incredibly food-friendly. Their bitterness and carbonation cleanse the palate, while the malt sweetness complements savory dishes.

Grilled & Roasted Meats
- Grilled Chicken: Citrus and pine hops match well with lemon-herb marinades.
- Burgers: Sharp cheese, grilled onions, and smoky bacon are lifted by the beer's bitterness.
- Pork Ribs: Malt sweetness echoes BBQ sauce; hops add a refreshing bite.

Spicy Foods
- Mexican Cuisine: APA pairs beautifully with tacos, enchiladas, and chili. Citrus hops accentuate lime and cilantro, while bitterness tames the heat.
- Beef Birria & Quesabirria: Hop bitterness cuts through rich, spicy meat; malt elevates umami flavors.
- Pambazos (Chorizo & Potato Sandwiches): APA balances fried richness and spicy chorizo with refreshing bitterness.

Savory & Rich Dishes
- Sausages & Bratwurst: Spice complements hop character, especially with mustard or sauerkraut.
- Buffalo Chicken Dip & Pizza: Hoppy bitterness cuts through creamy or cheesy richness.
- Pale ales are the Swiss Army knife of beer pairings—adaptable, flavorful, and always ready to elevate your meal.

Beer Can Chicken

Pale ales have a balanced profile, with a touch of malt sweetness, mild hop bitterness, and often subtle fruity or citrus notes. These elements complement the smoky, savory flavors of grilled or roasted chicken beautifully. Unlike darker or hoppier beers, pale ales don't overwhelm the chicken's natural taste, allowing the seasoning and crispy skin to shine through. Pale ale's lighter body and moderate alcohol content make it ideal for this process. When served alongside the finished dish, pale ale acts as a refreshing counterpoint to the richness of the chicken. Its crisp finish helps cleanse the palate between bites. If the chicken has a smoky char or spicy rub, the citrus and herbal notes in many pale ales can elevate those flavors without clashing.

Ingredients:
1 Tbsp. dark brown sugar
1 Tbsp. kosher salt
2 tsp. dried thyme
2 tsp. paprika
1 tsp. freshly ground black pepper
1 tsp. garlic powder
1/8 tsp. cayenne pepper
1 (3 1/2- to 4-lb.) whole chicken
1 (12-oz.) can beer

Instructions:
1. Prepare a grill for high heat; close the top and preheat for 10 minutes.
2. In a bowl, combine brown sugar, salt, thyme, paprika, black pepper, garlic powder, and cayenne.
3. Remove neck and giblets (if any) from the chicken. Season chicken all over with spicy rub, reaching under the skin of breasts and thighs.
4. Lift and slide chicken legs side down over a beer can. The legs should be able to touch a flat surface.
5. At medium-low heat, place chicken on the coolest part of the grill. Cover and grill 40 minutes. Rotate chicken 180°, then cover and continue to grill breast registers 165° about 20 minutes more.
6. Using large tongs in one hand and a wad of paper towels in the other, carefully remove the chicken to a clean baking sheet or platter. Discard beer.
7. Let the chicken rest for at least 10 minutes, then carve and serve.

Classic Chimichurri Sauce
1 cup fresh parsley
3–4 cloves garlic, minced
2 Tbsp. fresh oregano
½ cup olive oil
2 Tbsp. red wine vinegar
1 Tbsp. lemon juice
½ tsp. red pepper flakes, salt and black pepper to taste

Finely chop parsley, garlic, and oregano. Combine in a bowl. Stir in olive oil, vinegar, lemon juice, red pepper flakes, salt, and pepper. Allow to sit for 15–30 minutes at room temperature, so flavors meld.

Also Pairs With

Witbeir	Amber Ales	Stouts & Porters

American Pale Ale

American Pale Ales have enough hoppiness to complement the spice flavors present in most BBQ, as well as enough malt to hold up to stronger, more savory flavors. An American Pale Ale will also have enough bright flavor notes to be refreshing and cleanse the palate. Complement the lighter elements of foods like seared scallops and oil-cooked garlic shrimp, while adding a refreshing flavor contrasts burgers and pork.

American Pale Ale: Key Characteristics		Notable American Pale Ales:
Attribute	**Description**	Indeed, Day Tripper Pale Ale
Color	Golden to amber	Sierra Nevada Pale Ale
ABV	Typically, 4.3% – 6%	Oskar Blues Dale's Pale Ale
IBU	Moderate bitterness (30–50 IBU)	Half Acre Daisy Cutter
Body	Medium	3 Floyds Zombie Dust
Aroma	Citrus, pine, floral, or fruity (especially in American versions)	
Finish	Crisp, balanced, slightly dry	

Taste: Hoppy | Citrusy | Malty
Food Pairings: Salty Snacks | Beef | Spicy

Food Pairing Guide for American Pale Ale
American Pale Ales shine when paired with bold, savory, and spicy dishes. Their bitterness cuts through the richness, while the malt adds depth.

Grilled & Roasted Meats:
- Grilled Chicken: Citrus hops complement lemon-herb marinades
- Burgers: Sharp cheese, grilled onions, and smoky bacon are lifted by the beer's bitterness
- Pork Ribs: Malt sweetness echoes BBQ sauce; hops refresh the palate

Spicy & Hearty Dishes:
- Beef Birria & Quesabirria: APA's carbonation and bitterness soothe chili heat and enhance umami-rich beef
- Pambazos (Chorizo & Potato Sandwiches): APA balances spicy chorizo and heavy bread with refreshing bitterness
- Mexican Cuisine: Tacos, enchiladas, and chili benefit from APA's citrusy hops and palate-cleansing bitterness

Savory Comfort Foods:
- Sausages & Bratwurst: Spice and fat are balanced by hops; great with mustard or sauerkraut
- Buffalo Chicken Dip & Pizza: APA cuts through creamy richness and complements spicy toppings
- American Pale Ales are the ultimate dinner companion—bold enough to stand up to spice and richness, yet balanced enough to enhance delicate flavors

Pan Fried Pork Chops

Pan-fried pork chops pair well with an American pale ale because of the light, crisp, and refreshing nature of pale ales, which complements the richness of the pork. The hops in pale ales help balance the flavors of grilled meats like pork chops, making them a great accompaniment. Pale ales are often low in alcohol content, allowing them to be easily consumed alongside the savory flavors of pork chops, enhancing the overall dining experience.

Ingredients
2 lbs. lean boneless pork chops, about 1.5 inches thick
1 tsp. garlic powder
½ tsp. kosher salt
½ tsp. freshly cracked black pepper
2 Tbsp. avocado oil
2 Tbsp. salted butter
½ tsp. minced fresh thyme or rosemary

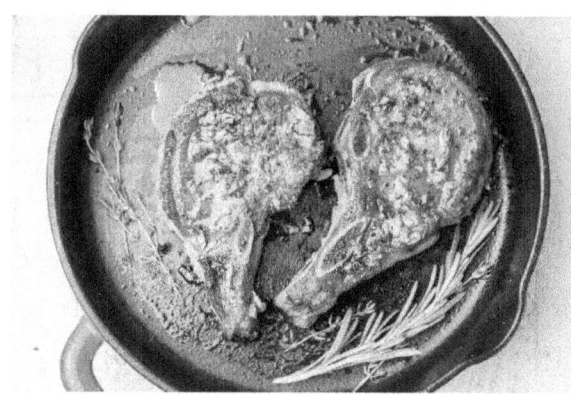

Instructions:
1. Rinse the pork chops and pat them dry with paper towels. Season both sides of the pork chops evenly with garlic powder, salt, and pepper.
2. Heat oil in a large cast-iron skillet over medium-high heat. Cook pork chops until the bottom side is golden brown and seared for about 1 to 2 minutes. Make sure your skillet is good and hot before adding the oil and then the pork chops to ensure a good sear!
3. Flip the pork chops and cook on the other side for about 1 to 2 minutes more before flipping once again. Repeat flipping the chops until they are deep golden brown and an instant-read meat thermometer inserted into the thickest part of the pork chop reaches 130°F. Total cooking time will be about 7 to 9 minutes, depending on the thickness of the chops.
4. Once the pork chops reach the desired temperature, add the butter and thyme. Continue cooking for 2 to 3 minutes more, while spooning butter on top of the pork chops until they reach an internal temperature of 145°F.
5. Place the pork chops on a serving plate and spoon the butter-sauce from the pan over the pork chops. Lightly cover the pork chops with foil and let them rest for 5 minutes, then serve. Letting them rest is an important step and will allow them to become fully relaxed, becoming much more tender and juicier.

Brandied Carrots Recipe
1 lb. carrots, peeled and sliced into ¼-inch rounds
2 tbsp unsalted butter
2 tbsp brown sugar (or honey for a floral twist)
¼ cup brandy
½ tsp salt and ground black pepper, to taste

ALso Pairs With:

Fruit Lambrics	Dunkels	Altbiers

Bring a pot of saltwater to boil. Add carrots and cook for 3–4 minutes until just tender. Drain and set aside. In a large skillet, melt butter over medium heat. Stir in the brown sugar and cook until it bubbles. Carefully pour in the brandy (it may flame briefly—stand back!). Stir and let it simmer for 2–3 minutes to reduce slightly. Add the carrots to the skillet, tossing to coat evenly. Cook for another 5–7 minutes, stirring occasionally, until the glaze thickens and the carrots are glossy. Sprinkle with salt and pepper. Garnish with herbs if desired.

Bitter (ESB)

Strong, British, and traditional cask-conditioned. Regional preferences create some maltier, stronger ales and some that are more aggressively hopped and carbonated. Expect caramel, toasty, and biscuit-like notes that provide a sweet backbone. Balanced bitterness: Earthy and floral hop character complements the malt without overpowering it. Fruity esters: Yeast contributes subtle fruitiness, adding complexity to the flavor. Aged or hard cheeses, chicken and pork and anything wrapped in bacon.

ESB (Extra Special Bitter): Key Characteristics		Notable American Bitter (ESB)
Attribute	Description	Robinsons Trooper Day Of The Dead
ABV	4.5–7.0% — stronger than Ordinary or Best Bitter	Minnesota Special Bitter
IBU (Bitterness)	20–40 — moderate bitterness, balanced by malt sweetness	Public Ale
Color (SRM)	8–18 SRM — deep gold to copper	Echo Sierra Bravo
Body	Medium — smooth and rounded	True Brit IPA
Carbonation	Low to moderate — often served on cask for a creamy texture	Calico
Finish	Balanced and clean, with subtle hop and malt interplay	Lord Admiral Nelson

Taste: Malty | Earthy | Biscuity
Food Pairings: Salty Snacks | Beef | Spicy

Food Pairing Guide for ESB
ESBs are all about balance—making them ideal for dishes that are rich, savory, or subtly sweet.

Classic British Pub Fare
- Fish & Chips: Malt sweetness complements the crispy batter; bitterness cuts through the oil
- Steak & Ale Pie: Rich gravy and tender beef match beautifully with ESB's toasty malt and subtle hops
- Bangers & Mash: Savory sausages and creamy potatoes are lifted by the beer's earthy bitterness
- Ploughman's Lunch: Cold cuts, pickles, crusty bread, and sharp cheese play off ESB's complexity

Cheese Pairings
- Aged Cheddar: Nutty and tangy flavors enhance ESB's caramel and toffee notes
- Red Leicester: Slightly sweet and nutty, it mirrors the malt profile for a harmonious match

Hearty & Savory Dishes
- Roast Chicken or Pork: Caramelized crust complements malt sweetness; hops refresh the palate
- Fried Foods: ESB's carbonation and bitterness "cut" through oil and fat, cleansing the palate

Surprising Sweet Pairings
- Toffee Pudding or Caramel Desserts: ESB's malt echoes the dessert's sweetness without clashing

Chicken Fried Chicken Recipe

Fried chicken is indulgent—crispy batter, juicy meat, often seasoned with salt and spices. ESBs have a moderate bitterness that acts like a palate cleanser, slicing through the fat and refreshing your taste buds between bites. The carbonation in beer helps lift the richness off your tongue, making each bite feel lighter and more enjoyable. If your chicken fried chicken comes with gravy, the ESB's earthy bitterness can contrast beautifully with the creamy sauce, adding depth and complexity to each mouthful.

Ingredients:

For the chicken
2 large chicken breasts
2 cups buttermilk
1 tsp. salt
1 tsp. black pepper
1 egg

To Cook
1 cup vegetable oil

For the seasoned flour
1 ½ cups all-purpose flour
1 tsp. ground black pepper
1 tsp. salt
1 tsp. paprika
½ tsp. smoked paprika
½ tsp. cayenne pepper
½ tsp. onion powder
½ tsp. baking soda
½ tsp. baking powder

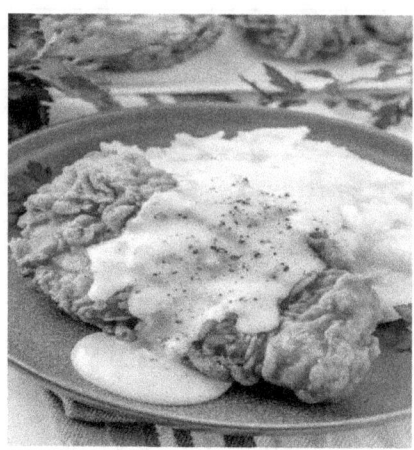

Instructions:
1. Prepare the chicken. Mix the buttermilk in a non-metallic bowl, with salt and black pepper: 2 cups buttermilk, 1 tsp. salt, 1 tsp. black pepper.
2. Lay your chicken breast flat on the board, then keeping your knife parallel to the chopping board, use a large sharp knife to cut sideways through the breast. Continue cutting through the chicken breast, keeping the knife flat until you have two plump fillets. Repeat with the second chicken breast.
3. Cover the chicken with parchment paper or plastic wrap and then use the smooth side of a meat mallet or a heavy-bottomed pan, to flatten the chicken to an equal thickness.
4. Add the chicken to the buttermilk and let it sit at room temperature for 30 minutes to an hour.
5. Dredge chicken breasts in seasoned flour.
6. Heat oil in a large saucepan to 350 degrees. Fry chicken, turning frequently, until golden brown, about 15 to 20 minutes.

Chicken-Fried Chicken Gravy (White Pepper Gravy)
2 tbsp pan drippings (from frying the chicken)
2 tbsp all-purpose flour
1½ cups whole milk (warm)
Salt & pepper to taste
Pinch of cayenne or smoked paprika for a kick

Also Pairs With		
Hefeweizen	Brown Ales	Gose

In the same skillet used for frying (leave about 2 tbsp of drippings), sprinkle in the flour. Whisk constantly over medium heat until it turns golden brown—about 2 minutes. Gradually pour in warm milk while whisking to avoid lumps. Keep whisking until it goes smoothly. Let it bubble gently for 3–5 minutes until thickened. Season with salt and lots of black pepper.

Imperial Pale Ale

Imperial India pale ale is darker in color than the American IPA, more bitter, and higher in alcohol by volume. The imperial India pale ale features high hop bitterness, flavor, and aroma that pair with strong spices and meats like brisket and lamb.

Imperial Pale Ale Key Characteristics		Notable American Imperial Pale Ale
Attribute	Description	Pliny the Elder
ABV	7–11% — significantly stronger than standard pale ales	Heady Topper
IBU (Bitterness)	60–100+ — intense bitterness, often resinous or citrusy	90 Minute IPA
Color (SRM)	6–14 SRM — deep gold to copper	Double Jack
Body	Medium to full — rich, sometimes warming	Hopslam Ale
Carbonation	Medium to high — helps lift bold flavors	Dreadnaught Imperial IPA
Finish	Dry to slightly sweet, with lingering hop bitterness	

Taste: Hoppy | Malty | Carmel
Food Pairings: Salty Snacks | Beef | Vegetables

Food Pairing Guide for Imperial Pale Ale

Imperial Pale Ales demand bold, flavorful dishes that can stand up to their intensity. Think rich, spicy, fatty, or umami-packed foods.

Spicy & Bold Dishes
- Indian Curries (Madras, Vindaloo): Bitterness cools the heat; hops complement spices like coriander and cardamom
- Buffalo Wings: IPA's bitterness cuts through the heat and fat; malt echoes the caramelized skin
- Mexican Street Tacos (Al Pastor, Chorizo): Citrus hops enhance lime and spice; bitterness balances fatty meats

Rich & Umami-Heavy Meats
- Grilled Ribeye or NY Strip Steak: Charred crust and juicy fat match the beer's bold malt and hop punch.
- Pulled Pork or Brisket: Smoky, sweet BBQ flavors pair beautifully with caramel malt and hop bitterness.
- Burgers with Blue Cheese or Bacon Jam: Funky cheese and sweet-savory toppings are tamed by the beer's intensity.

Salty & Aged Cheeses
- Aged Gouda or Sharp Cheddar: Salt and umami amplify hop bitterness and malt depth.
- Blue Cheese: Funky richness meets its match in the beer's bold hop profile.

Fried & Fatty Foods
- Fried Chicken or Cheese Curds: Salt and fat mellow the bitterness; carbonation cleanses the palate.
- Loaded Fries or Nachos: Rich toppings like sour cream, bacon, and jalapenos are balanced by hops and malt.
- Imperial Pale Ales are not subtle—but that's their charm. Pair them with dishes that are equally expressive, and you'll unlock a whole new level of flavor synergy.

Bacon Smash Burger

A bacon smash burger is rich, salty, smoky, and fatty. It's got crispy edges, melty cheese, and that umami punch from seared beef and bacon. You need a beer that can stand up to all that—and an Imperial Pale Ale brings the muscle. With higher alcohol and intense hop character, it doesn't get drowned out. The bitterness from the hops cuts through the richness of the burger like a knife through butter. It scrubs your palate clean after each bite, making the next one just as satisfying.

Ingredients:
2 pounds ground chuck (80/20), formed into 1/3-pound balls
2 white onions, thinly sliced
1/2-pound bacon, crispy and chopped
Salt, pepper, garlic for seasoning
Yellow mustard for cooking
Pepper jack cheese slices
Brioche Burger buns
Avocado oil for cooking
Bacon Jam

Smash Sauce
1/2 cup mayo
2 Tbsp. ketchup
2 Tbsp. mustard
1 Tbsp. Worcestershire sauce
1 Tbsp. apple cider vinegar
1 Tbsp. all-purpose rub
1 Tbsp. red pepper flakes

Instructions:
1. Form ground chuck into 1/3-pound balls and chill for 30 minutes.
2. Slice the onions thinly using a mandolin, squeeze out water and refrigerate.
3. Cook bacon until crispy, chop and set aside.
4. Mix mayo, ketchup, mustard, bacon, Worcestershire, vinegar, rub and pepper flakes. Chill.
5. Heat griddle, add oil, place meatballs, top with onions and smash. Season and cook 3-4 minutes.
6. Add mustard, flip, add cheese and cook 3 minutes until it melts.
7. Toast buns, coat one bun with bacon jam and the other with smash sauce, stack double burgers with some sauce between the burgers.

Also Pairs With		
Belgium Ales	Rich Stouts	Ranchbier

English Pale Ale

An English Pale Ale is a classic beer associated with the city of Burton-upon-Trent in England, a region known for its hard water, rich in calcium sulfate. This water quality enhances hop bitterness and contributes to beer clarity. English Pale Ales can vary in color, falling anywhere between golden and reddish amber. Aromas and flavors are a delightful mix of fruity notes, hoppy elements, earthy tones, hints of butteriness, and malt sweetness.

English Pale Ale: Key Characteristics		Notable English Pale Ales
Attribute	**Description**	Boddingtons Pub Ale
ABV	4.5–5.5% — moderate strength, ideal for session drinking	Bass Pale Ale
IBU (Bitterness)	20–40 — gentle bitterness, more earthy than sharp	Old Speckled Hen
Color (SRM)	8–14 SRM — golden to copper hues	Organic Pale Ale
Body	Medium — smooth and rounded mouthfeel	Fuller's London Pride
Carbonation	Low to moderate — often served on cask for a creamy texture	
Finish	Balanced — subtle hop bitterness and malt sweetness linger	

Taste: Fruity | Malty | Earthy | Sweet
Food Pairings: Beef | Grilled Sausages & Veggies | Cold Cuts

Food Pairing Guide for English Pale Ale
English Pale Ales are all about balance, so pair them with dishes that complement their malt sweetness and earthy hops without overpowering them.

Classic British Fare
- Steak & Kidney Pie / Pork Pie: Rich, savory fillings and buttery pastry match the malt depth and are refreshed by the beer's bitterness
- Roast Beef or Pork with Crackling: Umami-rich meats and crispy textures are elevated by the ale's caramel notes and dry finish
- Chicken & Mushroom Pie: Earthy mushrooms & creamy sauce pair beautifully with floral hops

Cheese Pairings
- Aged Cheddar: Sharpness balances malt sweetness
- Red Leicester: Nutty and slightly sweet, echoing the beer's toasty notes
- Stilton: Bold blue cheese matches the earthy hop character

Hearty & Savory Dishes
- Grilled Sausages & Mash: Savory sausage and creamy potatoes are lifted by bitterness and carbonation
- Shepherd's Pie: Ground lamb or beef with mashed potatoes and gravy pairs well with malt-forward beers

Lighter Options
- Ploughman's Lunch: Cold cuts, pickles, crusty bread, and cheese—perfect with the ale's balanced profile
- Grilled Veggie Sandwiches: Earthy vegetables and toasted bread mirror the beer's herbal and biscuity notes

Spiced Pork Chops with Apple Chutney

English Pale Ales have a moderate bitterness and earthy hop character that balances beautifully with the sweet-tart profile of apple chutney and the warm spices on the pork. The hops cut through the richness, while the malt complements the chutney's caramelized notes. Malty backbone that enhances savory depth with flavors of biscuit, toast, and subtle caramel, the malt in English Pale Ale mirrors the seared crust of the pork and adds depth to the dish without overpowering it.

Ingredients:
Chutney
1 Tbsp. butter
5 cups cubed peeled apples
1/4 cup dried cranberries
3 Tbsp. brown sugar
3 Tbsp. cider vinegar
2 tsp. minced ginger
1/4 tsp. salt
1/4 tsp. dry mustard
1/8 tsp. allspice

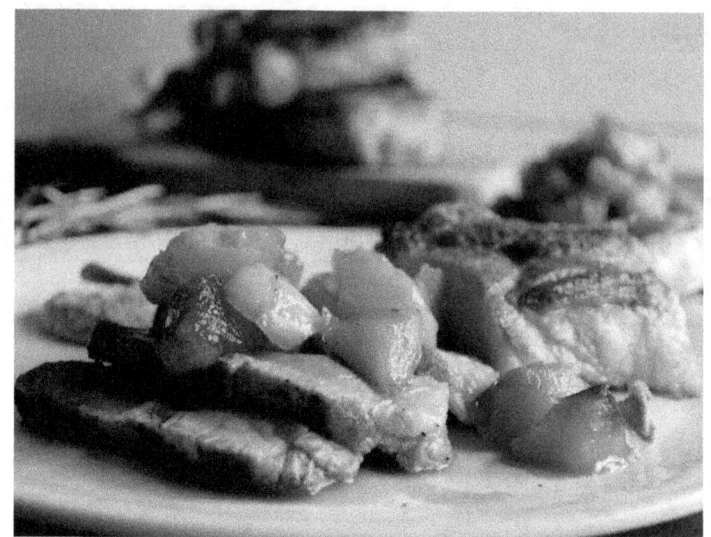

Pork Chops
3/4 tsp. ground chipotle chili pepper
1/2 tsp. salt
1/2 tsp. garlic powder
1/2 tsp. ground coriander
1/4 tsp. black pepper
4 boneless center-cut pork loin chops, trimmed

Instructions:
For Chutney
1. Melt butter over medium-high heat.
2. Add apples, sauté 4 minutes or until lightly browned.
3. Add the remaining 7 chutney ingredients; bring to a boil.
4. Reduce heat and simmer 8 minutes, or until the apples are tender, stirring occasionally.

For Pork
1. Combine the 5 spices and sprinkle over pork.
2. Grill either on an outdoor grill or a grill pan, cooking approximately 4 minutes on each side.
3. Serve with a dollop chutney on top of the chop.

Also Pairs With

Farmhouse Ales	Imperial Pale Ale	Rich Stouts

Belgian Golden Strong Ale

A Belgian Golden Strong Ale shimmers with a radiant golden hue, enticing the eye. It's complex and fruity, boasting a symphony of flavors—think fruity esters, spicy phenols, and a touch of alcohol warmth. Expect robust alcohol content, typically ranging from 7.5% to 10.5%. These ales finish dry and crisp with hints of clove, pepper, and other delightful spices dance on the palate.

Belgian Golden Ale: Key Characteristics		Notable Belgian Golden Ales
Attribute	Description	Damnationplex
ABV	7.5–10.5% — high alcohol, often hidden behind a smooth body	Curieux
IBU (Bitterness)	20–35 — low to moderate; bitterness is subtle and balanced	Golden Monkey
Color (SRM)	4–7 SRM — pale straw to deep gold	La Fin du Monde
Body	Light to medium — surprisingly crisp given the strength	Salvatio
Carbonation	High — champagne-like effervescence	Hennepin
Finish	Dry and warm, with lingering fruit and spice	

Taste: Fruity | Light | Floral | Smooth
Food Pairings: Beef | Grilled Sausages & Veggies | Cold Cuts

Food Pairing Guide for Belgian Gloden Strong Ale

These beers are complex and refined—ideal for dishes that highlight their fruity, spicy, and dry qualities.

Cheese & Charcuterie
- Aged Gouda: Nutty and caramel notes echo the malt sweetness
- Gruyère: Creamy texture contrasts with the beer's spice and carbonation
- Triple Cream Brie: Rich and buttery, it softens the alcohol warmth and lets fruity esters shine

Poultry & White Meats
- Roast Chicken with Herbs: Herbal notes complement the yeast spice; dry finish cuts through fat
- Duck with Apricot Glaze: Fruit and spice in the beer mirror the glaze's sweetness
- Pheasant or Goose: Gamey meats pair well with the beer's strength and complexity

Rich & Spiced Dishes
- Lasagna or Bolognese Pasta: Malt sweetness contrasts saltiness; carbonation lifts the richness
- Moroccan Lamb Tajine (Mrouzia): Spices like cinnamon, saffron, and ginger resonate with yeast-driven flavors
- Sweet & Sour Chinese Dishes: Fruity esters and dry finish balance bold sauces

Desserts
- Oven-Baked Pears or Apples: Fruit-forward desserts echo the beer's esters.
- Shortbread with Orange Glaze: Citrus and buttery notes pair with the beer's dry, spicy finish.
- Belgian Golden Strong Ales are like champagne with a Belgian twist—refined, expressive, and perfect for elevating your meal.

BBQ Brisket Nachos

Belgian Golden Ales are deceptively light in body but pack a punch in flavor—think fruity esters, subtle spice, and a dry finish. That makes them a great contrast to the rich, smoky, fatty brisket piled on nachos. The high carbonation in Belgian Golden Ales lifts the heaviness of melted cheese, sour cream, and brisket fat off your palate, keeping each bite fresh and lively. These ales often have hints of pear, apple, clove, or white pepper. Those flavors play beautifully with the smoky depth of brisket and the sweet-spicy kick of salsa or jalapenos.

Ingredients:
1 to 2 cups leftover shredded BBQ Brisket
¼ cup favorite BBQ Sauce
Tortilla Chips
1/4 cup sour cream
2 cups shredded cheese, (Colby Jack, Cheddar, or any Mexican blend)

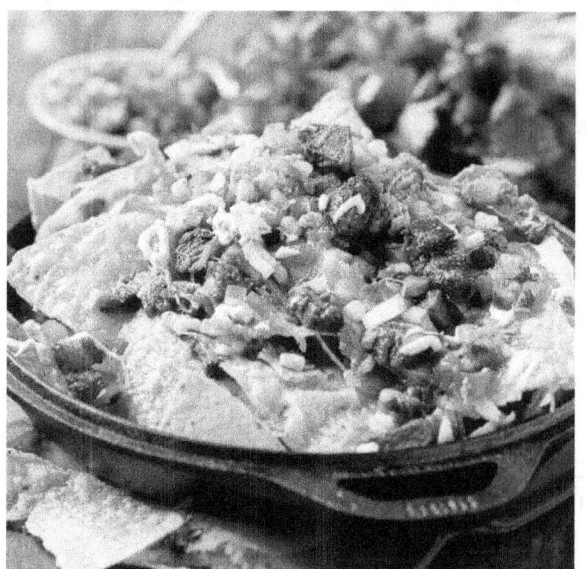

Cowboy Caviar or favorite Bean and Corn Salsa
1/2 cup corn
1/2 cup finely chopped red onion
1/2 cup finely diced tomatoes
½ cup black-eyed peas
½ Cup Black Beans
1/2 cup Pico de Gallo
2 Tbsp. chopped fresh cilantro

Instructions:
1. Preheat oven to 375 degrees.
2. If BBQ Brisket is dry or doesn't have much sauce, toss it with a little BBQ Sauce.
3. Spread tortilla chips out on a baking sheet or cast-iron pan.
4. Top with brisket, corn, and cheese. Place it in the oven until the cheese is melted.
5. To serve, top with Cowboy Caviar, Pico de Gallo, cilantro, and sour cream.

Pico De Gallo
1 cup white onion, diced
1 jalapeno , diced
¼ cup lime juice
¾ tsp of sea salt
1 1/3 cups of Roma tomatoes, diced
½ cup cilantro

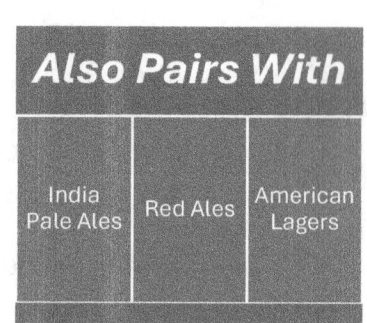

Also Pairs With: India Pale Ales, Red Ales, American Lagers

Mix in a bowl and let it marinate for at least 15 minutes in the refrigerator for the flavors to meld.

Belgian Pale Ale

A lighter type of Belgian beer that forgoes the booziness and has a more muted, yeast-driven flavor profile. These beers are maltier and have a hop finish. Soft, creamy, not too sweet, or too dry, easy to drink but also subtly complex. India pale ales work perfectly with barbecue steaks; mozzarella sticks and ribs.

Belgian Pale Ale: Key Characteristics		Notable Belgian Pale Ale
Attribute	**Description**	Saison Dupont
ABV	4.8–5.5% — moderate, ideal for session drinking	XX Bitter
IBU (Bitterness)	20–30 — restrained bitterness, often earthy or herbal	St. Feuillien Blonde
Color (SRM)	8–14 SRM — amber to copper, with excellent clarity	Palm Speciale
Body	Medium — smooth and slightly creamy	
Carbonation	Medium to high — lively but not aggressive	
Finish	Mildly dry to balanced, with soft malt and yeast interplay	

Taste: Malt Sweetness | Gentle Hops Bitterness | Spicy
Food Pairings: Grilled Pork | Spicy | Cheese

Food Pairing Guide
Belgian Pale Ales are all about balance—making them ideal for dishes that highlight subtle sweetness, gentle spice, and savory depth.

Poultry & Pork
- Roast Chicken or Turkey: Malt sweetness enhances roasted flavors; hops refresh the palate.
- Grilled Pork Chops or Tenderloin: Cuts through fat and complements spice rubs.
- Duck with Fruit Glaze: Apricot or orange glazes mirror the beer's esters.

Savory & Spiced Dishes
- Lasagna or Bolognese: Malt sweetness balances tomato acidity and meat richness.
- Moroccan Tagine (Lamb or Chickpea): Cinnamon, saffron, and ginger resonate with yeast-driven spice.
- Belgian Pale Ales are versatile and elegant—ideal for cozy dinners or refined pairings.

Cheese & Charcuterie
- Soft Cheeses: Brie, Camembert — creamy textures contrast with crisp bitterness.
- Semi-Hard Cheeses: Gouda, Gruyère — nutty and caramel notes echo the malt profile.
- Blue Cheese: Sharp and pungent flavors are mellowed by the beer's fruity esters.
- Charcuterie: Prosciutto, salami, chorizo — savory and smoky meats complement the beer's spice and bitterness.

Seafood
- Grilled Shrimp or Scallops: Light, sweet seafood pairs well with the beer's dry finish.
- White Fish with Herbs: Subtle flavors are elevated by yeast spice and floral hops.

Cedar Planked Salmon

Belgian Pale Ales typically have a gentle malt backbone with hints of biscuit, caramel, or toast. These flavors complement the smoky, woodsy notes from the cedar plank and the natural richness of the salmon. Many Belgian Pale Ales carry subtle spice notes from the yeast (like clove or white pepper), which can mirror or enhance any herb rub or glaze on the salmon—especially if you're using ingredients like thyme, mustard, or maple. The ale's crisp carbonation and dry finish help cut through the salmon's natural oils, keeping your palate refreshed and ready for the next bite.

Ingredients:
3 (12-inch) untreated cedar planks
⅓ cup soy sauce
⅓ cup vegetable oil
1 ½ Tbsp. rice vinegar
1 tsp. sesame oil
¼ cup chopped green onions
1 Tbsp. grated fresh ginger
1 tsp. minced garlic
2 (2-pound) salmon fillets, skin removed

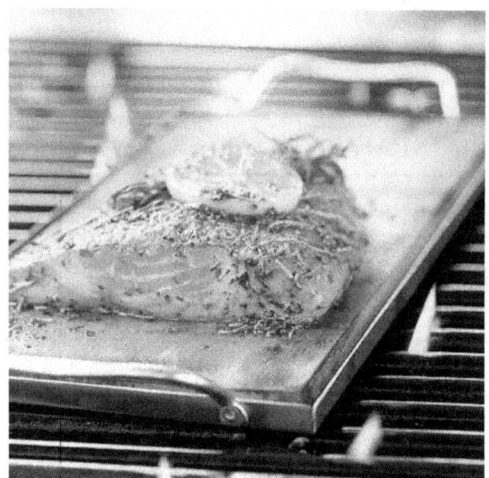

Instructions:
1. Soak cedar planks for at least 1 hour in warm water. Soak longer if you have time.
2. Stir soy sauce, vegetable oil, rice vinegar, sesame oil, green onions, ginger, and garlic together in a shallow dish.
3. Place the salmon fillets in the soy mixture and turn to coat. Cover and marinate for at least 15 minutes, or up to 1 hour refrigerated.
4. Preheat an outdoor grill to medium heat. Place planks on the grill grate. Heat planks until they start to smoke and crackle just a little.
5. Remove the salmon from the marinade and place it on planks; discard the marinade.
6. Close grill cover. Grill salmon until it flakes easily with a fork, about 20 minutes; salmon will continue to cook after you remove it from the grill. Serve with the dressing below.

Creamy Cucumber Dill Sauce
1 cup plain Greek Yogurt
½ English Cucumber, grated
¼ cup fresh dill, chopped
1 tsp fresh lime juice
1 clove garlic minced
Dash of Salt and Pepper

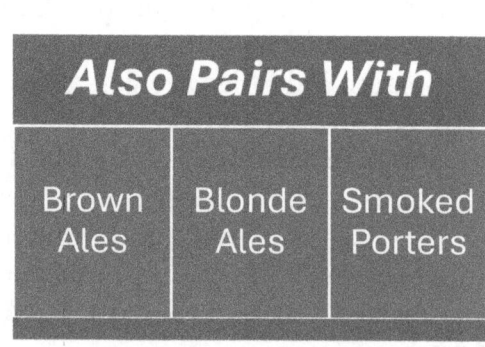

Also Pairs With

Brown Ales	Blonde Ales	Smoked Porters

Place the cucumber in a fine-mesh sieve and squeeze out as much water as possible. Combine all the remaining ingredients and refrigerate for at least 15 minutes.

Dubbel

Strong, malt beer with a notable fruitiness, heavy body, and low bitterness. A stronger version of brown beer. Dubbel pairs with chocolate, coffee, fried meat, cinnamon, and pepper-flavored dishes. Nicely paired nicely with steaks like a porterhouse, rib roast or most barbecue beef.

Dubbel: Key Characteristics		Notable Dubbel
Attribute	Description	Chinmay Premiere Red
ABV	6.0–7.6% — moderately strong, with gentle warmth	La Trappe Dubbel
IBU (Bitterness)	15–25 — low to moderate; bitterness is subtle	Rochefort 6
Color (SRM)	10–17 SRM — deep reddish-copper to dark amber	Achel 8 Bruin
Body	Medium to medium-full — smooth and rounded	Grimbergen Dubbel
Carbonation	Medium-high — creamy, mousse-like head	
Finish	Moderately dry — despite rich malt and fruit character	

Taste: Rich | Carmel | Fruity | Low Hop | Malty
Food Pairings: Grilled Pork | Spicy | Cheese

Food Pairing Guide
Dubbel is a rich, malty Belgian ale with deep roots in the Trappist brewing tradition. It's a style that balances complexity, warmth, and drinkability, making it a favorite among those who appreciate layered flavors.

Cheese & Charcuterie
- Aged Gouda or Gruyère: Nutty and caramel notes echo the malt richness
- Blue Cheese (Stilton, Gorgonzola): Funky and salty flavors contrast beautifully with dark fruit esters
- Prosciutto or Smoked Meats: Savory and smoky elements balance the beer's sweetness

Roasted & Braised Meats
- Beef Stew or Short Ribs: Deep umami and caramelized crust match the beer's malt depth
- Duck with Cherry or Fig Sauce: Fruit-forward sauces mirror the esters in the beer
- Lamb Tagine or Braised Pork: Spiced and slow-cooked dishes resonate with the yeast-driven spice

Rich & Spiced Dishes
- Moussaka or Eggplant Parmesan: Earthy vegetables and creamy textures pair well with the beer's body
- Sausage with Lentils or Beans: Heartiness and rustic flavors are lifted by carbonation and malt sweetness

Desserts
- Bread Pudding with Raisins: Echoes the beer's fig and toffee notes
- Chocolate Torte or Flourless Cake: Bittersweet chocolate complements the beer's richness
- Caramel Flan or Crème Brulé: Silky textures and burnt sugar match the malt profile

Braised Beef Short Ribs

Dubbels is known for their deep malt character—think caramel, toffee, and dark fruit. These flavors mirror the slow-cooked richness of braised short ribs, especially if the dish includes ingredients like onions, tomato paste, or a touch of brown sugar. The yeast in Dubbels produces esters like fig, raisin, or plum, which add a layer of sweetness and depth that plays off the savory, umami-packed meat. It's like adding a splash of port or balsamic glaze to the dish—without overpowering it. Dubbels has a smooth, velvety mouthfeel that matches the tender texture of braised short ribs. The gentle carbonation lifts the richness without being too aggressive.

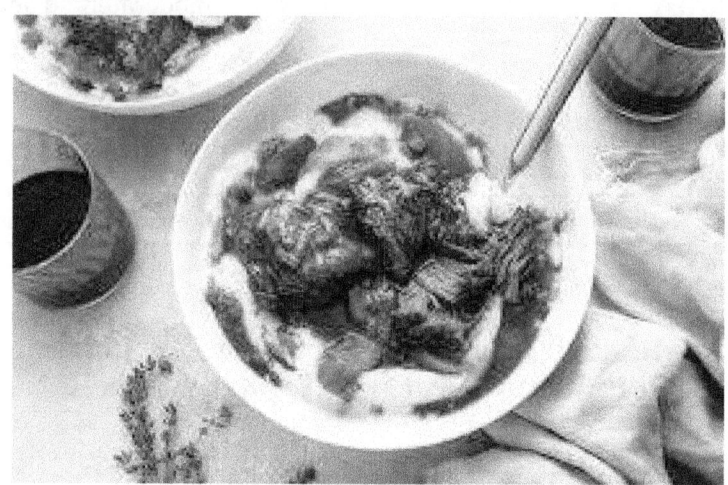

Ingredients:
4 pounds beef short ribs, about 8 ribs, bone-in
1/2 tsp. salt
1/2 tsp. black pepper
3 Tbsp. olive oil
1/2 cup diced white onion
3 cloves minced garlic
1 cup beef broth
1 cup red wine
1/4 cup Worcestershire sauce
1 sprig fresh rosemary

Instructions:
1. Preheat oven to 350 degrees Fahrenheit. Season all sides of the short ribs with salt and pepper.
2. Heat a heavy, oven-safe pot (with lid, for later use) over high heat. Add olive oil and heat it briefly. Sear short ribs in olive oil, about 1 minute per side, to render fat. Remove from the pot and set aside.
3. Add onion and sauté 3 to 5 minutes until softened. Add garlic and sauté 1 minute more.
4. Pour in beef broth, red wine (if using) and Worcestershire sauce. Bring to a simmer. Return the short ribs to the pan. Place a rosemary sprig on top.
5. Cover with a lid and transfer to a preheated oven to braise for about 2.5 hours until the meat is tender and easily shredded with a fork. Be sure the lid is sitting properly to avoid having your liquids evaporate through steam escaping the pot.

Discard the rosemary and serve hot with additional salt and pepper, to taste.

Red Wine Sauce
Some added water and red wine if necessary to make a cup.

Strain all liquids from the pot, pressing all juices out of the onions and carrots, returning to the pot. Add ½ cup of water and a little more wine if you've got little liquid, so it adds up to about a cup. Bring the pot to a simmer, add salt and pepper to taste, reduce by half and pour over the beef.

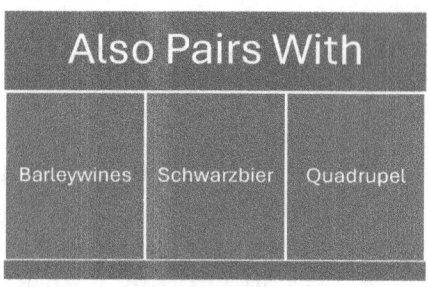

Also Pairs With: Barleywines | Schwarzbier | Quadrupel

Saison | Farmhouse Ale

These fun brews have a tart and complex flavor with balanced bitterness that will balance well with the sweeter or oily flavors in chicken and seafood. These pair nicely with Texas-style BBQ, and anything grilled or smoked, especially chicken and seafood.

Saison	Farmhouse: Key Characteristics		Notable Saison
Attribute	Range / Description		Saison Dupont
Base Ingredient	Local grains (barley, wheat, rye), herbs, spices		Blaugies Saison d'Epeautre
ABV	4.4–8.4% — ranges from sessionable to strong		Fantôme Saison
IBU (Bitterness)	25–45 — moderate; bitterness is balanced by yeast and spice		Saison Voisin
Color (SRM)	5–7 SRM — pale gold to light amber		
Body	Light to medium — crisp and refreshing		
Carbonation	High — effervescent, champagne-like		
Finish	Dry — often with peppery or citrusy snap		

Taste: Fruit | Tart | Peppery | Can Be Spicy
Food Pairings: Grilled Pork | Spicy | Cheese

Food Pairing Guide for Saison | Farmhouse Ale
Saison is a brewer's canvas—wild, expressive, and endlessly customizable.

Cheese & Charcuterie
- Goat Cheese or Chèvre: Tangy and creamy, perfect with the beer's acidity and spice
- Washed-Rind Cheeses (Taleggio, Époisses): Funky cheeses match the beer's wild yeast character
- Prosciutto or Country Pâté: Savory and fatty meats are lifted by carbonation and dry finish

Poultry & Pork
- Roast Chicken with Herbs: Thyme, rosemary, and sage echo the beer's herbal notes
- Grilled Pork Chops: Mild sweetness and char pair well with fruity esters and peppery spice
- Duck Confit or Cassoulet: Rich, rustic French dishes match the beer's farmhouse roots

Vegetables & Salads
- Beet & Goat Cheese Salad: Earthy beets and tangy cheese complement the beer's brightness
- Grilled Asparagus or Artichokes: Bitter greens are softened by fruity and spicy notes
- Mushroom Tart or Quiche: Earthy and creamy flavors pair beautifully with dry, effervescent ales

Seafood
- Mussels in White Wine & Garlic: Classic Belgian pairing; beer's spice and dryness enhance the broth
- Grilled Shrimp or Scallops: Light, sweet seafood matches the beer's delicate fruit and spice

Light Desserts
- Lemon Tart or Shortbread: Citrus and buttery notes echo the beer's crisp finish
- Poached Pears or Apple Galette: Fruit-forward and subtly sweet—great with a fruity Saison

Crock-Pot Dr. Pepper Shredded Beef

The beef is slow-cooked with Dr. Pepper, which adds a sweet, caramelized depth alongside savory spices and umami-rich meat. Farmhouse ales—especially Saisons—are typically dry, effervescent, and slightly tart. This cuts through the richness and sweetness of the beef, cleansing the palate between bites. Farmhouse ales often have earthy, peppery, and herbal notes from wild or Saison yeast strains. These flavors echo the spices in the beef and enhance its complexity. The soda contains a mix of flavors like cherry, licorice, and clove, which resonate with the subtle spice and funk of a farmhouse ale.

Ingredients
1 onion, sliced
2-3 pound chuck roast
1 tsp. onion powder
1 tsp. garlic salt
1 tsp. smoked paprika
1 tsp. black pepper
1 clove garlic, minced
1 Tbsp. Worcestershire sauce
12-ounce can of Dr. Pepper
1 cup barbecue sauce
hamburger buns (for serving)

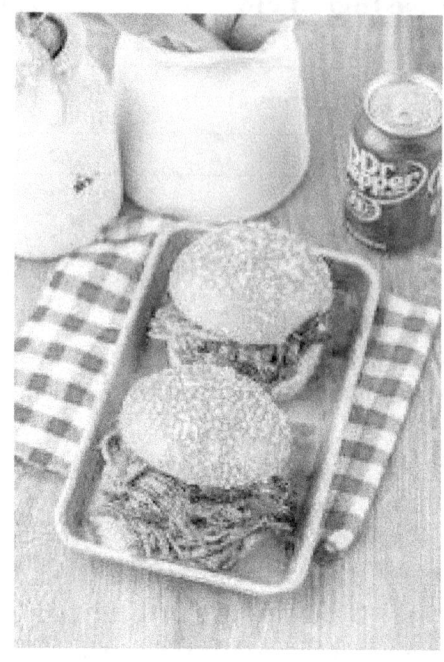

Instructions
1. Add 1 onion, sliced, to the bottom of a 6-quart slow cooker.
2. Place the 2–3-pound chuck roast on top of the sliced onions.
3. Season the roast with 1 tsp. onion powder, 1 tsp. garlic salt, 1 tsp. smoked paprika, 1 tsp. black pepper and 1 clove garlic, minced.
4. Cook for 6-8 hours on low.

Special Sauce for Dr. Pepper Shredded Beef
1 cup beef broth (from the crock pot or fresh)
½ cup Dr. Pepper
¼ cup ketchup
2 Tbsp. apple cider vinegar
1 Tbsp. Worcestershire sauce
1 Tbsp. brown sugar
1 tsp. smoked paprika
½ tsp. garlic powder
½ tsp. onion powder
¼ tsp. cayenne pepper (optional for heat)
Salt and black pepper to taste

Also Pairs With		
Amber Ale	East Coast Hazy IPA	Sour Ale

In a small saucepan, combine all ingredients. Bring to a simmer over medium heat, stirring occasionally. Let it reduce for 10–15 minutes until slightly thickened. Taste and adjust seasoning—more vinegar for tang, more sugar for sweetness, more cayenne for heat. Pour over shredded beef or serve on the side for dipping.

Blonde Ale

It has a light-bodied taste, with a sweet and bready biscuit flavor to it. Not too hoppy and not too malty, blonde ales give a balanced flavor that pairs smoothly with smoked or charred pulled pork or BBQ ribs. Pairs perfectly with sweet, hot, or spicy foods, including Asian dishes, chili, or jalapeno salsa. These pair nicely with Texas-style BBQ, brats, and spicy chicken.

Blonde Ale: Key Characteristics		Notable Blonde Ales
Attribute	Description	Central Waters Honey Blonde Ale
ABV	4.1–5.1% — sessionable and smooth	805 Blonde Ale
IBU (Bitterness)	15–25 — low to moderate; subtle hop presence	Dallas Blonde
Color (SRM)	3–7 SRM — pale yellow to light gold	Summer Love
Body	Light to medium — soft and rounded	Baby Genius
Carbonation	Medium to high — refreshing and lively	NOLA Blonde Ale
Finish	Clean and short — no lingering bitterness	

Taste: Light | Earthy | Sweet | Spicy
Food Pairings: Chicken | Cheese | Sugary Snacks | Fruit Tarts

Food Pairing Guide for Blonde Ale

Blonde Ale is the easygoing charmer of the beer world—light, crisp, and approachable, yet flavorful enough to keep things interesting. It's a great entry point for new craft beer drinkers and a refreshing staple for seasoned palates.

Poultry & Light Meats
- Grilled Chicken or Turkey: Mild malt sweetness complements charred skin and herbs
- Chicken Salad with Grapes or Apples: Fruity esters in the beer echo fresh ingredients
- Pork Tenderloin with Mustard Glaze: Blonde ale's crispness balances sweet-savory sauces

Seafood
- Grilled Shrimp or Scallops: Light, sweet seafood pairs well with the beer's clean finish
- Fish Tacos with Lime & Cilantro: Citrus hops enhance bright toppings; malt softens spice
- Crab Cakes or Lobster Rolls: Rich seafood is lifted by carbonation and subtle bitterness

Cheese & Appetizers
- Mild Cheeses (Havarti, Monterey Jack): Creamy textures match the beer's smooth body
- Bruschetta or Caprese Salad: Tomato, basil, and mozzarella are enhanced by floral hops
- Soft Pretzels with Mustard or cheese dip: Malt sweetness complements salty snacks

Vegetarian Dishes
- Quiche or Veggie Frittata: Egg-based dishes pair well with light malt and carbonation
- Grilled Veggie Skewers: Roasted flavors match the beer's toasty grain notes
- Spinach & Strawberry Salad: Fruity esters echo fresh berries and vinaigrette

Light Desserts
- Lemon Bars or Shortbread Cookies: Citrus and buttery notes mirror the beer's crisp finish
- Vanilla Panna Cotta or Cheesecake: Creamy and delicate desserts pair with blonde ales

Shrimp Tacos with Mango Salsa

Blonde ales are known for their smooth malt profile and mild bitterness. That clean finish makes them ideal for delicate proteins like shrimp, letting the seafood shine without overwhelming it. The light malt sweetness in a blonde ale pair beautifully with the juicy, tangy mango salsa, enhancing the fruit's natural sugars and balancing the acidity from lime or vinegar. If your tacos include creamy elements like avocado or a spicy aioli, the carbonation in the ale lifts the richness, keeping your palate refreshed.

Ingredients:
For the shrimp
2 tsp. olive oil
1 1/4 pounds shrimp, peeled, deveined and tails removed
chili powder and salt to taste

For the mango salsa
1 cup mango, finely diced
½ cup red bell pepper, finely diced
1/2 jalapeno pepper minced, seeded
juice for 1 lime
½ cup cilantro leaves, finely chopped

For the creamy cilantro lime sauce
1 cup sour cream
½ cup cilantro leaves, chopped
2 tsp. lime juice
1 1/2 tsp. honey
¼ cup prepared green salsa
salt and pepper to taste

For assembly
1 cup shredded purple cabbage
8 corn or flour tortillas

Instructions:
1. For the shrimp: Heat the olive oil over high heat in a large pan. Season both sides of the shrimp with chili powder and salt to taste. Place the shrimp in a single layer in the pan and sear for 2-3 minutes per side until the shrimp are pink and cooked through. Alternately grill shrimp.
2. For the mango salsa: Combine all the ingredients in a bowl, add salt to taste. Cover the bowl and place it in the refrigerator for at least 15 minutes, up to 4 hours.
3. For the creamy cilantro sauce: Place all ingredients in the food processor; process until the sauce is smooth and creamy. Add salt and pepper to taste.
4. To serve: Warm the tortillas. Add a spoonful of sauce, a handful of cabbage and place the shrimp on top of the cabbage. Top with mango salsa and serve immediately.

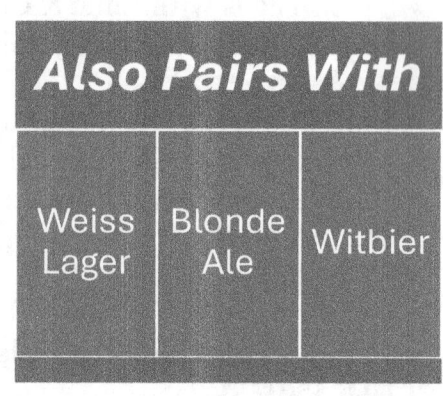

Also Pairs With

| Weiss Lager | Blonde Ale | Witbier |

Tripel

Belgian Tripel is a beer that is made with three times the normal amount of malt. Round malt flavor, robust bitterness, and a plethora of scents ranging from deep yellow to deep gold, these beers are effervescent, and their foam is long-lasting, creamy, and white.

Tripel: Key Characteristics		Notable Tripel
Attribute	Description	New Belgium Trippel
ABV	8.0–12.0% — strong, but often masked by smooth body and carbonation	Westmalle Tripel
IBU (Bitterness)	20–40 — moderate; bitterness balances sweetness	Tripel Karmeliet
Color (SRM)	4–7 SRM — bright golden to deep yellow	Chinmay Tripel
Body	Medium to full — creamy yet dry thanks to sugar fermentation	St. Bernardus Tripel
Carbonation	High — champagne-like effervescence	
Finish	Dry and warm, with lingering fruit and spice	

Taste: Bubbly | Fruity | Sweet | Spicy
Food Pairings: Grilled Pork | Spicy Foods| Muscly | Crab Cakes |Turkey

Food Pairing Guide for Tripel

Tripel is a bold and elegant Belgian ale that combines high alcohol, complex yeast character, and deceptive drinkability. It's a style born from monastic brewing tradition and refined over centuries. Here's a full breakdown tailored to your flavor-savvy, data-driven palate.

Cheese & Charcuterie
- Triple Cream Brie or Camembert: Rich and buttery cheeses contrast spice and carbonation
- Aged Gouda or Gruyère: Nutty and caramel notes echo the malt profile
- Prosciutto or Smoked Meats: Savory and salty meats balance the sweetness and warmth

Poultry & White Meats
- Roast Chicken with Herbs: Herbal notes complement yeast spice; dry finish cuts through fat
- Duck with Orange or Apricot Glaze: Fruit-forward sauces mirror the beer's esters
- Turkey with Sage Stuffing: Earthy herbs and mild meat pair well with the beer's complexity

Seafood
- Mussels in Garlic & White Wine: beer's spice and dryness enhance the broth
- Grilled Shrimp or Scallops: Light, sweet seafood matches the beer's fruity and spicy notes
- Crab Cakes or Lobster Rolls: Rich seafood lifted by carbonation and dry finish

Spiced & Rich Dishes
- Moroccan Tagine: Cinnamon, saffron, and dried fruit resonate with yeast-driven flavors
- Thai Curry (Yellow or Massaman): Coconut and spice balance the beer's warmth and sweetness
- Butternut Squash Ravioli Sage: Sweet and savory flavors echo the malt & spice

Desserts
- Poached Pears or Apple Tart: Fruit-forward desserts mirror esters and balance alcohol
- Lemon Shortbread or Citrus Cheesecake: Acidity and buttery textures pair with a dry finish
- Spiced Bread Pudding: Cinnamon and raisin notes complement the Tripel's depth

Santa Fe Pork Medallions with Peach Salsa

Pork medallions, especially when seared or grilled Santa Fe–style, have a savory, slightly fatty richness. A Tripel's lively carbonation lifts that weight off your palate, keeping each bite fresh and vibrant. Tripels often highlight fruity esters like pears, apples, bananas, or apricots, which beautifully mirror and enhance the sweet-tart brightness of peach salsa. It's like adding a layer of tropical harmony to the dish. The subtle spice notes from the yeast (think clove, white pepper, coriander) resonate with the chili rubs, cumin, and smoky paprika often found in Santa Fe–style pork. The dry, crisp finish of a Tripel keeps the dish from becoming cloying or overly spicy, offering a refreshing contrast.

Ingredients:
1 lb. pork tenderloin

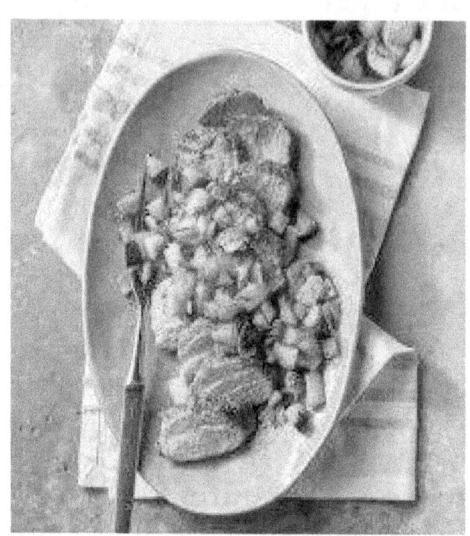

For Seasoning Paste
1 (4-ounce) can chopped green chilies
1 Tbsp. chili powder
1 Tbsp. ground cumin
1 1/2 tsp. black pepper
1/2 tsp. cayenne pepper
1/2 tsp. salt
1 tsp. onion powder
1 tsp. minced garlic
1 tsp. olive oil
2 Tbsp. chopped fresh cilantro

For the Peach Salsa
2 medium-firm fresh peaches, peeled, pitted, and coarsely chopped
1/2 cup canned black beans, rinsed and drained
2 tsp. balsamic vinegar
1 fresh jalapeno , stemmed, seeded, and chopped
1 Tbsp. finely chopped red bell pepper
1 1/2 Tbsp. chopped fresh cilantro
1 lime wedge
1/2 tsp. sugar

Instructions:
1. Trim the tenderloin of fat, etc.
2. Cut the pork tenderloin into medallions about ¾ inch thick.
3. Mix green chilies, chili powder, ground cumin, black pepper, cayenne, salt, onion powder, garlic, olive oil, and cilantro; process in a blender or food processor until it becomes a smooth paste.
4. Rub each side of the medallion with paste and allow it to rest at room temperature for approximately 30 minutes.
5. Meanwhile, mix peaches, black beans, balsamic, jalapeno , red bell pepper, cilantro, and sugar.
6. Squeeze in lime juice and adjust jalapeno and sugar flavorings to taste.
7. Grill pork medallions over medium mesquite, cooking about 4-5 minutes per side, or until meat is cooked through.
8. Alternatively, smoke at 225 for 2-3 hours until medallions reach 145 degrees.
9. Serve salsa spooned over medallions.

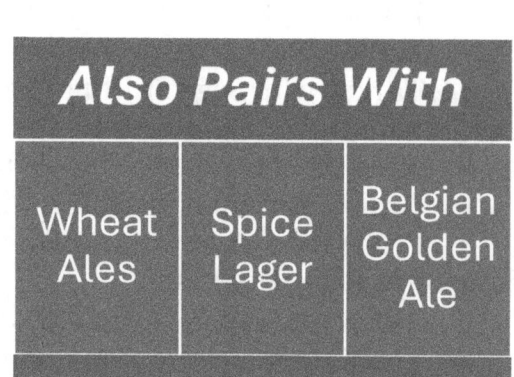

Also Pairs With

| Wheat Ales | Spice Lager | Belgian Golden Ale |

Quadrupel

Quadruple—often called "Quad"—is the boldest and richest of the Belgian Trappist-style ales. It's a beer that doesn't whisper; it roars with complexity, warmth, and depth. Carmel undertones pair nicely with slow-cooked barbecues.

Quadrupel: Key Characteristics		Notable Quadrupel
Attribute	**Description**	Boulevard Bourbon Barrel Quad
ABV	9.1–14.2% — very strong; warming but smooth2	Westvleteren 12
IBU (Bitterness)	20–35 — low to moderate; bitterness plays a supporting role	St. Bernardus Abt 12
Color (SRM)	12–22 SRM — deep amber to garnet brown	Rochefort 10
Body	Medium to full — rich, creamy, and velvety	Chinmay Blue (Grande Reserve)
Carbonation	Medium-high — effervescent but not sharp	
Finish	Moderately dry to slightly sweet; warming alcohol lingers	

Taste: Sweet | Coffee | Rich | Bready
Food Pairings: Grilled Pork | Spicy | Cheese

Food Pairing Guide for Quadrupel
It's a beer that doesn't whisper; it roars with complexity, warmth, and depth.

Cheese & Charcuterie
- Aged Gouda or Parmesan: Nutty, salty, and crystalline textures match the beer's richness
- Blue Cheese (Stilton, Roquefort): Funky and bold flavors contrast beautifully with dark fruit esters
- Smoked Meats or Pâté: Savory and fatty elements are lifted by carbonation and balanced by sweetness

Roasted & Braised Meats
- Beef Short Ribs or Pot Roast: Deep umami and caramelized crust echo the malt profile
- Duck Breast with Cherry Reduction: Fruit-forward sauces mirror esters and spice
- Lamb Shank or Osso Buco: Rich, slow-cooked meats pair perfectly with the beer's depth

Hearty & Spiced Dishes
- Moroccan Tagine (Lamb or Chickpea): Cinnamon, dried fruit, and saffron resonate with yeast-driven spice
- Mole Poblano Chicken or Pork: Chocolate and chili complexity matches the beer's layered sweetness
- Wild Mushroom Risotto: Earthy and creamy textures complement the malt and fruit notes

Decadent Desserts
- Sticky Toffee Pudding or Bread Pudding: Caramel and raisin flavors echo the beer's core profile
- Chocolate Truffles or Flourless Cake: Bittersweet chocolate balances sweetness and alcohol warmth
- Fig Tart or Poached Pears:

Grilled Leg of Lamb With Garlic and Lemon

Quadrupel are deep, malty, and complex—think caramel, molasses, fig, raisin, and dark chocolate. These flavors stand up to the robust, earthy character of grilled lamb, especially when it's kissed by smoke and char. The lamb's seasoning—pungent garlic and bright lemon—gets a flavor boost from the Quadruples' dried fruit esters. The beer's sweetness softens the garlic's bite and plays beautifully against the citrus' acidity. Quadrupel typically clock in at 9–12% ABV, which brings a warming sensation that enhances the richness of the lamb and adds a luxurious finish to each bite.

Ingredients:
½ cup extra-virgin olive oil
¼ cup freshly squeezed lemon juice plus more lemons, halved, for serving
4 garlic cloves, finely chopped
1 Tbsp. dried oregano
2 tsp kosher salt
1 tsp. freshly ground black pepper
1 (4½–5 lb.) butterflied boneless leg of lamb, trimmed of fat

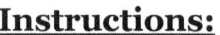

Instructions:
1. Combine all ingredients except the leg of lamb in a sealable plastic bag, shake well. Then add butterflied boneless leg of lamb, trimmed of fat, and seal bag, pressing out air. Turn bag to coat lamb, then put a bag in a shallow baking pan and marinate, chilled, turning bag occasionally, at least 8 hours and up to 24.
2. Remove the lamb from the refrigerator about 1 hour before grilling. Prepare the grill for cooking over direct heat with medium-hot charcoal (moderate heat for gas)
3. Remove lamb from marinade (discard marinade) and run 3 or 4 skewers lengthwise through lamb about 2 inches apart. Grill on a lightly oiled grill rack, covered only if using a gas grill, turning over occasionally and moving around on the grill to avoid flare-ups, until thermometer registers 125–128°F, to your desired doneness.
4. Transfer the lamb to a cutting board and remove the skewers. Let lamb stand, loosely covered with foil, 20 minutes. (Internal temperature will rise to 135°F while meat stands.)
5. Grill extra lemons, halved, cut side down, over direct heat until lightly charred and juices caramelize, about 4 minutes.
6. Cut the lamb across the grain into slices and serve with grilled lemons for squeezing.

Mint Chimichurri Recipe
½ cup fresh mint leaves
½ cup fresh parsley leaves
2 cloves garlic
1 small shallot
2 tbsp red wine vinegar or lemon juice
½ tsp red pepper flakes, to taste
½ cup olive oil
Salt and black pepper, to taste

Also Pairs With

English Pale Ale	Red Ale	Kolsch

Chop herbs finely by hand for a rustic texture or pulse in a food processor. Mince finely or pulse with the herbs. Add red pepper flakes, salt, and black pepper. Stir olive oil until emulsified and glossy.

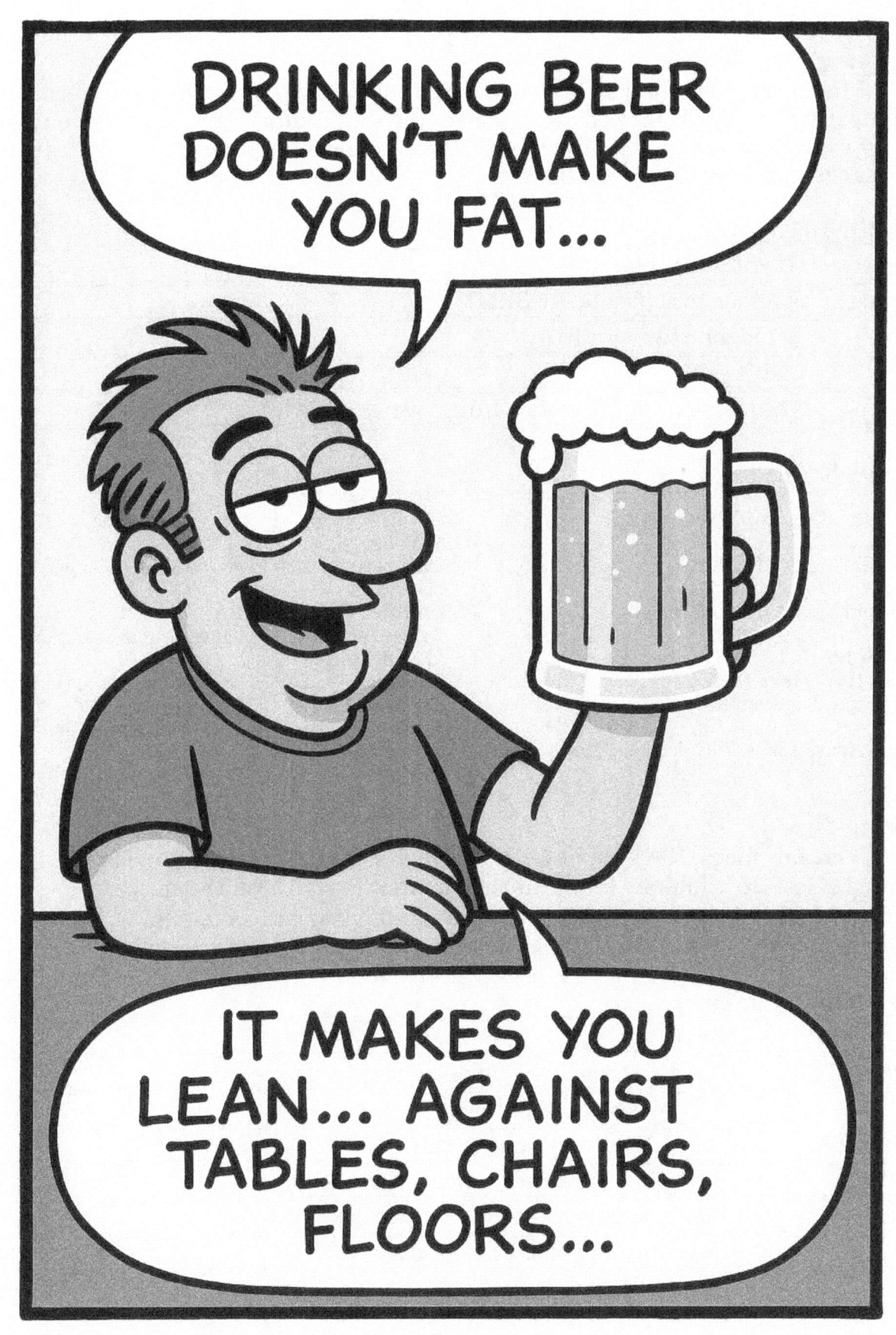

IPA's

What Is an IPA?
IPA stands for India Pale Ale, a beer style known for its bold hop character, higher bitterness, and aromatic complexity. Originally brewed in England in the 18th century, IPAs survived long voyages to India by using extra hops as a preservative. Today, IPAs are the most popular style in craft brewing, with countless substyles and flavor variations.

Flavor Profile Breakdown

Characteristic	Typical Range
Color	Golden to copper (4–16 SRM)
Bitterness	Moderate (20–50 IBU)
ABV	3.0% – 8%
Aroma	Citrus, pine, floral, earthy, fruity (varies by style)

IPA Styles by Region

English IPA
Flavor: Earthy, floral hops with balanced malt
ABV: 5–7%
Examples: Samuel Smith's India Ale

American IPA
Flavor: Citrus, pine, resin, bold bitterness
ABV: 6–7.5%
Examples: Stone IPA, Bell's Two Hearted Ale

New England IPA (Hazy IPA)
Flavor: Juicy, tropical, low bitterness
ABV: 6–8%
Examples: Tree House Julius, The Alchemist Heady Topper

West Coast IPA
Flavor: Dry, crisp, high bitterness, piney
ABV: 6.5–7.5%
Examples: Russian River Pliny the Elder, Green Flash West Coast IPA

Double / Imperial IPA
Flavor: Intense hops, higher alcohol, sweet malt backbone
ABV: 8–10%
Examples: Dogfish Head 90 Minute IPA, Hopslam Ale

Session IPA
Flavor: Light body, hop-forward, low alcohol
ABV: 3.5–5%
Examples: Founders All Day IPA

Food Pairing Tips
- Fatty or creamy foods: IPA bitterness cuts through richness like a palate cleanser.
- Spicy cuisines: Hops interact with chili heat to intensify and layer the spice.
- Citrusy or herbal dishes: Match the beer's aroma with similar food notes.
- Fruity IPAs (like hazy or New England styles) pair surprisingly well with light desserts.

Awesome Food Pairings

IPA Style	Best Pairings
English IPA	Roast chicken, aged cheddar, shepherd's pie
American IPA	Spicy wings, burgers, tacos
New England IPA	Sushi, Thai curry, mango salsa
West Coast IPA	BBQ ribs, grilled steak, sharp cheeses
Double IPA	Blue cheese, pork belly, rich desserts
Session IPA	Fish and chips, salads, light pasta

American IPA

American IPAs are pale gold in color. They highlight fruity, citrusy, and piney hop aromas and flavors. The perception of hop bitterness is medium to high. American IPAs typically have an ABV of 5% to 8%. If you're a hop enthusiast looking for bold flavors, American IPAs are the way to go.

American IPA: Key Characteristics		Notable American Pale Ales
Attribute	**Description**	Stone IPA
ABV	5.5% – 7.5% (some go higher)	Dogfish Head 60 Minute IPA
IBU	40 – 70 (moderate to high bitterness)	Lagunitas IPA
Color	Medium gold to light amber	Julius
Aroma	Citrus, pine, resin, tropical fruit, floral	Two Hearted Ale
Finish	Medium body, smooth texture, dry finish	90 Minute IPA

Taste: Hoppy | Bitter | Fruity
Flavor: Spicy Foods | Buffalo Wings | BBQ | Rich Dishes

Food Pairings for American IPAs
American IPAs pair best with foods that match their intensity, contrast their bitterness, or highlight their hop flavors:

Spicy & Bold Dishes
- Buffalo Wings: Bitterness cools heat; citrus hops enhance tangy sauce.
- Thai Curry: Juicy IPAs (like NEIPAs) complement coconut and spice.
- Spicy Tacos: West Coast IPAs cut through fatty meats and salsa heat.

Grilled & Roasted Meats
- BBQ Ribs: Resinous hops balance sweet, smoky sauces.
- Smoked Brisket: Double IPAs stand up to bold, charred flavors.
- Pulled Pork Sandwiches: Citrusy hops brighten rich, savory meat.

Cheese Pairings
- Sharp Cheddar: Bitterness contrasts richness; citrus notes add lift.
- Blue Cheese: Funky cheese meets its match in bold IPAs.
- Goat Cheese: NEIPAs with tropical fruit notes complement tangy cheese.

Vegetarian Options
- Grilled Veggie Tacos: Hops enhance charred flavors and spice.
- Falafel Wraps with Harissa: Bitterness balances spice and herbs.
- Roasted Cauliflower with Curry Spices: Juicy IPAs echo warm spice notes.

Dessert Pairings
- Carrot Cake: Spices and sweetness play well with citrusy hops.
- Citrus Tart: Mirrors the hop profile in fruity IPAs.
- Dark Chocolate: Bitterness meets bitterness—especially with a Double IPA.

Fish Tacos

Whether your fish is battered and fried or grilled with spices, the assertive bitterness of an American IPA slices through the richness, refreshing your palate and keeping the flavors crisp. American IPAs often burst with citrus-forward hop notes—think grapefruit, orange, or lime zest. These flavors mirror classic taco toppings like lime juice, cilantro, and salsa, creating a vibrant harmony. Fish tacos often come with spicy slaw, pickled onions, or jalapenos. The intensity of an IPA stands up to these bold ingredients, enhancing the heat and complexity without getting lost.

Ingredients

1-1/2 pounds white fish fillets or your Fishing catch
1 Lime
3 Tbsp. Lime Juice
1 Tbsp. Chipotle Powder
1 Tbsp. Canned Jalapeno
¼ cup Coriander
2 Garlic Cloves
4 Tbsp. Olive Oil
Pepper to taste

Pickled Cabbage
4 cups Red Cabbage
3 Green Onion Stems
2 Tbsp. red wine vinegar
½ tsp. Salt

Pink Sauce
¾ cup Sour Cream
3 Tbsp. Sriracha

12 Small Tortillas
Wedges of Lime

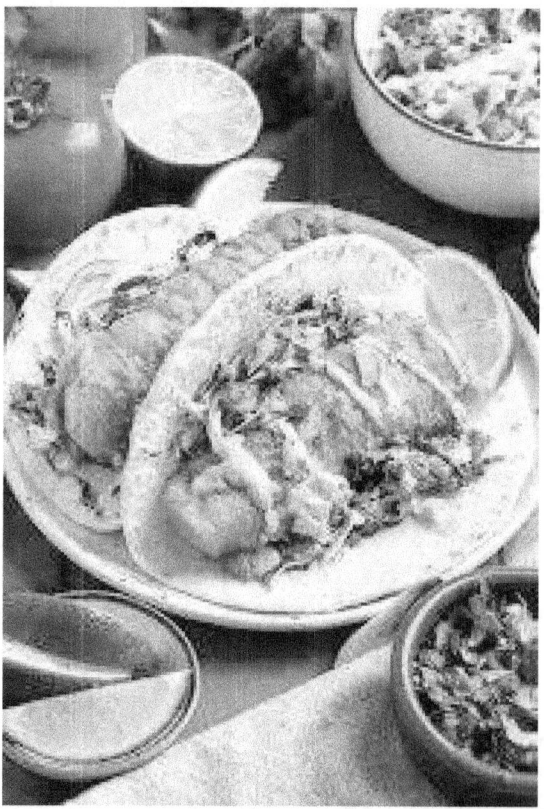

Instructions

1. Marinate fish: Combine Fish Marinade ingredients in a Ziplock bag. Set aside for 20 minutes to marinate - no longer than 1 hour.
2. Pickled Cabbage: Place Pickled Cabbage ingredients in a bowl. Toss to combine and set aside for 30 minutes. Drain excess liquid, scrunch cabbage with your hands (to help soften). Set aside.
3. Pink Sauce: Mix to combine.
4. Cook fish: Heat oil in a skillet over high heat. Cook fish for 2 minutes on each side, or until golden and cooked.
5. Remove the fish from the plate and then flake it into large pieces.
6. To assemble tacos, top with cabbage and then fish, a dollop of sour cream and a squeeze of lime juice.

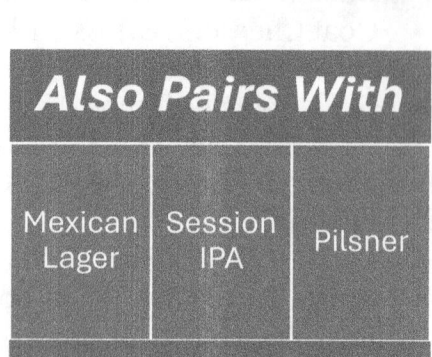

Also Pairs With

Mexican Lager	Session IPA	Pilsner

East Coast IPA

An East Coast IPA, also known as a New England IPA (NEIPA), is a style of beer that has gained popularity in recent years. East Coast IPAs are characterized by their hazy appearance. Unlike crystal-clear West Coast IPAs, these beers often have a cloudy, unfiltered look. East Coast IPAs are less bitter compared to their West Coast counterparts. Expect bursts of juicy, fruity flavor. These beers often highlight tropical fruit notes like mango, pineapple, and citrus. While hops play a significant role, the malty sweetness doesn't take a back seat. It's a bittersweet balance. East Coast IPAs are smoother on the palate.

East Coast IPA: Key Characteristics		Notable East Coast IPAs
Attribute	**Description**	SKA The Tropical Hazy IPA
ABV	Typically, 6–7.5% — moderate to strong	Green State Conehead
IBU (Bitterness)	30–50 — softer bitterness than West Coast IPAs	Maine Beer Lunch
Color (SRM)	4–8 SRM — pale gold to hazy straw	Tree House Julius
Body	Medium to full — creamy mouthfeel from oats or wheat	Hill Farmstead Abner
Carbonation	Medium — smooth and rounded	
Finish	Juicy and slightly sweet; bitterness is restrained	

Taste Pairings: Fruity | Some Sweetness | Juice-Like
Food Pairings: Spicy Seafood | BBQ with Sweet Sauce |

Food Pairing Guide for East Coast IPAs
East Coast IPAs are all about juicy intensity and soft bitterness—perfect for dishes that highlight spice, fat, and umami.

Spicy & Bold Dishes
- Thai Curry: Coconut milk and chili heat are balanced by tropical hops and creamy texture
- Buffalo Wings: Juicy hops tame the spice and echo the tangy sauce
- Spicy Tacos: Citrus and pineapple notes complement bold meats and salsas

Rich & Savory Meats
- Pulled Pork or Brisket: Sweet BBQ sauce and smoky meat match the beer's fruit and malt
- Fried Chicken Sandwiches: Crispy, fatty textures are lifted by carbonation and hop brightness
- Burgers with Bacon or Avocado: Juicy beef & creamy toppings pair with beer's lush mouthfeel

Cheese & Snacks
- Sharp Cheddar or Pepper Jack: Bold flavors match the hop intensity
- Nachos with Guac & Salsa: Juicy hops enhance fresh toppings and cut through richness
- Soft Pretzels with Beer Cheese Dip: Malt sweetness and creamy texture echo the dip

Vegetarian & Vegan Options
- Grilled Veggie w/ Tahini/Citrus Dressing: Bright, earthy flavors match beer's fruit and spice
- Falafel Wraps with Harissa: Spicy and herbaceous elements are balanced by juicy hops
- Sweet Potato Fries: Natural sweetness complements tropical fruit notes

Fruity Desserts
- Citrus Sorbet or Mango Cheesecake: Echoes the beer's juicy esters and soft finish
- Pineapple Upside-Down Cake: Sweet and tangy flavors pair beautifully with tropical hops

The Best Ever Cheeseburger

East Coast IPAs (especially New England-style) are known for their hazy, juicy hop character—think tropical fruit, citrus, and stone fruit. These flavors complement the savory, umami-rich beef and add a bright contrast to the melted cheese. East Coast IPAs have a subtle malt sweetness that pairs beautifully with the toasted bun and the caramelized crust of a grilled patty, creating a warm, cohesive flavor bridge. The smooth, almost creamy mouthfeel of a hazy IPA mirrors the melty cheese and juicy beef, making each bite and sip feel indulgent and satisfying.

Ingredients:
2 pounds ground beef, 80/20
Kosher salt, to taste
freshly ground black pepper, to taste
garlic powder, to taste
1 Tbsp. canola oil
6 slices American cheese

for the burger sauce
½ cup mayonnaise
¼ cup ketchup
3 Tbsp. dill pickle relish
1 Tbsp. Dijon mustard

for serving
Brioche hamburger buns
Romaine or shredded lettuce
Sliced tomato
Sliced red onion
Dill pickle chips

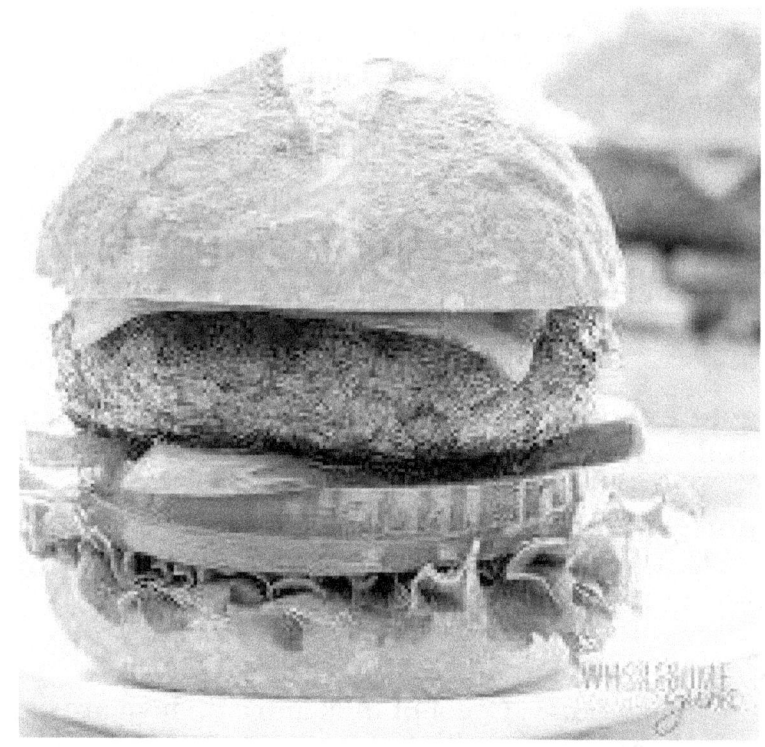

Instructions:
1. In a large bowl, combine beef, 1 1/2 tsp. salt and 1 1/2 tsp. pepper. Using a wooden spoon or clean hands, stir until well combined. Gently form into 6 1-inch-thick patties, about the size of the hamburger buns.
2. Heat canola oil in a large cast-iron skillet over medium-high heat. Working in batches, add patties and cook until lightly charred or until desired doneness, about 3-5 minutes per side; top with cheese.
3. Serve immediately in hamburger buns with burger sauce and desired toppings.

Burger Sauce
In a small bowl, whisk together mayonnaise, ketchup, dill pickle relish and Dijon.

Also Pairs With

Belgium Pale Ale	Rauchbier	Milk Stout

West Coast IPA

The term originated because most West Coast IPAs were brewed in states along the Pacific Ocean. West Coast IPAs proudly highlight their hoppy bite. Expect bold, hoppy aromas and flavors. Think pine forests, citrus groves, and tropical fruit baskets about its hop Aroma. These beers often feature citrus notes (like grapefruit and orange) and piney resin undertones. West Coast IPAs have a dry and crisp finish, leaving your palate refreshed.

West Coast IPA: Key Characteristics		Notable West Coast IPAs
Attribute	Description	Liquid Gravity IPA
ABV	Typically, 6.5–7.5% — bold but not overpowering	Steambarrel IPA
IBU (Bitterness)	50–80+ — assertive, lingering bitterness	Destihl Deadhead Westcoast IPA
Color (SRM)	6–14 SRM — pale gold to deep amber	Pliny the Elder
Clarity	Crystal clear — no haze here	Union Jack IPA
Body	Medium-light to medium — dry and crisp	Head Hunter IPA
Carbonation	Medium to high — refreshing and snappy	
Finish	Bone-dry with a clean, bitter snap	

Taste: Hoppy | Some Sweetness | Clean Taste | Citrus | Floral
Food Pairings: Smoked Foods | Spicy BBQ Sauces | Grilled Veggies

Food Pairing Guide for West Coast IPA
West Coast IPAs were born in California and brewed to challenge the palate. Breweries like Stone, Russian River, and Firestone Walker helped shape the style into a global phenomenon.

Spicy & Bold Dishes
- Buffalo Wings/Spicy Fried Chicken: Bitterness cools the heat; citrus hops enhance tangy sauces
- Spicy Tacos (Carne Asada, Chorizo): Charred meat and spice are lifted by piney hops
- Indian Curries balance bitterness, chili heat and complement earthy spices

Grilled & Roasted Meats
- BBQ Ribs or Brisket: Smoky, sweet sauces contrast beautifully with hop bitterness
- Grilled Steak with Chimichurri: Herbal sauce and charred meat match the beer's intensity
- Burgers with Sharp Cheese or jalapenos: Rich toppings are cut by bitterness and carbonation

Cheese & Savory Snacks
- Aged Cheddar or Pepper Jack: Sharp, salty cheeses enhance hop bite
- Nachos with Salsa & Guac: Bright toppings echo citrus hops; bitterness balances richness
- Charcuterie with Pickled Veggies: Fatty meats and acidic sides pair well with crisp bitterness
- **Vegetarian Options**
- Grilled Veggie Skewers (Zucchini, Bell Peppers): Roasted flavors match piney hops
- Falafel Wraps with Harissa or Tahini: Spice and earthiness balance the beer's dryness
- Stuffed Portobello Mushrooms: Umami-rich and hearty enough to stand up to hops

Dessert
- Dark Chocolate Bark with Sea Salt: Bitterness complements cocoa; salt enhances hop flavor
- Grapefruit Sorbet: Echoes citrus notes and refreshes the palate

Cioppino (Fisherman's Stew)

The IPA's hops slice through the tomato broth's umami and the seafood's natural oils, cleansing the palate. The grapefruit and lemony notes echo the acidity of the tomato base and enhance the briny sweetness of shellfish. The bubbles lift and lighten the stew's heavier textures, making each bite feel vibrant. Cioppino is bold and layered, and West Coast IPAs are no wallflowers—they stand up to the dish without overpowering it.

Ingredients:
¼ cup + 2 Tbsp. extra-virgin olive oil, divided
⅔ cup finely chopped shallots, from about 3 shallots
3 cloves garlic, minced
1 cup white wine
1 (28 oz) can crushed tomatoes
2 (8 oz) bottles clam juice
2 tsp. sugar
1¾ tsp. salt, divided
½ tsp. crushed red pepper flakes
½ tsp. dried oregano
7 sprigs fresh thyme, plus 1 tsp. freshly chopped thyme
1½ pounds firm-fleshed fish fillets, such as halibut, cod, Your Catch of the Day, cut into 2-inch pieces
3 Tbsp. unsalted butter
1½ pounds (about 18) littleneck clams, scrubbed
1½ pounds extra-large raw shrimp, peeled and deveined
Freshly chopped Italian parsley, for garnish

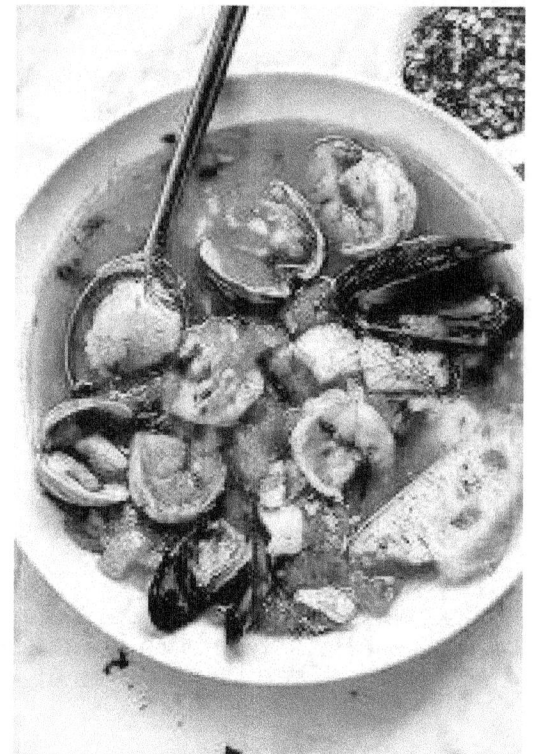

Instructions:
1. Preheat the oven to 400°F and set an oven rack in the middle position. Line a baking sheet with aluminum foil and set aside.
2. In a large pot, heat ¼ cup of the oil over medium heat. Add the shallots and cook, stirring frequently, until soft and translucent, about 5 minutes. Add the garlic and cook, stirring constantly, for 1 minute more. Do not brown.
3. Add the wine and increase the heat to high. Boil until the wine is reduced by about half, 3 to 4 minutes.
4. Add the crushed tomatoes, clam juice, sugar, 1 tsp. of salt, red pepper flakes, oregano, thyme sprigs, and 1 cup of water. Bring to a boil; reduce the heat and simmer, covered, for 25 minutes.
5. Meanwhile, while the stew is simmering, toss the fish with the remaining 2 Tbsp. oil and remaining ¾ tsp. salt. Arrange the fish on the prepared baking sheet and bake for about 10 minutes, or until just cooked through. Cover and keep warm until ready to serve.
6. When the stew is done simmering, remove and discard the thyme sprigs and stir in the butter. Add the clams and bring the stew back to simmer. Cover and cook for about 6 minutes, until the clams have mostly opened. Gently stir in the shrimp and bring the stew back to a simmer; cover and cook until the shrimp are just cooked through and the clams are completely opened, about 5 minutes. Discard any unopened clams. Add the chopped thyme, then taste the stew and adjust the seasoning.
7. Divide the warm fish into serving bowls. Ladle the stew over top, dividing the clams and shrimp evenly among the bowls. Garnish with parsley, if using, and serve with garlic bread, focaccia, or a baguette for sopping up the broth. Set out a second bowl of shells and plenty of napkins.

Also Pairs With

Farmhouse Ale	Fruited Sour Lambric	Belgian Witbier

Triple IPA

Triple IPA, also known as a Triple India Pale Ale (TIPA), is a beer style that has gained popularity in recent years. Triple IPAs are high-gravity, high-alcohol beers brewed with a significant amount of malt and hops. Their alcohol content typically falls between 10% and 12% ABV, although some examples can even reach 15% ABV. The result is a beer that is incredibly hoppy, bitter, and aromatic. Descriptors of the hop aroma often include fruity, floral, or piney notes.

Triple IPA: Key Characteristics		Notable Triple IPA
Attribute	**Description**	Lupulin Sexxxy Hops
ABV	9–13%+ — very high alcohol content; often warming on the finish	DDH Triple IPA
IBU (Bitterness)	60–100+ — intensely bitter, but can be balanced by malt sweetness	Green Bullet
Color (SRM)	8–14 SRM — deep gold to copper	Hopfetti
Body	Full-bodied; rich and sometimes syrupy	Simtra Triple IPA
Carbonation	Medium to high — helps lift the heavy flavors	Dire Wolf IPA
Finish	Lingering bitterness, Bone-dry with a clean, bitter snap with a warming alcohol presence	

Taste: Hoppy | Pine | Floral | Malty
Food Pairings: BBQ | Smoked Sausages

Food Pairing Guide for Triple IPAs

Triple IPA is the heavyweight champion of the IPA family—bold, boozy, and bursting with hops. If you're chasing intensity, this is where the hopheads go to play.

Pub Food
- Buffalo Wings or Nashville Hot Chicken: Heat and fat are tamed by bitterness and alcohol
- Spicy Thai or Indian Curries: Coconut milk and chili balance the beer's hop punch
- Mexican Street Tacos (Al Pastor, Chorizo): Citrus hops enhance lime and spice; malt sweetness complements charred meats

Rich & Umami-Heavy Meats
- Grilled Ribeye or NY Strip Steak: Charred crust and juicy fat match malt and hop intensity
- Pulled Pork or Brisket: Smoky, sweet BBQ flavors pair with caramel malt and bitterness
- Burgers with Blue Cheese or Bacon Jam: Funky cheese and sweet-savory toppings are tamed by the beer's power

Salty & Aged Cheeses
- Aged Gouda or Sharp Cheddar: Salt and umami amplify hop bitterness and malt depth
- Blue Cheese: Funky richness meets its match in the beer's bold hop profile

Fried & Fatty Foods
- Loaded Fries or Nachos: Sour cream, bacon, and jalapenos are balanced by hops and malt
- Fried Chicken/Cheese Curds: Salt and fat mellow the bitterness; carbonation cleanses the palate

Dessert
- Bittersweet Chocolate Cake or Brownies: Cocoa and caramel echo malt sweetness and contrast hop bite
- Carrot Cake with Cream Cheese Frosting: Spice and richness complement the boozy warmth

Crispy Smoked Pork Belly Recipe

This pairing is all about balance through contrast: the beer's bitterness and alcohol tame the pork's richness, while its sweetness and body echo the dish's smoky depth. The aggressive hops in a triple IPA slice through the pork belly's richness, cleansing your palate and keeping each bite exciting. Many triple IPAs have a malty backbone that complements the smoky-sweet glaze or rub on the pork belly. The higher ABV enhances the pork's savory notes and adds a warming contrast to the cool, fatty texture. Smoked pork belly is no delicate dish—it demands a beer that can stand up to its boldness, and a triple IPA delivers.

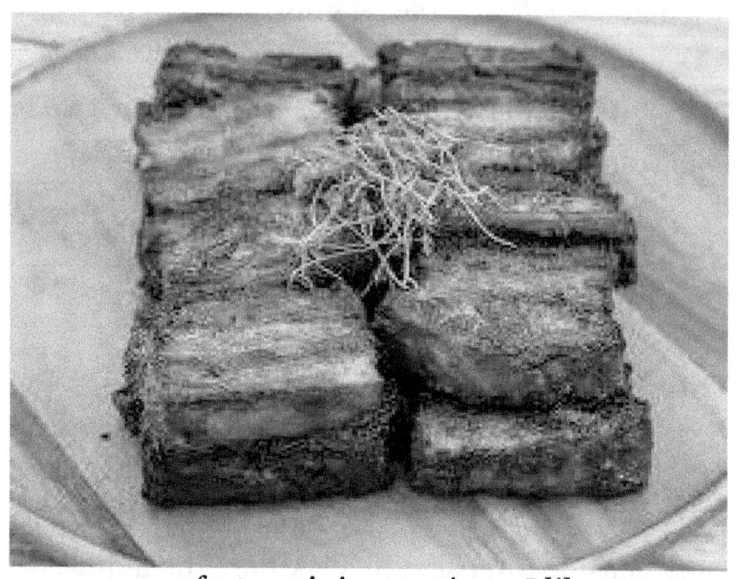

Ingredients:
1 3 to 3-1/2- pound section of pork belly
3 tbsp mustard
Freshly ground salt & pepper to taste
1/2 tsp. ground white pepper
1/2 tsp. cayenne pepper
1/2 Tbsp. ground black pepper
1/2 Tbsp. mustard powder
1 Tbsp. granulated garlic
1 Tbsp. chili powder
1 Tbsp. ground cumin
2 Tbsp. kosher salt
2 Tbsp. sugar
2 Tbsp. sweet paprika

Instructions: Preheat your smoker to 250°F as per your manufacturer's instructions. I like to use a mix of cherry and hickory wood.

1. With a sharp knife, remove the top layer of fat on the pork belly. Score the fat in 1-inch squares. You don't want to cut all the way through the pork belly, only go around a ¼ inch deep. I like to cut into square planks so that all sides get maximum flavor from the rub.
2. In a medium-sized bowl, mix cayenne, chili powder, cumin, garlic, mustard powder, paprika, sugar, salt, and pepper.
3. Dab any excess moisture off the pork belly with a paper towel. Then, apply the mustard binder. Then, rub the dry rub over the top, bottom and sides of the pork belly. Don't be scared to get in there with your hands and make sure everything is covered.
4. Once the smoker is up to temperature, smoke, the pork belly, fat side down, until it is bronzed with smoke. You are looking for an internal temperature of 165°F. This should be around 2–3 hours; however, Check after 2.5 hours and adjusting accordingly.
5. At 165°F, wrap your pork in foil with apple juice.
6. Once the internal temperature gets to 200°F, remove the foil and allow the skin to crisp up.
7. Once the skin is crispy (10-15 minutes) remove the piece of pork from the smoker and allow it to rest for at least 10 minutes.
8. Slice into desired portion sizes, typically ½ inch thick squares bites.

Also Pairs With

Robust Porter	Oatmeal Stout	Amber Ale

Black IPA

A Black IPA, also known as a Cascadian Dark Ale, is a style of beer that combines the bitterness of an IPA with the roasted malt flavors of a stout or porter. It occupies a perplexing spot in the beer universe, sitting at the intersection of a dry Irish stout and a West Coast IPA. Imagine a beer that pours out dark, like a stout or porter, but drinks with the body and hop-forwardness of an IPA. Darker malts dominate, but without the astringency associated with stouts or porters.

Black IPA: Key Characteristics		Notable Black IPA
Attribute	Description	Three Black Bouquet
ABV	Typically, 5.5–9.0% — moderate to strong alcohol content	Wookey Jack
IBU (Bitterness)	50–90 — assertive hop bitterness balanced by roasted malt	Sublimely Self-Righteous
Color (SRM)	25–40 SRM — deep brown to pitch black, often with ruby highlights	Black Witch
Clarity	Usually clear despite the dark color; dry-hopped versions may be hazy	Black IPA
Head	Tan to light brown, persistent foam	Hop in the Dark CDA
Body	Medium — smooth with a dry finish	
Finish	Crisp and bitter, with lingering roast and hop notes	

Taste: Bold | Coffee | Hoppy | Malty | Chocolate
Food Pairings: BBQ | Spicy Ribs | Vegetables | Salty Snacks

Food Pairing Guide for Black IPAs
Black IPA—also known as Cascadian Dark Ale or India Black Ale—is a fascinating hybrid that merges the roasty depth of dark malts with the bold hop character of American IPAs

Spicy & Charred Dishes
- Blackened Fish or Cajun Chicken: Charred crust echoes roasted malt; hops cut through spice
- Spicy Tacos (Carne Asada, Chipotle Pork): Smoky meats and bold salsas match hop bitterness
- Grilled Sausages with Mustard: Earthy spice and fat are lifted by piney hops

Roast & Smoked Meats
- BBQ Brisket or Burnt Ends: Smoky sweetness complements dark malt and hop bite
- Grilled Lamb Chops: Gamey richness pairs well with roasted malt and herbal hops
- Pulled Pork with Coffee Rub: Roast and bitterness mirror the beer's profile

Cheese & Savory Snacks
- Aged Cheddar or Smoked Gouda: Sharp and smoky flavors enhance malt complexity
- Blue Cheese or Stilton: Funky richness contrasts with hop bitterness
- Charcuterie with Pickled Veggies: Fat and acid balance the beer's boldness

Vegetarian Options
- Grilled Portobello Burgers: Earthy mushrooms match roasted malt and piney hops
- Stuffed Bell Peppers with Black Beans: Smoky and spicy fillings complement the beer's depth
- Roasted Root Veggies with Balsamic Glaze: Sweet and earthy notes play off bitterness

Dessert Pairings
- Bittersweet Chocolate Tart or Brownies: Cocoa and roast echo the beer's malt profile
- Espresso Gelato or Mocha Cheesecake: Coffee and cream balance hop intensity

Slow Cooker Short Ribs

The hops in a Black IPA slice through the richness of the ribs, cleansing your palate between bites. The dark malt flavors mirror the smoky, caramelized crust of the ribs, creating a seamless flavor bridge. These bright hop notes lift the dish, preventing it from feeling too heavy or one-note. Both the beer and the dish are bold and complex—either gets lost or overpowers the other.

Ingredients:
8-10 beef short ribs
salt and pepper
1 Tbsp. olive oil
5 large carrots sliced
1 cup beef broth
3 cloves garlic minced
1/4 cup tomato paste
1 Tbsp. Worcestershire Sauce
1 Tbsp. Italian Seasoning

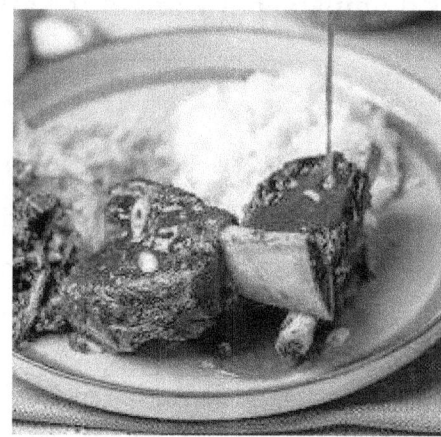

Instructions:
1. Salt and pepper the beef short ribs. Heat a large skillet with the olive oil over medium-high heat. Add the short ribs and sear each side for 1-2 minutes or until they have a golden-brown crust. Remove from skillet and add to the slow cooker and add the carrots on top.
2. In a small bowl, whisk the beef broth, garlic, tomato paste, Worcestershire sauce and Italian seasoning. Add to the slow cooker.
3. Cook on low for 8-9 hours or high 4-5 hours.

Garlic Mashed Potatoes
2 lbs. Yukon Gold or Russet potatoes, peeled and cut into chunks.
4–6 cloves garlic, peeled
½ cup whole milk or heavy cream
¼ cup unsalted butter
Salt and freshly ground black pepper to taste
¼ cup sour cream or cream cheese for extra creaminess
chopped chives or parsley

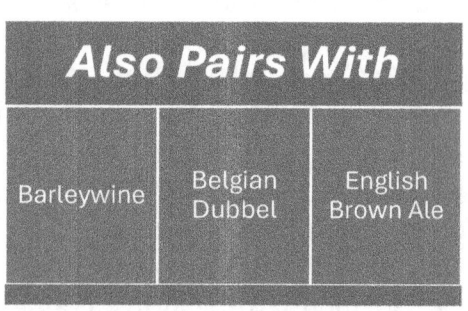

Also Pairs With

Barleywine	Belgian Dubbel	English Brown Ale

Place the potatoes and garlic cloves in a large pot. Cover with cold water and add a generous pinch of salt. Bring it to a boil, then reduce it to a simmer. Cook until the potatoes are fork-tender (about 15–20 minutes). Drain the potatoes and garlic well. Return them to the pot or a large bowl. Mash using a potato masher, ricer, or electric mixer for desired texture. Warm the milk and butter together until melted (microwave or stovetop). Pour into the mashed potatoes and mix until smooth. Stir in sour cream or cream cheese if using. Season with salt and pepper to taste. Spoon into a serving bowl and top with extra butter or fresh herbs.

Belgian IPA

A Belgian IPA marries the hop-forwardness of American IPAs with the distinctive characteristics of Belgian ales. Belgian IPAs are often considered too hoppy by traditional Belgian beer drinkers. These beers use various malts but finish with Belgian yeast strains (often bottle-conditioned). Expect a cleaner bitterness compared to American IPAs, along with a pronounced dry edge reminiscent of an IPA crossed with a Belgian Tripel. Belgian IPAs typically have an ABV ranging from 6.0% to 11.0%.

Belgian IPA: Key Characteristics		Notable Belgian IPAs
Attribute	Description	Unibroue Ce N'est Pas La Fin Du Monde
ABV	6.2–9.5% — often stronger than standard IPAs	Raging Bitch by Flying Dog Brewery
IBU (Bitterness)	50–100 — high bitterness, but balanced by yeast esters	Houblon Chouffe by Brasserie d'Achouffe
Color (SRM)	5–15 SRM — pale gold to amber	Green Flash Le Freak by Green Flash Brewing Co.
Body	Medium — with a dry to medium-dry finish	
Carbonation	Moderate to high — lively and effervescent	
Clarity	Fair to hazy — depending on yeast and dry hopping	

Taste: Fruity | Spicy | Dry | Toasty | Hop Forward
Food Pairings: Grilled Pork | Spicy | Cheese | Barbecue

Food Pairing Guide For Belgian IPAs
Belgian IPAs are still a developing style, but they've carved out a niche for drinkers who want hop-forward beers with yeast-driven depth.

Spicy & Bold Dishes
- Thai Curry: Coconut and chili heat are balanced by fruity esters and hop bitterness
- Spicy Sausage or Chorizo: Fat and spice are lifted by carbonation and yeast spice
- Tandoori Chicken or Paneer: Charred edges and bold spices match the hop and yeast profile

Roasted & Grilled Meats
- Herb-Rubbed Pork Tenderloin: Rosemary, thyme, and sage echo the beer's herbal notes
- Grilled Lamb Chops: Gamey meat with herbs pairs beautifully with Belgian yeast and hops
- Duck Breast with Orange Glaze: Fruit-forward sauces mirror esters and balance bitterness

Cheese & Fermented Foods
- Washed-rind cheeses, Funky and creamy cheeses match the beer's wild yeast character
- Aged Gouda or Alpine Cheeses: Nutty and caramel notes echo malt sweetness
- Kimchi or pickled veggies: Acid and spice contrast beautifully with the beer's complexity

Vegetarian Options
- Grilled Veggie Skewers: Roasted flavors and herbal brightness match yeast and hops
- Mushroom Risotto or Tart: Earthy umami complements malt and yeast spice
- Falafel Wraps with Yogurt Sauce: Creamy, tangy, and herbaceous elements balance dry finish

Dessert Pairings
- Pear Tart or Apple Galette: Fruit-forward desserts mirror esters and enhance the finish
- Spiced Shortbread or Biscotti: Clove and nutmeg echo yeast phenols
- Lemon Poppyseed Cake: Bright citrus and subtle sweetness pair well with hop bitterness

Roast Chicken with Rosemary and Lemon

This pairing is all about elevated balance. The beer's complexity enhances the chicken's brightness and depth without overwhelming it. It's refined, flavorful, and just a little unexpected. The rosemary's piney notes echo the hop bitterness and herbal tones in the Belgian IPA. Lemon in the chicken amplifies the citrusy hop character, creating a zesty bridge between food and drink. The yeast-driven spice in the beer complements the garlic and pepper often used in roast chicken seasoning. The beer's carbonation and dry finish cut through the chicken's richness, refreshing your palate with each sip.

Ingredients:
1 (3 lb.) chicken, washed and dried, fat removed
1/2 onion, chopped into large chunks
2 cloves garlic, smashed
1 lemon, halved
3 sprigs fresh rosemary
1 tbsp dried Herbs de Provence, (Thyme, Oregano, Basil, Marjoram, Fennel, Rosemary, Savory)
kosher salt and fresh pepper

Instructions:
1. Heat oven to 425F. Season the chicken inside and out with salt, pepper, and herbs de Provence.
2. Squeeze half of the lemon on the outside of the chicken and stuff the remains of the lemon along with onion, garlic, and rosemary sprigs inside the chicken. Transfer to a sheet pan and tie the chicken by taking kitchen twine and plumping up the breast, then coming around with the string to lasso the legs and tie them together. Don't forget to tuck the wing tips under themselves so they don't burn.
3. Roast the chicken until the juices run clear and the internal temperature is 160°F, about 50-60 minutes.
4. Let the bird rest for 10 minutes, tenting with foil before carving.
5. Serve chicken, either breast, or one thigh/drumstick; skin is optional.

Creamy Cilantro Lime Sauce
1 cup fresh cilantro, chopped
½ cup sour cream or Greek yogurt
¼ cup mayonnaise
2 Tbsp. fresh lime juice (about 1 lime)
1 clove garlic
1–2 Tbsp. olive oil
½ tsp. salt
½ jalapeno (seeded for less heat)

Also Pairs With		
Weizen	Hefeweizen	Berliner Weisse

Add all ingredients to a blender or food processor. Blend until smooth and creamy. Scrape down sides as needed. Taste and adjust: more lime for tang, more cilantro for freshness, more mayo for richness. Chill for 15–30 minutes to let the flavors meld.

Sessions IPA

The most widely known session beer, session IPAs are lighter-bodied, lower ABV versions of their IPA counterparts. Session IPAs keep the citrusy, hoppy punch and aromatic complexity but aren't as filling or high in alcohol. It's designed for "session" drinking, meaning you can enjoy a few without overwhelming your palate or your liver.

Sessions IPA: Key Characteristics		Notable Sessions IPAs
Attribute	**Description**	All Day IPA
ABV	3.8–5.0% — significantly lower than standard IPAs	Go To IPA
IBU (Bitterness)	30–50 — moderate bitterness, often balanced by citrus or floral hops	DayTime IPA
Color (SRM)	4–8 SRM — pale gold to light amber	Easy Jack
Body	Light to medium — crisp and refreshing	Citra Session IPA
Carbonation	Medium to high — enhances drinkability	Pinner Throwback IPA
Finish	Clean and dry, with lingering hop notes	Brew Free! Or Die Session IPA

Taste: Citrus | Fruit | Floral | Biscuity
Food Pairing: Grilled Chicken | Vinaigrette Salads | BBQ | Citrus Tacos

Food Pairing Guide for Sessions IPA
Session IPAs are built for versatility—great with grilled foods, spicy bites, and picnic-style dishes.

Spicy & Zesty Dishes
- Buffalo Wings or Spicy Chicken Tenders: Bitterness cools the heat; citrus hops enhance tangy sauces
- Fish Tacos with Lime & Jalapeno : Bright toppings echo citrus hops and balance spice
- Spicy Falafel Wraps with Harissa: Herbal and spicy elements match the beer's hop profile

Grilled & Fried Favorites
- Grilled Burgers or Brats: Charred meat and savory toppings pair well with crisp bitterness
- Fried Chicken Sandwiches: Crunchy, fatty textures are lifted by carbonation and hops
- BBQ Pulled Pork Sliders: Sweet and smoky flavors contrast beautifully with hop bite

Cheese & Snacks
- Sharp Cheddar or Pepper Jack: Bold cheeses match hop intensity
- Soft Pretzels with Mustard or cheese dip: Malt sweetness complements salty snacks
- Nachos with Guac & Salsa: Fresh toppings and spice are balanced by citrusy hops

Light & Fresh Dishes
- Grilled Veggie Skewers: Roasted flavors match piney hops
- Cobb or Caesar Salad: Rich dressings and bacon are cut by bitterness and carbonation
- Caprese Salad with Balsamic Glaze: Tomato and basil echo herbal hop notes

Casual Desserts
- Lemon Bars or Citrus Sorbet: Bright acidity complements hop character
- Shortbread Cookies or Biscotti:

Grilled Chicken Thighs

The hops in a Session IPA cut through the richness of the chicken thighs, keeping each bite from feeling heavy. Lemon or orange notes in the beer brighten the charred edges of the chicken, adding contrast and complexity. The bubbles cleanse the palate, especially helpful when the chicken is seasoned with bold spices or sauces. Session IPAs are flavorful but not overpowering—just like grilled chicken thighs. They complement without competing.

Ingredients:
2 pounds bone-in chicken thighs
2 tsp. brown sugar
1 ½ tsp. smoked paprika
1 tsp. salt
1 ½ tsp. garlic powder

Instructions:
1. Clean and grease the grill or grill pan. Preheat grill to 450 degrees Fahrenheit or grill pan over medium heat.
2. In a small bowl, combine the spices for seasoning.
3. While the grill is preheating, trim the thighs of any trim-able fat and extra skin if there is any. Blot the thighs dry with a paper towel. This is to make sure you get that crispy skin.
4. Rub the seasoning over the thighs and cover entirely. Let rest at room temperature until the grill is preheated.
5. Place the thighs on the grill with the skin side up. Grill for 10 minutes and then flip onto the other side. Grill for an additional 10 minutes with the skin side down. They are done at 165°F, but we like to grill to 180-185°F so the part around the bone isn't bloody. They will not dry out.
6. Remove from grill and allow it to rest for 5 minutes to allow the juices to redistribute into the meat and give you juicy chicken thighs.

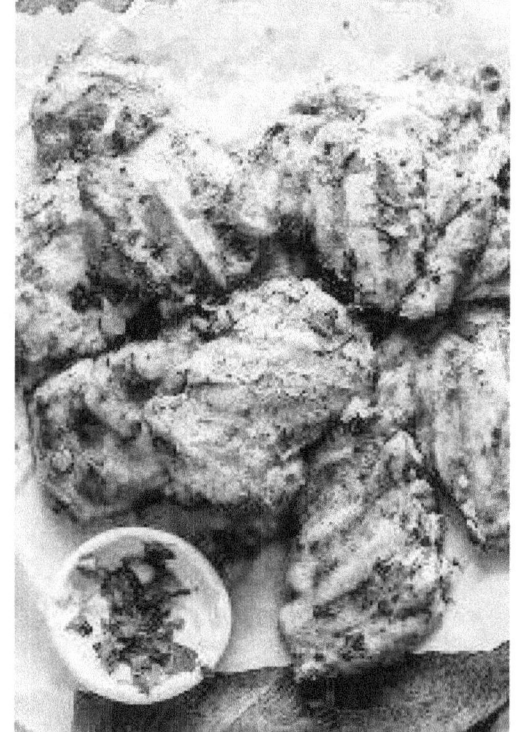

Creamy Mustard Sauce
½ cup Dijon Mustard
½ cup heavy Cream
Dash white pepper

Stir in saucepan on low heat until mixed and thickened.

Also Pairs With

Choc Stout	West Coast IPA	Triple IPA

Double IPA

Double IPA should be hop-centric and assertive both in aroma and flavor and have a higher alcohol content than a standard IPA (not "double," per se, just higher), achieved by adding more malt. Pairs nicely with sausage and rich spicy barbecue beef.

Double IPA: Key Characteristics		Notable Double IPA
Attribute	Description	Beast of Both Worlds IPA
ABV	7.5–10%+ — high alcohol, often warming on the finish2	Double Dust
IBU (Bitterness)	60–120 — intense bitterness, especially in West Coast styles	Trainwreck Hazy DIPA
Color (SRM)	6–14 SRM — deep gold to copper	Port Mongo Double IPA
Body	Medium to full — rich, sometimes syrupy	Just One Thing…Nelson!
Carbonation	Medium to high — helps lift heavy flavors	DDH Hazy DIPA
Finish	Dry to slightly sweet, with lingering hop bitterness	RuinTen IPA

Taste: Boozy | Hoppy | Juicy | Malty | Carmel | Biscuit
Food Pairings: Smoked Meats | Spicy BBQ | Dark Chocolate Desserts | Roast Meats

Food Pairing Guide for Double IPA

Double IPA—also known as Imperial IPA—is the bold, boozy beast of the hop world. It's where brewers go all-in on hops, malt, and alcohol, creating a beer that's intense yet surprisingly drinkable.

Spicy & Bold Dishes
- Buffalo Wings or spicy fried chicken: Bitterness cools the heat; hops enhance tangy sauces
- Thai Curry (Green or Red): Coconut and chili balance the beer's hop punch
- Spicy Tacos (Al Pastor, Chorizo): Citrus hops echo lime and pineapple; malt softens spice

Grilled & Roasted Meats
- BBQ Ribs or Brisket: Smoky, sweet sauces contrast beautifully with hop bitterness
- Grilled Steak with Chimichurri: Herbal sauce and charred meat match the beer's intensity
- Pulled Pork with Spicy Rub: Fat and spice are lifted by carbonation and alcohol warmth

Cheese & Savory Snacks
- Aged Cheddar or Blue Cheese: Sharp, funky flavors stand up to bold hops
- Smoked Gouda or Gruyère: Nutty and smoky notes complement malt sweetness
- Loaded Nachos or Fries: Rich toppings like bacon, jalapenos, and cheese balance bitterness

Vegetarian Options
- Stuffed Portobello Mushrooms: Earthy umami matches roasted malt and piney hops
- Grilled Veggie Skewers with Garlic & Herbs: Roasted flavors and herbal brightness pair well

Dessert Pairings
- Bittersweet Chocolate Cake: Cocoa and caramel echo malt sweetness and contrast hop bite
- Carrot Cake with Cream Cheese Frosting: Spice and richness complement boozy warmth
- Grapefruit Sorbet or Citrus Tart:

Grilled Ham and Cheese Sandwich

This pairing is all about contrast and complementing the beer's bitterness and alcohol tame the richness, while its malt sweetness plays nice with the savory layers. The hops in a Double IPA cut through the cheese's creaminess and the buttery bread, refreshing your palate between bites. The saltiness of the ham enhances the perception of hop flavors, making the beer taste even more vibrant. The slight sweetness in the beer's malt base complements the ham's cured richness, and the caramelized crust of the sandwich. A Double IPA is no wallflower—it stands up to the intensity of grilled cheese and salty ham without getting lost.

Ingredients:

Sandwich
Thick sliced bread
Deli Ham
Sliced Provolone cheese
2 or 3 onions, grilled
Butter, for grilling

For the Grilled Onions:
3/4 tsp. salt
1 tsp. sugar
1 tbsp. honey
2 tsp. apple cider vinegar
1/2 tsp. coarse ground black pepper

For Mayo Dip:
1/2 cup mayonnaise
2 tbsp. chili garlic sauce
1 tbsp. apple cider vinegar
2 tbsp. honey
1/2 tsp. coarse black pepper

Instructions:

For Mayo Dip:
1. Combine all the ingredients in a small bowl and mix. Taste for seasoning. Set aside.

For the Grilled Onions:
1. Slice the onions very thin.
2. Heat a large cast iron pan. Place the onions in the heated pan and sprinkle with salt and sugar.
3. Allow the onions to get a nice golden color and become very soft.
4. Place the onions in a small bowl and add the apple cider vinegar, black pepper, honey, and toss. Set aside.

Building the Sandwich:
1. Place about 2 slices of cheese and ham on each slice of bread.
2. Place the onions on one side of the bread and then close the sandwich.
3. Heat a large cast-iron frying pan.
4. Place a few pats of butter on one side of the closed sandwich and place in the heated pan.
5. Cover the sandwich with another heavy pan to press the sandwich down. Grill the sandwich for about 3 minutes until golden.
6. Place butter pats on the ungrilled side and carefully turn the sandwich over to grill; place a heavy pan on top of the sandwich once again.
7. Finish grilling for about 3 minutes.

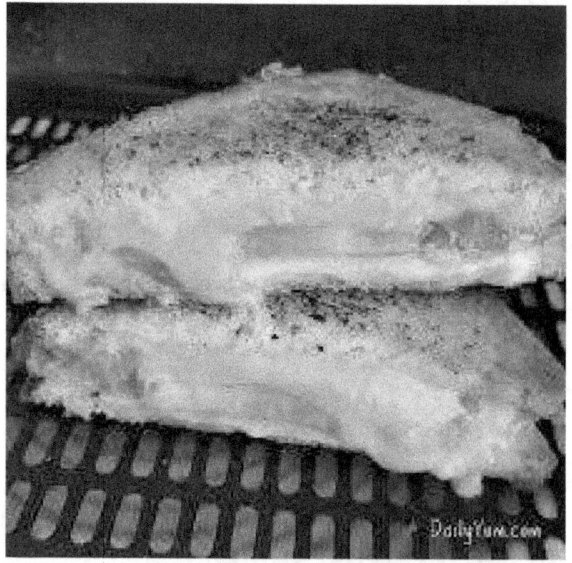

Also Pairs With

English Brown Ale	Amber Ale	Pilsner

Sour Ales

What Is a Sour Ale?
Sour ales are beers intentionally brewed to have a tart, acidic, or funky flavor profile. Unlike most modern beers, which are fermented with controlled yeast strains, sour ales often use wild yeasts and bacteria—like *Lactobacillus*, *Pediococcus*, and *Brettanomyces*—to create their signature tang. Some are barrel-aged for months or even years, while others use faster methods like kettle souring.

Flavor Profile Breakdown

Characteristic Typical Range

Color	Pale straw to deep red or brown
Acidity	Mild to intense tartness
ABV	3% – 8% (some go higher)
Aroma	Fruity, funky, earthy, vinous, spicy

Types of Sour Ales by Region

Style	Origin	Flavor Profile
Berliner Weisse	Germany	Light, tart, low ABV; often served with fruit syrup
Gose	Germany	Salty, citrusy, with coriander spice
Lambic	Belgium	Funky, dry, often blended with fruit (e.g., cherry for Kriek)
Flanders Red Ale	Belgium	Deep red, vinous, aged in oak barrels
Oud Bruin	Belgium	Brown, malty, with gentle sourness
American Wild Ale	USA	Experimental, often fruit-forward or funky
Kettle Sour	Global	Quick souring method; bright and clean acidity

Food Pairing Tips
- Use Acidity to Cut Through Richness
- Match Fruit with Fruit
- Balance Funk with Bold Flavors
- Contrast Tartness with Sweet or Spicy

Awesome Food Pairings

Sour Ale Style	Best Pairings
Berliner Weisse	Soft cheeses, fruit tarts, ceviche
Gose	Grilled shrimp, goat cheese, watermelon salad
Lambic (Kriek, Framboise)	Duck breast, dark chocolate, berry desserts
Flanders Red	Charcuterie, roast pork, aged Gouda
American Wild Ale	BBQ, funky cheeses, mushroom risotto

Wild

Sour beers, also labeled "wild," are made by intentionally inoculating the wort (sugary liquid that turns into beer) with wild yeast strains. These beers can range from slightly tart to massively sour. Tangy, stinky cheese, fresh fruit, seafood with lemon and/or drawn butter, egg dishes, cured pork and other salty meats or anything with a vinegar-based sauce.

Wild Beer: Key Characteristics		Notable Wilds
Attribute	Description	Destihl Wild Sour Dragonfruit Mango
ABV	Typically, 6–10%, but can vary widely depending on the base style	The Bruery Terreux
IBU (Bitterness)	5–30 — usually low, as sourness and funk dominate the profile	Funkatorium
Color	Highly variable — from pale gold to deep amber or even darker	La Roja
Body	Light to medium — often lighter than expected because of acidity	Coolship Resurgam
Carbonation	Moderate to high — effervescent and lively	
Finish	Dry to tart, often with lingering funk or fruit notes	

Taste: Fruity | Floral | Earthy | Funky | Sour
Food Pairings: Charcuterie boards | Grilled Pork | Cheese | Smoked Meats

Flavor Profiles of Wild Beers
Wild-style beer—often referred to as American Wild Ale or simply wild ale—is a boundary-pushing category that embraces unpredictability, fermentation funk, and microbial magic.

Cheese Pairings
- Goat Cheese & Brie: Their creamy tang complements sour ales beautifully
- Washed-rind Cheeses: Match the funk of Brett-heavy beers

Light & Fresh Dishes
- Salads with Vinaigrette: Acidity in both beer and dressing creates harmony
- Ceviche or Sushi: Bright, citrusy beers enhance delicate seafood flavors

Rich & Hearty Fare
- Charcuterie & Smoked Meats: Earthy wild ales balance the salt and smoke
- Roasted Game Meats: Venison, elk, or duck pair well with dry, funky brews

Desserts
- Fruit Tarts or Lemon Bars: Sour beers echo the tartness and refresh the palate
- Cheesecake with Berry Compote: Funky beers contrast the richness and highlight the fruit

Ceviche

The tartness of wild ale mirrors the citrus in ceviche, amplifying the dish's brightness without clashing. The earthy, funky notes in wild ale add depth to the clean, oceanic flavors of the seafood. Wild ales are often highly carbonated, which scrubs the palate and keeps the ceviche tasting crisp and vibrant. If the wild ale has stone fruit or citrus notes, it can echo the ceviche's ingredients like mango, lime, or chili.

Ingredients:
1 1/4 lbs. medium shrimp, peeled, deveined and tails removed
1/3 cup fresh lime juice
1/3 cup fresh lemon juice
2 medium Roma tomatoes, diced (1 cup)
3/4 cup chopped red onion
1/2 cup chopped cilantro
1 medium jalapeno pepper, diced
Salt and pepper, to taste
1/2 medium cucumber, peeled and diced (about 1 cup)
1 medium avocado, diced

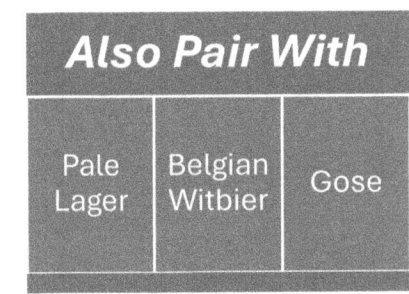

Instructions:
1. Bring a pot of water to a boil. Meanwhile, fill up a medium bowl with ice water, set aside.
2. Add shrimp to boiling water and cook just until pink and opaque, about 1 minute.
3. Drain the shrimp in a colander and then transfer them to ice water to cool for a few minutes. Drain well, then chop the shrimp into small pieces (about 1/2-inch).
4. In a medium non-reactive bowl (you can use the same bowl that was previously filled with ice water) combine shrimp, lime juice, lemon juice, tomatoes, onion, cilantro, jalapeno pepper and season with salt and pepper to taste.
5. Transfer to the refrigerator and let rest 30 minutes to 1 hour.
6. Toss in cucumber and avocado and serve (if desired, you can strain off some juices). It's delicious with tortilla chips or over tostada shells.

Fried Sweet Plantains (Maduros)
2 ripe plantains (yellow with black spots—soft but not mushy)
2–3 Tbsp. vegetable oil (or coconut oil for extra flavor)
Pinch of salt (optional)

Also Pair With		
Pale Lager	Belgian Witbier	Gose

Cut off the ends of the plantain. Score the peel lengthwise and remove it. Slice diagonally into ½-inch-thick pieces for more surface area and caramelization. In a large skillet, heat oil over medium heat until shimmering. Add plantain slices in a single layer. Fry for 2–3 minutes per side until golden brown and caramelized. Flip carefully with tongs or a spatula. Transfer to a towel-lined plate. Sprinkle with a pinch of salt if desired.

Lambic

Lambic differs from most other beers because it is fermented through exposure to wild yeasts and bacteria native to the Zenne valley, as opposed to exposure to carefully cultivated strains of brewer's yeast. This process gives the beer its distinctive flavor: dry, vinous, and cidery, often with a tart aftertaste, and pairs with vinegar-based sauces.

Lambic: Key Characteristics		Notable Lambics
Attribute	**Description**	Lindeman's Framboise
ABV	2–8% — varies by style and age	Thumbprint Nectar Ale
IBU (Bitterness)	0–10 — very low; sourness replaces bitterness	Coolship Series
Color (SRM)	Pale gold to deep red — depending on fruit additions	Beatification
Body	Light to medium — often dry and tart	Gueuze 100% Lambic
Carbonation	Low to high — varies by substyle (e.g., Gueuze is sparkling)	Hommage
Finish	Dry, tart, funky, and sometimes vinous or cider-like	Oude Lambiek

Taste: Funky | Fruit | Sour |
Food Pairings: Grilled Pork | Spicy | Cheese

Food Pairing Guide for Lambic

Lambic beers—Belgium's wild-fermented treasures—offer a stunning range of flavors from tart and fruity to earthy and funky. Use lambic's tartness to cut through fat and richness.

Cheese Pairings
- Goat Cheese (Chèvre): Enhances the citrus and barnyard notes of Greuze lambics.
- Triple Cream Cheeses (Brillat-Savarin, Camembert): Their richness is cut beautifully by the tartness and effervescence of fruit lambics like kriek or framboise.
- Aged Gouda or Comté: Nutty and firm cheeses pair well with the earthy depth of unfruited lambics.

Meat & Savory Dishes
- Duck Confit or Pork Belly: Lambic's acidity slices through the richness of fatty meats.
- Mussels with Garlic & Herbs: A classic Belgian pairing, especially with Greuze.
- Charcuterie Boards: Funky lambics complement cured meats and pickled vegetables.

Desserts
- Fruit Tarts (Cherry, Raspberry): Perfect with fruit lambics like kriek or framboise.
- Lemon Bars or Cheesecake: The tartness of lambic balances creamy, citrusy desserts.
- Apple Galette or Peach Cobbler: Match with muscat or peach lambics for a layered fruit experience.

Light Fare & Snacks
- Fresh Berries or Stone Fruits: Serve alongside fruit lambics to echo their flavors.
- Salads with Vinaigrette: Acidity in both beer and dressing creates harmony.
- Toasted Nuts or Olives: Earthy snacks that play well with funky lambics.

Smoked Chicken Wrap

Lambic's tartness slices through the creamy sauces and smoky meat, keeping the wrap from feeling heavy. The earthy, wild-yeast character complements the charred, smoky chicken in a way that's complex and satisfying. Fruited Lambics add a sweet-tart contrast to the savory wrap, especially if there's a spicy or herbaceous element. The effervescence scrubs the palate clean, making each bite feel fresh and vibrant.

Ingredients:
12 ounces cooked, shredded chicken
3 ounces shredded cheddar cheese
3 ounces roasted tomatoes, diced
6 ounces spring mix or mixed greens
1 ounce honey
1/2-ounce sriracha
2 drops liquid smoke
4 ounces olive oil
3 twelve-inch whole-wheat flour wraps

Instructions:
1. Make the filling: In a large bowl, whisk together honey, sriracha, liquid smoke, and olive oil. Add shredded chicken, cheddar cheese, roasted tomatoes, and spring mix. Toss to combine.
2. Assemble the wraps: Lay out a whole wheat wrap on a flat surface. Place a third of the filling on the bottom edge of the wrap. Top with Roast Pepper Aioli below.
3. Roll the wraps: Fold the bottom of the wrap over the filling, then fold in the sides. Continue rolling to form a tight wrap.

Roasted Red Pepper Aioli
1 large roasted red pepper (jarred or freshly roasted, peeled and seeded)
½ cup mayonnaise
1 clove garlic
1 Tbsp. lemon juice
½ tsp. smoked paprika
Salt to taste
Optional: pinch of cayenne or chili flakes for heat

Blend all ingredients in a blender or food processor. Blend until smooth and creamy. Add more lemon juice for brightness, garlic for punch, or paprika for smokiness. Chill, Refrigerate for at least 30 minutes to let flavors meld. Add to wrap for next-level taste.

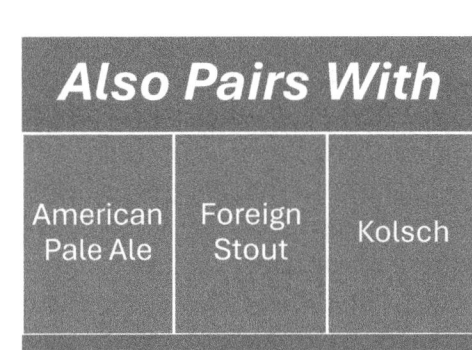

Also Pairs With		
American Pale Ale	Foreign Stout	Kolsch

Beliner Weisse

Berliner Weisse is a sour wheat beer that is produced only in Berlin, Germany. This brew is tart and bubbly, a combination that is not for everyone, but Berliners and most Germans love it! Pairs with tart fruit, fruit salads, light greens along with red berries, Kumquats, or tart melon. Perfect for fatty barbecue and heavily salted dishes.

Berliner Weisse: Key Characteristics		Notable Beliner Weisse
Attribute	**Description**	Modist Half Believing Gravity
ABV	2.8–3.8% — very low; designed for refreshment	Cherry Lime Berliner Weisse
IBU (Bitterness)	3–8 — extremely low; sourness replaces bitterness	Peach & Passion Fruit Berliner
Color (SRM)	2–4 SRM — pale straw to light gold	Boysenberry & Black Currant Berliner
Body	Light — crisp and dry	Valencia Orange Berliner Weisse
Carbonation	High — lively and sparkling	
Finish	Tart, dry, and slightly fruity or funky depending on fermentation	

Taste: Sour | Bready | Fruity | Earthy
Food Pairings: Grilled Pork | Beef | Chicken | Smoked Salmon | Fruit Salads | Charcuterie

Food Pairing Guide for Beliner Weisse
Berliner Weisse is a delightfully tart and effervescent German wheat beer—often called the **"Champagne of the North"** for its light body and sparkling acidity.

Cheese Pairings
- Fresh Goat Cheese: Tangy and creamy—perfect with the beer's acidity
- Ricotta or Mascarpone: Mild cheeses that let Berliner Weisse shine
- Young Brie or Camembert: Soft and buttery, balanced by the beer's tartness

Light Fare & Veggies
- Arugula Salad with Citrus Vinaigrette: Peppery greens and bright dressing echo the beer's profile
- Grilled Asparagus or Zucchini: Earthy veggies contrast the crispness
- Avocado Toast with Pickled Onions: Creamy, tangy, and fresh

Seafood Dishes
- Ceviche or Crudo: Acidic beer complements citrus-marinated fish
- Smoked Salmon on Rye: A nod to Northern European flavors
- Shrimp Cocktail: Bright and briny, with a refreshing finish

Poultry & Light Meats
- Lemon-Herb Chicken: Citrus and herbs match the beer's brightness
- Turkey Sandwich with Cranberry Relish: Tart meets savory
- Prosciutto-Wrapped Melon: Sweet, salty, and tangy—especially good with fruited Berliner Weisse

Desserts
- Lemon Bars or Key Lime Pie: Tart-on-tart pairing that sings
- Berry Pavlova or Sorbet: Light, fruity, and refreshing
- Crepes with Raspberry Syrup: Echoes traditional Berliner Weisse service

Bratwurst Stewed with Sauerkraut

The tartness of Berliner Weisse complements the fermented zing of sauerkraut, enhancing its brightness without clashing. The beer's acidity and carbonation slice through the richness of the bratwurst, refreshing your palate after each bite. Wheat and citrus notes in the beer echo the herbal spices in the sausage while contrasting the saltiness of the kraut. You get all the flavor without overwhelming the dish or your senses—perfect for a long afternoon meal.

Ingredients:
2 Tbsp. oil
2 pounds fresh bratwurst links
2 onions, chopped
2 garlic cloves, minced
3 cups chicken stock
1 Tbsp. paprika
1 Tbsp. caraway seeds
4 cups sauerkraut, drained
2 Tbsp. chopped fresh dill
1 baguette

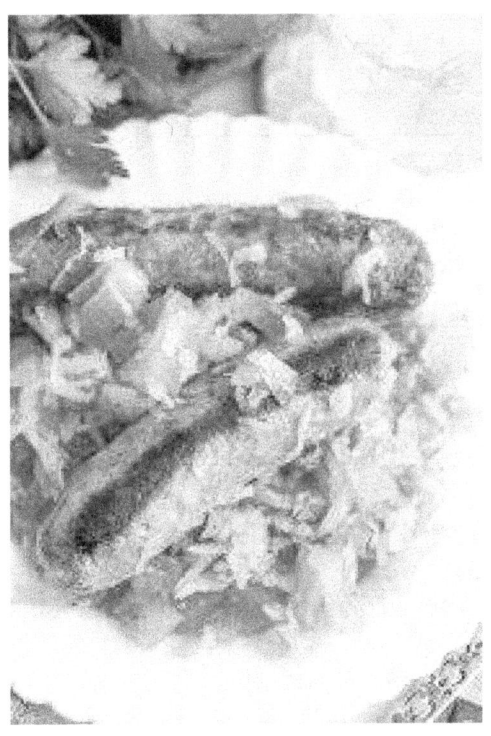

Instructions:
In a large pan, heat oil over high heat. Brown bratwurst in oil and reduce heat to medium. Add onions and garlic and cook until lightly caramelized. Add stock, paprika, caraway seeds, and sauerkraut and simmer for 45 minutes. Remove from the heat and stir in fresh dill. Serve on baguette.

Warm German Potato Salad
2 lbs. red or Yukon Gold potatoes
6 slices of thick-cut bacon
½ cup finely chopped onion
¼ cup apple cider vinegar
2 Tbsp. Dijon mustard
1 Tbsp. sugar
½ tsp. salt
¼ tsp. black pepper
2 Tbsp. chopped fresh parsley (optional garnish)

Also Pair With		
German Oilsner	Munich Helles	Dunkel

Scrub and boil whole potatoes in salted water until fork-tender (about 15–20 minutes). Drain, cool slightly, then slice into ¼-inch rounds or chunks. In a large skillet, cook bacon until crispy. Remove and crumble. Reserve 2–3 Tbsp. of bacon fat in the pan. In the skillet, add the chopped onion to the bacon fat and cook until soft and translucent (about 3–4 minutes). Stir in vinegar, mustard, sugar, salt, and pepper. Simmer for 1–2 minutes to blend flavors. Pour over the potatoes and gently mix to coat evenly.

Flanders

A Flanders red ale, also known as Flemish red-brown, is a style of sour ale brewed in West Flanders, Belgium. Flanders red ales undergo long periods of aging, often in oak barrels, to develop their distinctive flavor. Expect flavors of plum, prune, raisin, and raspberry are common, followed by orange and some spiciness. The sour and acidic taste can range from moderate to strong. Often Flanders is described as the most wine-like of all beers.

Flanders Red Ale: Key Characteristics		Notable Flanders
Attribute	**Description**	Duchesse de Bourgogne
ABV	4.6–6.5% — moderate, with a smooth warmth2	Rodenbach
IBU (Bitterness)	10–25 — low; acidity and tannins replace hop bitterness2	Vander Ghinste Roodbruin
Color (SRM)	10–16 SRM — deep red, burgundy, or reddish-brown	
Body	Medium — soft and rounded, often with a wine-like texture	
Carbonation	Low to moderate — gentle effervescence	
Finish	Dry, tart, and tannic — reminiscent of aged red wine	

Taste: Complex | Fruity | Acidic | Oaked Malty
Food Pairings: Grilled Pork | Spicy | Cheese

Food Pairing Guide for Flanders

Flanders Red Ale is a beer for contemplative sipping—layered, elegant, and deeply expressive. It's where beer meets wine in the best possible way.

Cheese Pairings
- Aged Gouda or Gruyère: Nutty and caramel-like, echoing the malt sweetness
- Blue Cheese (Gorgonzola, Stilton): Funk meets funk—intense and rewarding
- Washed-Rind Cheeses (Taleggio, Époisses): Earthy and pungent, perfect with the beer's acidity

Meat & Savory Dishes
- Braised Short Ribs or Beef Bourguignon: Rich meats meet the beer's acidity and depth
- Duck Breast with Cherry Reduction: Fruit and game are a classic match
- Charcuterie with Pickled Veggies: Salt, fat, and acid in harmony

Vegetables & Light Fare
- Roasted Root Vegetables: Earthy sweetness complements malt and oak
- Beet Salad with Goat Cheese: Tangy and vibrant, great with Flanders Red
- Grilled Mushrooms or Eggplant: Umami-rich and satisfying

Desserts
- Dark Chocolate Tart or Flourless Cake: Bitterness and richness balance the beer's acidity
- Cherry Clafoutis or Berry Cobbler: Fruit-forward desserts echo the beer's profile
- Caramel Flan or Bread Pudding: Sweet and creamy with a touch of tang

Smoked Ribeye

The tartness of the ale slices through the ribeye's richness, balancing each bite and keeping your palate refreshed. Cherry and berry notes in the beer play beautifully with the steak's smoky crust, adding contrast and intrigue. The ale's wine-like structure pairs well with the deep umami of aged, marbled beef—like a red wine, but with bubbles. The earthy undertones of the beer echo the grilled, caramelized edges of the steak, creating a layered flavor experience.

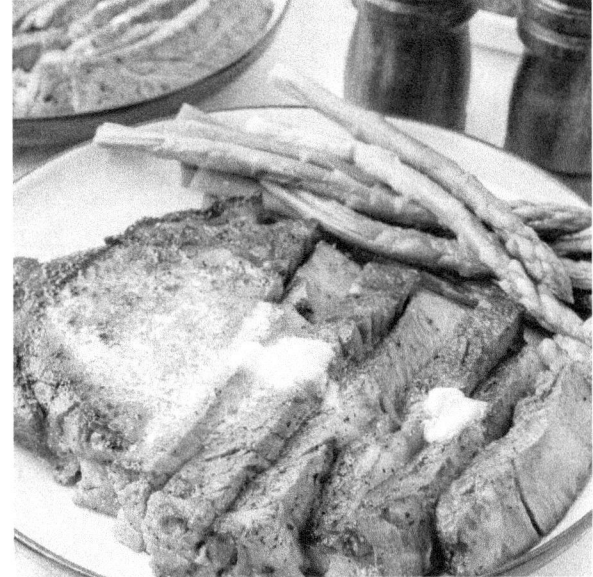

Ingredients:
1 Ribeye, 1–1 ½ inches thick
Coarse Salt
1 tsp. butter per steak

Instructions:
1. 60 minutes before smoking, salt your ribeye on both sides.
2. Preheat smoker to 220-225°F using your favorite wood chips.
3. Once your smoker is at temperature, place ribeye's in smoker and place the thermometer in the steak. Cook steaks until they reach an internal temperature of 110-115°F, then remove them from the smoker. About 25-30 minutes.
4. Heat the BBQ grill to 400°F, or a pan on the stovetop with 1 tbsp of oil until the oil shimmers and just smokes. Place the ribeye on the pan or grill and sear for 2-3 minutes, it is nicely seared, then flip and cook for another 2-3 minutes. Add a tsp. of butter to the steak after you flip it for extra flavor. Pull the steak off the heat when it reaches your desired doneness- it will cook faster.

Creamy Peppercorn Sauce
1 Tbsp. whole black peppercorns (crushed slightly)
1 Tbsp. unsalted butter
1 small shallot, finely minced
½ cup beef or vegetable broth
½ cup heavy cream
1 Tbsp. brandy or cognac (optional, for depth)
Salt to taste

Also Pairs With		
Robust Porter	Dry Stout	American Ale

In a skillet over medium heat, melt butter. Add crushed peppercorns and toast for 1 minute until fragrant. Add minced shallots and cook until soft and translucent (about 2–3 minutes). Add brandy or cognac (if using) and simmer for 30 seconds to burn off the alcohol. Scrape up any bits from the pan. Add the broth and simmer until reduced by half (about 3–5 minutes). Stir in heavy cream and simmer gently until thickened (another 3–5 minutes). Season with salt to taste. Pour over steak or add to a small dipping container.

Wheat Beer

Wheat beers are one of the most flexible beers when pairing. This comes in handy for barbecue meals. Some wheat beers are also very spicy. You must be keen when you are choosing the barbecue dish to pair it with, avoid the delicacy being too heavy. Since wheat has no flavor, many processes, therefore, add citrus to make it more enjoyable to drink. This works well with smoked salmon, Buffalo wings and a variety of seafood. Hefeweizens and wheat beers are great when combined with soups and grilled vegetable dishes. Wheat beers are one of the most flexible beers when pairing. It is because it can be paired with a variety of meals. This comes in handy for barbecue meals.

Wheat Beer: Key Characteristics	
Attribute	Description
ABV	2.8–5.6% — light to moderate strength
IBU (Bitterness)	10–35 — low to moderate; hops play a supporting role
Color (SRM)	2–8 SRM — straw to light amber
Body	Light to medium — creamy and smooth because of wheat proteins
Carbonation	Medium to high — lively and refreshing
Finish	Crisp, sometimes tart or fruity depending on style

Wheat beer is a refreshing, versatile style known for its smooth mouthfeel, hazy appearance, and **fruity-spicy character**. It's brewed with a significant proportion of wheat—usually 30–50% or more—which gives it its signature texture and flavor.

Flavor & Aroma Profile
- **Wheat**: Adds a soft, bready, and slightly tangy base
- **Yeast**: Often contributes banana, clove, bubblegum, or **citrus** notes (especially in German styles)
- **Hops**: Mild and subtle—herbal, floral, or citrusy depending on the region
- **Mouthfeel**: Creamy and smooth with excellent head retention

Popular Wheat Beer Styles

Style	Key Traits
German Hefeweizen	Unfiltered, hazy, with banana and clove from yeast
Belgian Witbiers	Brewed with coriander and orange peel; citrusy and spicy
American Wheat Beer	Cleaner yeast profile; often citrusy and hop-forward
Berliner Weisse	Tart and sour; often served with fruit syrups
Gose	Salty and sour with coriander spice
Dunkelweizen	Dark wheat beer with caramel and banana notes

Food Pairings
- Grilled chicken or fish — complements light seasoning
- Goat cheese or feta — acidity and creaminess match well
- Fruit desserts — echoes, esters and citrus notes
- Brisket burritos or salads — balances richness with refreshment

Wheat Ales

Wheat beers, also known as wheat ales, are a diverse category of beers brewed with a significant proportion of wheat besides malted barley. Wheat imparts a clean and unobtrusive grain flavor. Wheat beers offer a range of flavors, from light and refreshing to complex and spicy. Common flavor notes include citrus, banana, and spices.

Wheat Ale: Key Characteristics		Notable Wheat Ales
Attribute	Description	Vedett Extra White
ABV	4.5–5.5% — sessionable and smooth	Allagash White
IBU (Bitterness)	15–30 — low to moderate; hops are subtle but present	Live Oak Hefeweizen
Color (SRM)	3–6 SRM — pale gold to light amber	Stone & Wood The Gatherer
Body	Light to medium — soft and rounded because of wheat proteins	Alaskan White
Carbonation	Medium to high — refreshing and lively	Samuel Adams Summer Ale
Finish	Clean and dry, sometimes with a touch of citrus or spice	

Taste: Bready | Citrus | Herbal | Malt Sweetness
Food Pairings: Seafood | Grilled Veggies | Poultry

Wheat Ale—especially in its American Wheat Ale form—is a refreshing, easy-drinking style that blends the smooth texture of wheat with a clean, crisp finish. It's less yeast-driven than its German cousin (Hefeweizen) and more hop-friendly, making it a versatile canvas for brewers.

Food Pairing Guide for Wheat Ales
Cheese Pairings
- Fresh Goat Cheese or Ricotta: Tangy and mild, perfect with citrusy wheat ales
- Brie or Camembert: Soft and creamy, balanced by the beer's effervescence
- Havarti or Young Gouda: Mild and buttery, ideal for American wheat ales

Light Fare & Veggies
- Citrus-Dressed Salads: Echo the beer's brightness
- Grilled Asparagus or Zucchini: Earthy veggies contrast the light body
- Avocado Toast with Herbs: Creamy and fresh, especially with Witbiers

Seafood Dishes
- Grilled Shrimp or Scallops: Sweet and delicate, enhanced by wheat ale's acidity
- Fish Tacos with Mango Salsa: Tropical and spicy flavors pop with Belgian wit
- Smoked Salmon on Toast: Rich and briny, balanced by the beer's crispness

Poultry & Light Meats
- Lemon-Herb Chicken: Citrus and herbs match the beer's profile
- Turkey Sandwich with Cranberry Relish: Tart and savory pairing
- Prosciutto-Wrapped Melon: Sweet, salty, and refreshing

Desserts
- Citrus Sorbet or Lemon Bars: Tart-on-tart pairing that sparkles
- Banana Bread or Spice Cake: Especially with hefeweizen's banana-clove notes
- Berry Shortcake: Fruity and creamy, great with American wheat ales

Shrimp Po' Boy

A shrimp po'boy pairs beautifully with a wheat ale because the beer's light, citrusy, and effervescent character complements the sandwich's crispy, briny, and creamy richness in all the right ways. The fried shrimp in a po'boy are crunchy, salty, and slightly sweet. A wheat ale—with its soft carbonation and smooth mouthfeel—refreshes the palate and cuts through the fried coating, keeping each bite light and lively. Wheat ales often have citrus notes (like lemon, orange, or coriander) that brighten the shrimp's natural sweetness and play beautifully with any tangy remoulade or hot sauce. The beer's subtle fruitiness enhances the briny, oceanic flavor of the shrimp without overpowering it.

Ingredients:

For the Shrimp:
1 lb. medium shrimp, peeled and deveined
1 cup buttermilk
1 cup cornmeal
1 cup all-purpose flour
1 tsp paprika
1 tsp garlic powder
½ tsp cayenne pepper
Salt and pepper to taste
Vegetable oil for frying

For the Remoulade Sauce:
½ cup mayo
2 tbsp Dijon mustard
1 tbsp ketchup
1 tbsp chopped pickles or relish
1 tsp hot sauce
1 tsp paprika
1 clove garlic, minced
Salt and pepper to taste

For Assembly:
4 French rolls or baguette sections, split
Shredded lettuce
Sliced tomatoes
Pickles (optional)

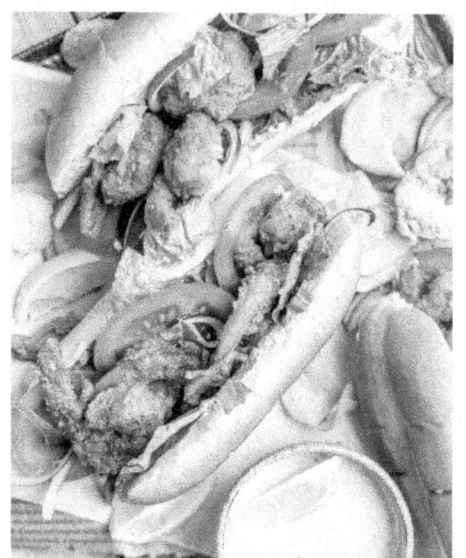

Instructions:
1. Marinate the Shrimp: Toss shrimp in buttermilk and let sit for 15–30 minutes.
2. Make the Remoulade: Mix all sauce ingredients in a bowl. Chill until ready to use.
3. Prepare the Coating: In a separate bowl, combine cornmeal, flour, paprika, garlic powder, cayenne, salt, and pepper.
4. Fry the Shrimp. Heat oil to 350°F (175°C). Dredge shrimp in the dry mixture. Fry in batches until golden and crispy (about 2–3 minutes). Drain on paper towels.
5. Assemble the Po'boy:
   - Spread remoulade on both sides of the bread.
   - Layer lettuce, tomatoes, and pickles.
   - Add fried shrimp generously.
   - Serve immediately while hot and crispy.

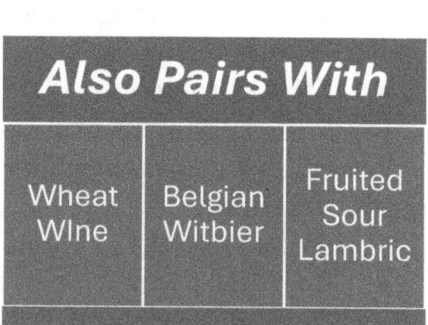

Also Pairs With

Wheat Wine	Belgian Witbier	Fruited Sour Lambric

Hefeweizen

These usually have a little heavier body compared to a Light Lager but are still refreshing and light enough for chicken and seafood. With these, you will find a delicate blend of fruit flavors (like banana, for example), lemon, cloves, coriander, and a hint of tartness. Classically paired with Weisswurst (white sausage); contrasts with pungent, intense aromatics such as mustard flavors, pickles, horseradish, and cured meats. Go to beer for smoked sausage and hot links and dry-rubbed ribs.

Hefeweizen: Key Characteristics		Notable Hefeweizen
Attribute	Description	Paulaner Hefeweizen
ABV	4.9–5.6% — moderate and sessionable	Ayinger Bräuweisse
IBU (Bitterness)	8–15 — very low; bitterness is subtle and balanced	Live Oak Hefeweizen
Color (SRM)	3–9 SRM — pale straw to amber; always hazy	Altstadt Hefeweizen
Body	Medium-light — creamy and smooth because of wheat proteins	Sierra Nevada Kellerweis
Carbonation	High — lively and effervescent with a thick, foamy head	Franziskaner Hefe-Weissbier
Finish	Dry and crisp, with lingering fruit and spice	

Taste: Fruity | Wheat | Banana | Bready | Floral | Creamy
Food Pairings: Grilled Pork & Seafood | Beef | Chicken | Brat Banana Bread

Food Pairing Guide for Hefeweizen

Hefeweizen is the classic German wheat beer that's all about cloudy charm, fruity spice, and creamy refreshment. It's a style that highlights yeast character more than hops or malt, and it's beloved for its smooth drinkability and expressive aroma.

Cheese Pairings
- Brie or Camembert: Soft and creamy, balanced by the beer's spice
- Goat Cheese: Tangy and fresh, complements fruity esters
- Mild Cheddar or Havarti: Smooth and mellow, ideal with wheat malt

Light Fare & Veggies
- Arugula Salad with Citrus Vinaigrette: Peppery greens and bright dressing echo the beer's zest
- Grilled Asparagus or Zucchini: Earthy veggies contrast the fruity-spicy profile
- Avocado Toast with Pickled Onions: Creamy, tangy, and refreshing

Seafood Dishes
- Grilled Shrimp or Scallops: Sweet and delicate, enhanced by banana and clove
- Smoked Salmon on Rye: Rich and briny, balanced by carbonation
- Fish Tacos with Pineapple Salsa: Tropical fruit notes play beautifully with the beer

Poultry & Light Meats
- Lemon-Herb Chicken: Citrus and herbs match the beer's brightness
- Turkey Sandwich with Cranberry Relish: Tart and savory pairing
- Prosciutto-Wrapped Melon: Sweet, salty, and refreshing

Desserts
- Banana Bread or Spice Cake: Echoes the beer's signature yeast character
- Apple Strudel or Peach Cobbler: Fruity and warmth, great with wheat malt
- Vanilla ice cream with caramel drizzle

Chicken Satay with Peanut Sauce

Chicken satay with peanut sauce pairs beautifully with a hefeweizen because the beer's fruity, spicy, and effervescent profile complements the dish's nutty, savory, and slightly sweet flavors in a way that's both refreshing and harmonious. Peanut sauce is creamy, earthy, and often slightly sweet or spicy. Hefeweizen—with its signature notes of banana, clove, and citrus—adds a bright, fruity contrast that lifts the richness of the sauce and keeps the palate refreshed. The grilled chicken brings smoky, caramelized flavors. The soft wheat malt backbone and light body balance the char without overpowering it, creating a smooth, mellow pairing.

Ingredients:

For the Chicken Satay:
1½ lbs. boneless, skinless chicken thighs or breasts, cut into thin strips
2 tbsp soy sauce
2 tbsp fish sauce
1 tbsp brown sugar
1 tbsp lime juice
1 tbsp vegetable oil
2 cloves garlic, minced
1 tsp ground coriander
1 tsp turmeric
½ tsp ground cumin
Bamboo skewers (soaked in water for 30 minutes)

For the Peanut Sauce:
¾ cup creamy peanut butter
1 tbsp red curry paste
1 tbsp soy sauce
1 tbsp brown sugar
1 tbsp lime juice
1 tsp fish sauce
½ cup coconut milk (more too thin if needed)
Optional: crushed peanuts and chopped cilantro for garnish

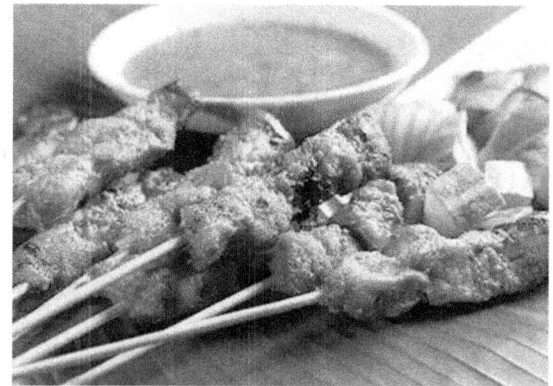

Instructions:

1. In a bowl, mix soy sauce, fish sauce, brown sugar, lime juice, oil, garlic, and spices. Add chicken strips and toss to coat. Marinate for at least 1 hour (or overnight for deeper flavor).
2. In a saucepan over medium heat, combine all sauce ingredients. Stir until smooth and heated through. Adjust the thickness with more coconut milk if needed. Set aside and keep warm.
3. Thread marinated chicken onto skewers. Grill over medium-high heat for 3–4 minutes per side, until cooked through and slightly charred.
4. Plate skewers with a side of peanut sauce. Garnish with crushed peanuts and cilantro.

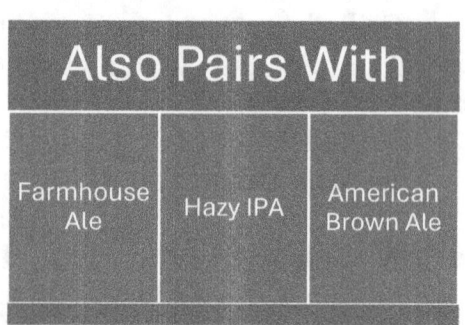

Also Pairs With: Farmhouse Ale | Hazy IPA | American Brown Ale

Gose

Gose is a warm fermented beer that originated in Goslar, Germany. It is usually brewed with at least 50% of the grain bill being malted wheat. Dominant flavors in Gose include lemon sourness, an herbal characteristic, and strong saltiness (the result of either local water sources or added salt). This beer goes well with barbecue side dishes, like coleslaw and potato salad.

Gose: Key Characteristics		Notable Gose
Attribute	**Description**	Anderson Valley Gose Blood Orange
ABV	4.0–5.0% — light and sessionable	Gose Gone Wild
IBU (Bitterness)	5–15 — very low; sourness replaces bitterness	Key Lime Pie Gose
Color (SRM)	3–6 SRM — pale straw to light gold	Druif Blanc
Body	Light — crisp and refreshing	All Roads Lead
Carbonation	Moderate to high — lively and effervescent	Mango Lassi Gose
Finish	Tart, salty, and slightly spicy	Gose Gone Wild

Taste: Complex | Sour | Acidic | Salty | Spicy
Food Pairings: Smoked Fish | Grilled Pork | Goat Cheese |

Food Pairing Guide for Gose Beers
Gose is a wonderfully quirky German beer style that defies convention with its salty, sour, and spicy profile.

Cheese Pairings
- Feta or Halloumi: Salty cheeses echo Goses' briny edge
- Fresh Mozzarella or Burrata: Creamy textures contrast the tartness
- Goat Cheese: Tangy and bright, perfect with citrus-forward Gose

Seafood Dishes
- Oysters or Clams: Salinity meets salinity—pure magic
- Ceviche or Shrimp Cocktail: Acidic beer complements citrus-marinated seafood
- Grilled Fish Tacos: Especially with lime crema or mango salsa

Light Fare & Veggies
- Watermelon & Feta Salad: Sweet, salty, and tangy—Gose loves this combo
- Cucumber Gazpacho: Cool and herbal, a refreshing match
- Roasted Beets with Citrus Vinaigrette: Earthy meets bright acidity

Meat & Mains
- Roast Chicken with Lemon & Herbs: Gose amplifies the citrus and cuts through fat
- Prosciutto-Wrapped Melon: Sweet, salty, and savory—Gose ties it all together
- Pork Schnitzel with Lemon: A nod to Gose's German roots

Desserts
- Key Lime Pie or Lemon Tart: Tart-on-tart pairing that sings
- Salted Caramel Ice Cream: Salty-sweet contrast with Goses' brightness
- Fruit Sorbets (Mango, Raspberry): Refreshing and complementary

Smoked Skirt Steak

The natural salinity of a Gose complements the smoky, seasoned crust of the steak, enhancing umami. The sourness refreshes your palate and balances the richness of the meat. If your steak has lime or citrus in the rub, the Gose amplifies those bright notes. The bubbles lift the flavors and keep the meal from feeling heavy.

Ingredients:
1 lb. skirt steak
kosher salt

Marinade
3 oranges juice of
3 lemons juice of
3 limes juice of
¼ cup olive oil
¼ cup Worcestershire sauce
2 tsp red pepper flakes
1 tsp ground cumin
2 garlic cloves minced

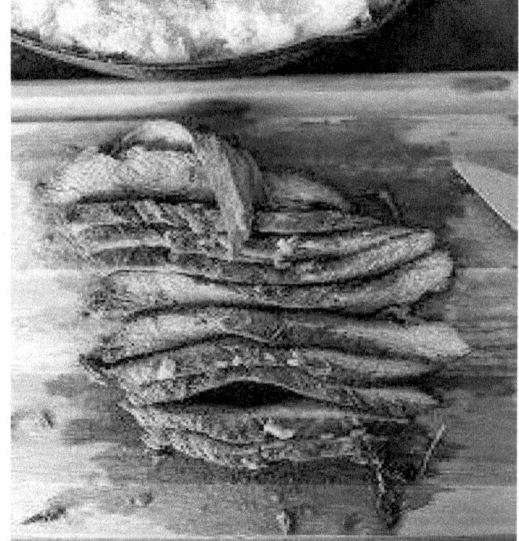

Instructions:
1. Start by dry brining the skirt steaks with about 1 tsp of kosher salt. Let the steaks brine in the refrigerator for 3-4 hours.
2. In a large bowl, combine the orange juice, lemon juice, lime juice, olive oil, Worcestershire sauce, red pepper flakes, cumin, and minced garlic. Mix the marinade ingredients well.
3. Place the skirt steak in a large resealable bag and pour the marinade over it. Seal the bag and massage the marinade into the meat. Marinate in the refrigerator for at least 1-2 hours, or overnight for maximum flavor.
4. Preheat your smoker to 225°F.
5. Remove it from the marinade and pat it dry with paper towels.
6. Season all sides of your skirt steak with your favorite dry rub.
7. Place the skirt steak on the smoker grates and smoke for 45 minutes, or until it reaches an internal temperature of 110°F.

Sear Meat choose one method
   1. Fire up a separate grill to 500°F or move indoors to sear the steaks on a hot cast-iron skillet. Sear for 1-2 minutes per side, until the internal temperature is 130°F (55°C). or
   2. Increase the smoker temperature to high heat, or around 450°F. Sear the skirt steak for 1-2 minutes per side, or until it reaches an internal temperature of 130°F.

8. Remove the skirt steak from the smoker and let it rest for 5-10 minutes before slicing it against the grain and serving.

Add meat to tacos, quesadillas, salads or roast veggies.

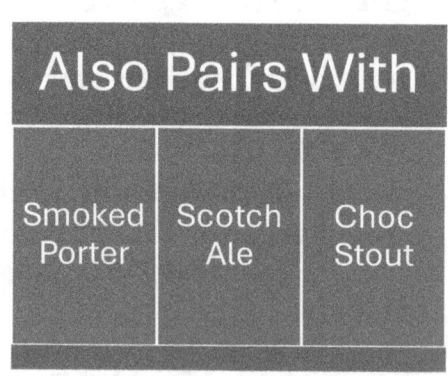

Also Pairs With		
Smoked Porter	Scotch Ale	Choc Stout

Dunkel

A German-style Dunkel, sometimes referred to as a Muncher Dunkel, should have an aroma composed of chocolate, roasted malt and bread or biscuit-like features that stem from the use of Munich malt. Despite the malt forward flavor profile, this beer does not offer an overly sweet impression. Rather, you will find a mild balance between the distinct character of malt and the refined touch of bitterness from noble hops. Pair well with Kansas City Style BBQ, sausages, and slow cooked meats.

Dunkel: Key Characteristics		Notable Dunkel
Attribute	Description	Hofbrau Dunkel
ABV	4.5–5.6% — moderate strength, highly sessionable2	Weihenstephaner Dunke
IBU (Bitterness)	16–25 — low to moderate; bitterness is subtle	Ayinger Dunkel
Color (SRM)	14–28 SRM — deep amber to dark brown	Spaten Dunkel
Body	Medium — smooth and rounded with a soft mouthfeel	Paulaner Dunkel
Carbonation	Moderate — creamy and refreshing	
Finish	Clean and malty, with hints of toast and chocolate lingering	

Taste: Balanced | Malty | Chocolaty | Toasty | Bready | Rich | Light
Food Pairings: Smoked & BBQ meats | Roast Chicken or Pork | Chocolate Desserts

Food Pairing Guise for Dunkel

Dunkel is the original Bavarian dark lager—smooth, malty, and steeped in centuries of tradition. It's a style that delivers depth without heaviness, making it a go-to for those who love rich flavor and a clean finish.

Cheese Pairings
- Aged Gouda or Emmental: Nutty and sweet, echoing the malt profile
- Smoked Cheddar: Adds depth and complements the beer's roast
- Gruyère or Fontina: Melty and savory, perfect for fondue or grilled cheese

Meat & Savory Dishes
- Bratwurst or Weisswurst: Classic Bavarian pairing—add mustard and pretzels
- Roast Pork or Pork Schnitzel: Rich meats balanced by Dunkel's smoothness
- Beef Stew or Sauerbraten: Deep, slow-cooked flavors match the beer's maltiness

Vegetables & Sides
- Red Cabbage or Sauerkraut: Sweet and sour sides that contrast nicely
- Roasted Root Vegetables: Earthy and caramelized—ideal with Dunkel's body
- Soft Pretzels with Mustard: A classic beer hall snack

Desserts
- Apple Strudel or Bread Pudding: Warm, spiced, and comforting
- Chocolate Cake or Brownies: Rich cocoa plays well with roasted malt
- Caramel Flan or Toffee Bars: Sweetness mirrors the beer's caramel notes

Beef Rouladen

Beef Rouladen—thinly sliced beef rolled with mustard, bacon, onions, and pickles—is braised until tender, developing deep, meaty flavors. Dunkel's offer toasty malt notes like bread crust, caramel, and mild chocolate, which echo the browned beef and savory fillings without overpowering them. The dish's onions and bacon bring sweetness and umami, while the mustard and pickles add tang. Dunkel's have a subtle malt sweetness and low bitterness, which balances the acidity and enhances the umami, creating a smooth, cohesive bite. Their moderate carbonation lifts the richness of the gravy and meat, keeping the pairing from feeling heavy.

Ingredients:
4 - ¼ inch thick slices of deli roast beef
Kosher salt and freshly ground black pepper
1/2 cup spicy brown mustard
2 dill pickles, sliced into thin spears
1 large onion, thinly sliced
1/2 cup chopped browned bacon
One 32-ounce carton beef stock
2 sliced potatoes,
1 cup all-purpose flour
1 cup butter, melted

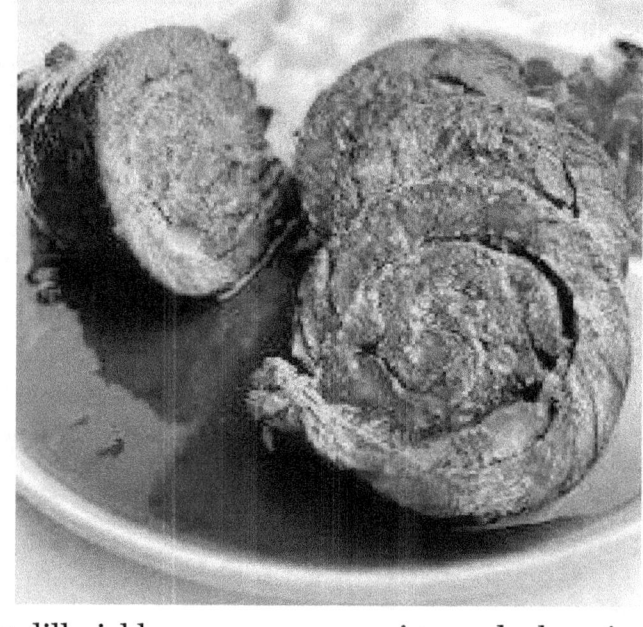

Instructions:
1. Preheat the oven to 375 degrees F.
2. Place each top round slice between wax paper and pound to tenderize; add salt and pepper and generously spread each with the spicy mustard.
3. On the wide part of each piece of meat, place about 5 dill pickle spears, some onion and a heaping Tbsp. of the browned bacon. Fold in the edges and roll up like a burrito.
4. Carefully brown the rolls on all sides in a frying pan. Place it in a large pot with beef stock.
5. Put a slice of the raw potatoes between each rolled roulade, making sure the pot is packed tight; the potato slices will hold the roulades together without having to use a string. Cover and bake for about 45 minutes.
6. Make your gravy from the drippings by mixing the flour and butter and adding it slowly into the beef stock until it reaches the desired consistency. Serve with red cabbage and potatoes or spaetzle. You can also serve the potatoes that have soaked up all the delicious juices and held together the roulade.

Also Pairs With		
Dortmunder	Octoberfest Lager	Doppelbock

Witbiers

Belgian unfiltered wheat beer. Spiced often with orange and coriander. Tangy and sharp from the wheat and high carbonation. Slightly hazy because of lack of filtration. Complement salads with light citrus dressings and feta or goat cheese and ceviche and other light, citrus-flavored dishes. Classic for smoked mussels and shellfish.

Witbiers: Key Characteristics		Notable Witbiers
Attribute	**Description**	Blue Moon Belgian White Belgian
ABV	4.5–5.5% — light and sessionable	Hoegaarden White
IBU (Bitterness)	8–20 — very low; bitterness takes a back seat	Allagash White
Color (SRM)	2–4 — pale straw to light gold, often cloudy	Kronenbourg 1664 Blanc
Body	Light to medium — creamy from wheat and oats	Bell's Oberon Ale
Carbonation	High, lively and effervescent, often bottle-conditioned	
Finish	Crisp, slightly tart, with lingering citrus and spice	

Taste: Fruity | Coriander | Orange Peel | Bready | Fruity
Food Pairings: Seafood | Grilled Pork | Roasted Chicken | Turkey

Food Pairing Guide for Witbiers

Witbiers—also known as Belgian White Ale—is a refreshing, hazy wheat beer that's as much about tradition as it is about spice and citrus flair

Cheese Pairings
- Goat Cheese or Ricotta: Tangy and fresh, echoing citrus notes
- Brie or Camembert: Soft and creamy, balanced with spice and bubbles
- Feta or Queso Fresco: Salty and bright, great with Witbiers acidity

Seafood Dishes
- Grilled Shrimp or Scallops: Sweet and delicate, enhanced by citrus and spice
- Ceviche or Crudo: Acidic and fresh, perfect with Witbiers' brightness
- Fish Tacos with Lime Crema: Zesty and creamy—an ideal match

Light Fare & Veggies
- Arugula Salad with Orange Vinaigrette: Peppery greens and citrus dressing echo the beer's profile
- Roasted Beets with Goat Cheese: Earthy and tangy, balanced by spice
- Avocado Toast with Pickled Shallots: Creamy, tangy, and refreshing

Poultry & Light Meats
- Lemon-Herb Chicken or Turkey: Citrus and herbs complement Witbiers zest
- Prosciutto-Wrapped Melon: Sweet, salty, and bright
- Grilled Sausages with Mustard: Especially with mild, herbal sausages

Desserts
- Orange Sorbet or Lemon Tart: Tart-on-tart pairing that sparkles
- Spice Cake or Ginger Cookies: Echoes coriander and clove notes
- Berry Shortcake or Pavlova: Fruity and creamy, great with Witbiers effervescence

Vietnamese Pork Banh Mi Sandwiches

Vietnamese pork Banh mi sandwiches pair beautifully with Witbiers because the beer's bright citrus, subtle spice, and creamy texture complement the sandwich's savory, tangy, and herbaceous layers in a way that's refreshing and harmonious. The crusty baguette of a Banh mi offers crunch and chew. Witbiers, brewed with wheat, have a soft, pillowy mouthfeel that balances the bread's texture without overwhelming it. The marinated pork is rich, slightly sweet, and often grilled or roasted. Witbiers bring orange peel and coriander notes that brighten the meat's richness and add a zesty contrast. Bánh mi toppings like pickled carrots, daikon, cucumber, cilantro, and jalapenos add tang, crunch, and heat. The beer's low bitterness and subtle spice cool the heat and echo the herbal freshness, while its creamy body softens the acidity.

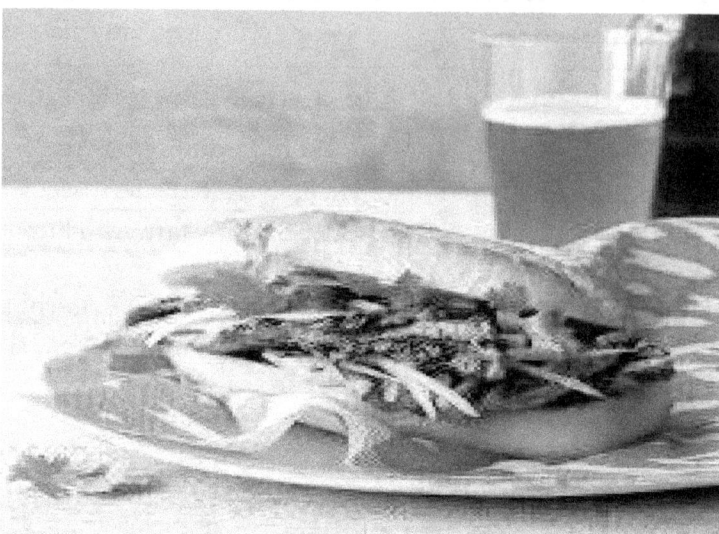

Ingredients:
2 pounds Chinese BBQ pork *
1 cup carrots
1 cup daikon
1 cup cucumber
2 fresh jalapeno peppers, sliced
1 cup rice vinegar
1 cup water
2 Tbsp. sugar
1 cup mayonnaise
4 Tbsp. Sriracha
4 French-style baguette loaves
1/2 cup cilantro, coarsely chopped

Instructions:
1. Prepare pork as stated below.
2. Peel carrots, daikon, and cucumber and cut them into small matchsticks.
3. Place the cut vegetables in a quart-sized canning jar along with the sliced jalapeno.
4. Combine vinegar, water and sugar and stir oil is dissolved.
5. Pour the mixture over the vegetables in the jar and seal (make sure all the vegetables are covered with the liquid). Refrigerate at least 10 minutes.
6. Combine mayonnaise and Sriracha. Slice the bread lengthwise, cutting down just one side (try not to cut all the way through; you will want to just slice it open, so it lays flat.
7. Spread the mayo mixture over the baguette.
8. Cut the pork into thin slices and place on bread.
9. Drain the vegetables and place them evenly over the pork.
10. Sprinkle a little cilantro over the top of the veggies and serve.

*Quick BBQ Pork**
3-pound Pork butt (will end up 2-pounds cooked)
½ cup brown sugar
1 jar Chines Char Sim Sauce

Cut the pork into thin strips, coating them with Char Sim sauce and then topping them with brown sugar. Let the meat sit overnight in a Ziplock bag. Heat grill to 375. Grill until the pork reaches 150°F. Shred.

Also Pairs With

Saison	Fruited Sour Lambric	Amber Ale

Brown Ales

Brown Ale is a style of beer known for its deep amber to dark brown color and rich malt-forward flavor. Originating in England in the late 17th century, brown ales are brewed with roasted and specialty malts that give them notes of caramel, toffee, chocolate, and nuts. They typically have moderate bitterness and a smooth, medium-bodied mouthfeel, making them one of the most approachable and food-friendly beer styles.

Brown Ale Characteristics Chart

Feature	English Brown Ale	American Brown Ale
Color (SRM)	Medium brown to dark amber (12–22 SRM)	Medium to dark brown (15–25 SRM)
ABV	4.2% – 5.4%	4.5% – 6.3%
Malt Flavor	Toasty, nutty, caramel, toffee, biscuit	Rich malt with chocolate, caramel, roasted notes
Hop Flavor	Low to moderate, earthy or floral	Moderate to high, often citrusy or piney
Bitterness (IBU)	20–30	25–45
Body	Medium-light to medium	Medium to full
Aroma	Malty with subtle fruit esters	Malt-forward with a noticeable hop aroma
Finish	Smooth, sometimes slightly sweet or dry	Balanced, can be dry or slightly bitter

Brown Ale Styles by Region

English Brown Ale
- **Flavor**: Nutty, slightly sweet, with hints of biscuit and toast
- **Examples**: Newcastle Brown Ale, Samuel Smith's Nut Brown Ale

American Brown Ale
- **Flavor**: Toasted malt with a noticeable hop presence (citrus, pine)
- **Examples**: Brooklyn Brown Ale, Big Sky Moose Drool

Food Pairing Tips
- Match with Roasted and Grilled Meats
- Pair with Nutty and Aged Cheeses
- Balance with Earthy Vegetables
- Enhance with Caramel and Chocolate Desserts

Awesome Food Pairings

Brown Ale Style	Best Pairings
English Brown Ale	Roast chicken, bangers and mash, aged cheddar
American Brown Ale	BBQ ribs, burgers, spicy chili

American Brown

American Brown Ales may let the hops peek out a little more aggressive, sometimes with fresh or citrusy flavors cutting into that richer malty quality. Bitterness from the hops will also likely be higher in American versions, often backed up by notes of toasty chocolate and caramel from the malt. Not a lot of fruit or esters here, and it should not get as hoppy as an IPA, but it will not be malty-sweet either. Pairs well with roasted pork, smoked sausage, and hearty foods; complement the nutty flavors of chicken satay, cashew chicken, pecan pie and peanut sauces. Also try grilled salmon, lean steaks, and classic grilled burgers.

American Brown Ale: Key Characteristics		Notable American Browns
Attribute	Description	Bald Man Tupelo Honey Brown Ale
ABV	4.3–6.2% — moderate strength, ideal for casual sipping	Moose Droo
IBU (Bitterness)	18–35 — balanced bitterness; more assertive than English versions	Brooklyn Brown Ale
Color (SRM)	18–35 SRM — deep amber to dark brown, often with ruby highlights	Naughty Brunette
Body	Medium to medium-full — smooth and rounded	Turmoil Brown Ale
Carbonation	Moderate to high — enhances drinkability and aroma release	Bender
Finish	Dry to slightly sweet, with lingering malt and hop notes	

Taste: Rich | Citrusy | Fruity | Biscuity | Nutty | Roasty
Food Pairings: Roasted Chicken | Cheese Sandwich | Meatloaf | Smoked BBQ

Food Pairing Guide for American Brown

American Brown Ale is a beer that rewards attention—robust, balanced, and full of character. It's perfect for those who love malt complexity but still crave a touch of hop brightness.

Cheese Pairings
- Smoked Gouda or Cheddar: Echoes the beer's roasted depth
- Blue Cheese: Bold funk meets earthy malt
- Aged Gruyère or Fontina: Nutty and savory, perfect with brown ale's richness

Meat & Savory Dishes
- Grilled Steak or Burgers: Charred flavors match the beer's roast and hops
- BBQ Pulled Pork or Ribs: Sweet and smoky sauces play well with caramel malt
- Roast Chicken with Herbs: Earthy and balanced, especially with citrusy hop notes

Vegetables & Sides
- Grilled Mushrooms or Eggplant: Umami-rich and earthy
- Sweet Potato Fries or Roasted Carrots: Sweetness complements malt
- Mac & Cheese: Creamy comfort food cut by bitterness and roast

Desserts
- Chocolate Cake or Brownies: Cocoa-on-cocoa pairing that sings
- Pecan Pie or Toffee Bars: Nutty and sweet, echoing malt complexity
- Coffee Ice Cream: Roasty and creamy, a perfect match

Smoked Brisket

Smoked brisket brings deep, savory, smoky notes from hours of slow cooking. American Brown Ale offers roasted malt flavors—think toasted nuts, cocoa, and caramel—that echo and enhance the smokiness of the meat. The beer's subtle hop bitterness adds just enough edge to cut through the richness without overpowering it. Brown ales bring caramel and toffee notes that mirror and elevate the sweet elements of sauces. The earthy, piney hops in many American brown ales subtly reinforce the wood smoke flavors in brisket.

Ingredients:
One 12 to 14 lb. whole packer brisket, trimmed with a ¼-inch fat cap
¼ cup each table salt, black pepper, brown sugar
3 Tbsp garlic powder
1½ Tbsp. smoked paprika
1½ Tbsp. garlic powder
1½ Tbsp. onion powder
1½ Tbsp. instant espresso powder (optional)
2 tsp. dry mustard
1 tsp. cayenne pepper

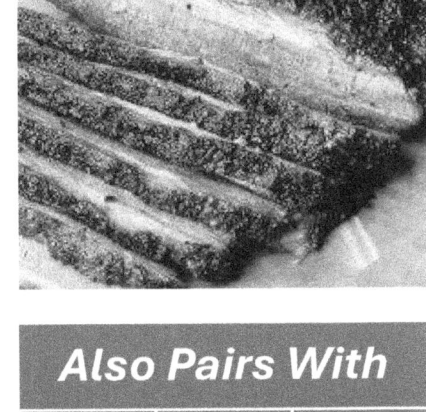

Instructions:
1. Preheat your smoker to 225°F Trim any excess fat off the brisket.
2. In a small bowl, spice and coat the brisket evenly on both sides. Allow the meat to sit for 10 to 15 minutes to "sweat" and absorb the rub, then coat the meat with the rest of the rub. Place the brisket on a rack over a baking sheet and refrigerate, uncovered, for 24 to 36 hours.
3. Place the brisket in the smoker, fat side up. If you use a digital meat thermometer with a wired probe, insert it into the thickest part of the meat to check the internal temperature continuously. Smoke for 6 to 8 hours, or until the internal temperature is 165°F to 170°F, and the bark is a nice mahogany color.
4. Cut 2 sheets of butcher paper or aluminum foil, each about 3 feet long, and overlap them on a large work surface. Using heat-proof gloves or oven mitts, remove the brisket from the smoker and place it lengthwise on the papers/foil, fat side down, about 1 foot from the bottom edge. Fold the bottom edge over the brisket and pull it tightly. Fold in the sides snugly, then continue rolling the brisket, keeping the wrap tight. Make sure the brisket is fully enclosed. Return it to the smoker, seam side down (it doesn't matter if the fat side is up or down at this point). If you use a thermometer with a wired probe, place it back through the paper/foil. Continue cooking until the internal temperature reaches 203°F, 4 to 6 hours more. The cooking time will vary with each piece of meat; the brisket is done when it reaches the proper temperature and the thermometer probe slides in and out of the meat with little resistance, like soft butter.
5. Place the wrapped brisket in an insulated cooler to rest for 1 to 3 hours, allowing the meat to relax and the juices to redistribute.
6. To serve the brisket, unwrap it over a sheet pan to catch any juices (you'll want those for serving). Transfer the brisket, lean side down, to a cutting board (preferably one with a well for collecting juices). Using a sharp carving knife or an electric carving knife, slice the meat against the grain. Start by slicing the flat cut ¼-inch thick if you're serving it chopped, then chop that slice for sandwiches. Arrange the slices on a platter or plates and spoon the reserved meat drippings over them. Serve barbecue sauce and other fixin's' on the side.

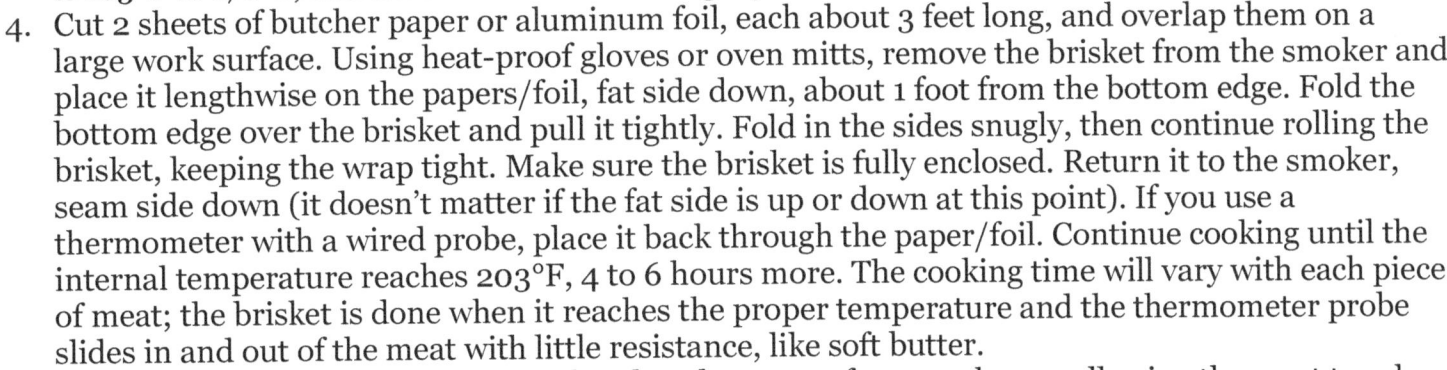

Also Pairs With

Foreign Stouts	Schwarzbeir	Barleywine

English Brown

The English Mild style (which may be more roasted or fruitier), means English Brown Ales highlight malt character, anything from toast, caramel, and toffee to chocolate, raisin, and coffee (and beyond). Hops are low here and not really meant to take part in the overall impression, which can be very dry or sweet, depending on the style. Famous for pairing well with about anything from roasted pork, smoked sausage, and hearty foods; complements the nutty flavors of chicken satay, cashew chicken, pecan pie and peanut sauces. Great with lamb and game meat on the grill.

English Brown Ale: Key Characteristics		Notable English Brown
Attribute	Description	Invictus James Maple Pecan Brown Ale
ABV	2.8–5.4% — low to moderate, ideal for session drinking	Newcastle Brown Ale
IBU (Bitterness)	15–25 — mild bitterness, hops play a supporting role	Wychwood Hobgoblin
Color (SRM)	12–22 SRM — coppery to dark brown, often with reddish hues	Fuller's London Pride
Body	Medium — smooth and sometimes creamy mouthfeel	Brains Dark
Carbonation	Moderate — enhances malt flavors without sharpness	Black Sheep Ale
Finish	Can be dry (Northern) or sweet (Southern), depending on regional style	

Taste: Rich | Nutty | Malty | Slightly Sweet |
Food Pairings: Chicken | Roast Beef or Lamb | Smoked Sausages | Creamy Desserts

Food Pairing Guide for English Brown

English Brown Ale is a pub classic—warm, inviting, and endlessly drinkable. It's a style that rewards slow sipping and pairs beautifully with comfort food.

Cheese Pairings
- Aged Cheddar or Red Leicester: Sharp and savory, matched by malt sweetness
- Stilton or Blue Cheese: Funky and bold, balanced by earthy hops
- Double Gloucester or Wensleydale: Creamy and nutty, echoing the beer's profile

Meat & Savory Dishes
- Roast Beef or Lamb: Classic pub fare—rich meats meet mellow malt
- Bangers & Mash: Sausage and gravy with a comforting brown ale
- Shepherd's Pie or Steak & Ale Pie: Hearty, savory, and deeply satisfying

Vegetables & Sides
- Roasted Root Vegetables: Caramelized sweetness complements malt
- Mushroom Risotto or Gravy: Earthy umami meets nutty roast
- Yorkshire Pudding or Soft Pretzels: Bready sides that echo the beer's grain character

Desserts
- Sticky Toffee Pudding: Rich caramel dessert with matching malt tones
- Nutty Brownies or Chocolate Cake: Cocoa and nuts play off the beer's roast
- Apple Crumble with Custard: Sweet, spiced, and creamy—perfect with a smooth brown ale

Pulled Pork Sandwich with Apple Slaw

Slow-cooked pork is rich and tender, often seasoned with sweet and smoky rubs or sauces. The caramel and toffee notes in English Brown Ale mirror the sweetness in the pork, while its roasty backbone enhances the smoky depth. Apple slaw adds a bright, acidic crunch that cuts through the richness of the meat. The beer's nutty malt character complements the apple's sweetness, and its low bitterness doesn't clash with the slaw's tang. Think of it as a sweet-savory-sour triangle: the pork brings savory and sweet, the slaw adds sour and crunch, and the beer ties it all together with warmth and depth.

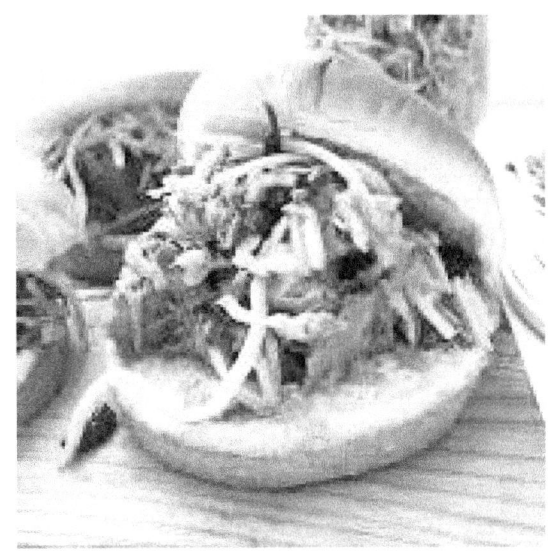

Ingredients:
Pork
1 tbsp mustard powder
12 round bread rolls
2 bay leaves
1 brown onion
1 Tbsp. of olive oil
2 garlic cloves
1 Cup sachet smoky chipotle cooking sauce
2-3 lb. boneless roast pork shoulder

Slaw
2 spring onions
1 Tbsp. white wine vinegar
2 Cups finely cut coleslaw
1 Tbsp. wholegrain mustard
1 Cup creme fraiche
2 Envy apples, cored

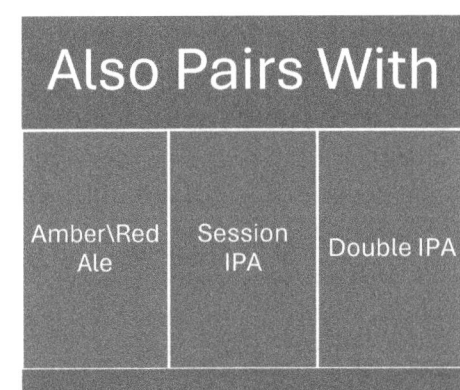

Also Pairs With

| Amber\Red Ale | Session IPA | Double IPA |

Instructions:
7. Trim any excess fat or glands from the pork.
8. In a small bowl, mix the spices and then coat the pork on all sides. Allow the meat to sit in the refrigerator, uncovered, for 24 to 36 hours.
9. Preheat your smoker to 225°F Place the pork in the smoker and spritz every 30 minutes. Smoke for 6 to 8 hours, or until the internal temperature is 165°F to 170°F, and the bark is a nice mahogany color.
10. Cut 2 sheets of butcher paper or aluminum foil, each about 3 feet long, and overlap them on a large work surface. Using heat-proof gloves or oven mitts, remove the pork from the smoker and place it lengthwise on the papers/foil, fat side down, about 1 foot from the bottom edge. Wrap the pork butt. Continue cooking until the internal temperature reaches 203°F, 4 to 6 hours more. The cooking time will vary with each piece of meat.
11. Place the wrapped pork in an insulated cooler to rest for 1 to 3 hours, allowing the meat to relax and the juices to redistribute.
12. Shred the pork with two forks and serve on sandwich buns.

Porters

Porter is a dark ale known for its roasted malt character, offering flavors of chocolate, coffee, caramel, and sometimes subtle smoke. Originating in London in the early 18th century, porter was one of the first beer styles to be mass-produced and widely exported. It was originally brewed for working-class laborers—especially porters—hence the name.

Flavor Profile Breakdown

Characteristic	Typical Range
Color	Deep brown to black
Aroma	Coffee, chocolate, caramel, toast
Body	Medium to full
Bitterness	Mild to moderate (20–50 IBU)
ABV	4% – 9% depending on style

Styles of Porter by Region

Style	Flavor Profile	ABV Range
English Porter	Balanced roast, mild bitterness, nutty and chocolatey	4–5.5%
Robust Porter	Bold roast, higher bitterness, coffee and cocoa	5.5–7%
Baltic Porter	Smooth, lager-fermented, rich and boozy	7–9.5%
American Porter	Roasty with a noticeable hop character	5–7%
Imperial Porter	Intense malt, high ABV, often barrel-aged	8%+

Food Pairing Tips

- Match with Smoked and Grilled Meats
- Enhance Chocolate and Coffee Desserts
- Balance with Salty and Umami-Rich Foods
- Contrast with Spicy Dishes

Awesome Food Pairings

Porter Style	Best Pairings
English Porter	Roast chicken, shepherd's pie, aged cheddar
Robust Porter	BBQ ribs, grilled steak, spicy chili
Baltic Porter	Smoked meats, mushroom risotto, dark chocolate
American Porter	Burgers, pulled pork, Gouda
Imperial Porter	Blue cheese, rich desserts, braised lamb shank

Baltic (English)

Baltic Porter is a dark porter that is cold-fermented and brewed with lager yeast. It is high in alcohol percentage and has a thick head with complex aroma notes. Pair well with almost any meat dish and a variety of cheeses and desserts. Best with barbecue, sausage, or anything grilled.

Baltic Porter: Key Characteristics		Notable Baltic Portes
Attribute	**Description**	Fortuna Komes Raspberry Porter
ABV	7% to 10% ABV	Sinebrychoff Porter
IBU (Bitterness)	Medium-low to medium hop bitterness,	Żywiec Porter
Color (SRM)	Deep brown to black	Koff Porter
Body	Medium to full — mouth-coating and luxurious2	Baltic Fire
Carbonation	Medium — supports aroma and texture without sharpness	Raven's Roost Baltic Porter
Finish	Medium to long — lingering malt and subtle fruit notes	Baltic Sunrise

Taste: Vanilla | Fruity | Spicy Finish | Coffee | Roasty | Malty
Food Pairings: Chicken | Beef | Chocolate | Stews | Smoked Meats | Root Vegetables

Food Pairing Guide for Baltic Porters
Baltic Porter is a fascinating hybrid—born from English porters, refined by continental brewing traditions, and often brewed with lager yeast for a smooth, rich finish.

Cheese Pairings
- Aged Gouda or Manchego: Nutty and caramel-like, echoing malt sweetness
- Blue Cheese (Stilton, Gorgonzola): Bold and funky, balanced by roast and sweetness
- Smoked Cheddar or Gruyère: Adds depth and complements the beer's smooth roast

Meat & Savory Dishes
- Smoked Brisket or BBQ Ribs: Deep char and sweet sauce match the beer's richness
- Roast Duck or Venison: Gamey meats pair beautifully with dark fruit and malt
- Beef Stroganoff or Short Ribs: Creamy and hearty dishes meet the beer's velvety texture

Vegetables & Sides
- Grilled Mushrooms or Eggplant: Earthy umami plays off roasted malt
- Sweet Potato Mash or Roasted Carrots: Sweetness complements toffee notes
- Lentil Stew or Mushroom Risotto: Hearty and savory, ideal with Baltic Porter's depth

Desserts
- Chocolate Torte or Flourless Cake: Cocoa-on-cocoa pairing that sings
- Bread Pudding with Caramel Sauce: Rich and comforting, echoing molasses
- Fig Tart or Plum Galette: Fruit-forward desserts match dark fruit esters

Smoked Ham and Grilled Cheese

Baltic Porter offers roasted malt notes—think dark chocolate, coffee, and toasted bread—that echo and enhance the smokiness without overwhelming it. Melted cheese (especially aged cheddar, Swiss, or Gruyère) adds creamy richness and umami. The beer's smooth, slightly sweet body balances the salt and fat, while its carbonation refreshes the palate between bites. If the sandwich is grilled or toasted, the caramelized crust mirrors the porter's toffee and molasses notes. The lager-clean beer finish keeps the pairing from becoming too heavy, making it satisfying, but not cloying.

Ingredients:
4 slices Artisan sourdough bread, sliced thick
4 tbsp unsalted butter, room temperature
4 slices of thick-cut ham
1 cup smoked Gouda, shredded
1 cup sharp cheddar, shredded
2 cloves garlic, grated

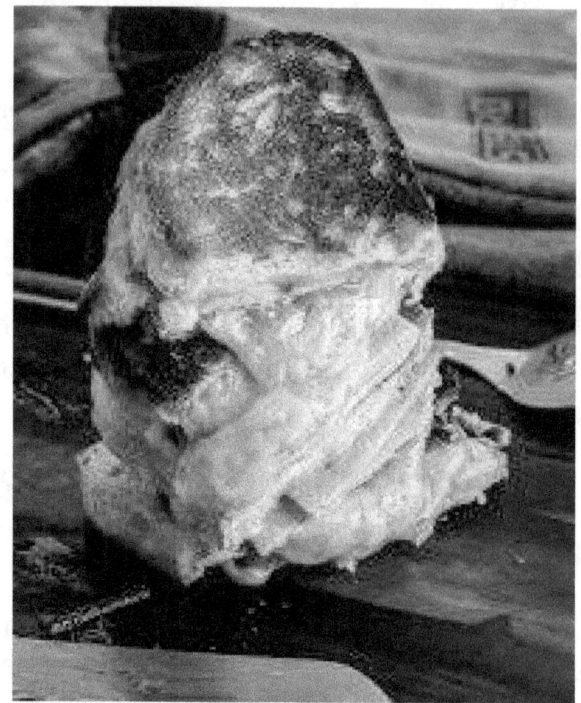

Instructions:
1. Preheat your grill or smoker to 350-375°F.
2. Place the skillet on the grill to preheat as well.
3. Mix the cheese and the grated garlic together. Place equal amounts of each cheese mix onto the sandwiches. Add slices of ham. Butter the outsides of the slices.
4. Place the sandwiches onto the hot skillet and press down. If you have a sandwich press, use it. Cook for about 3 minutes with the lid closed. Flip the sandwiches, and repeat. Cook longer if needed but be careful not to burn the bread.

Sweet & Tangy Ham Sauce
½ cup brown sugar
¼ cup Dijon mustard
¼ cup apple cider vinegar
2 Tbsp. honey or maple syrup
1 Tbsp. Worcestershire sauce
1 tsp. ground cloves or allspice
½ tsp. garlic powder
Pinch of salt and black pepper
Optional: 2 Tbsp. pineapple juice or orange juice for a fruity twist

Also Pairs With

Brown Ales	Scoth Ale	Belgian Witbeir

In a small saucepan, whisk together all ingredients until smooth. Bring to a gentle boil over medium heat, then reduce to low and simmer for 5–7 minutes until slightly thickened. Add more vinegar for tang, more sugar or honey for sweetness, or a splash of juice for brightness. Brush over baked ham during the last 20 minutes of roasting or serve warm on the side.

Robust (American)

Robust porters have a roast malt flavor, often reminiscent of cocoa, but no roast barley flavor. Their caramel and malty sweetness is in harmony with the sharp bitterness of black malt. Hop bitterness is evident. Features a bitter and roasted malt flavor than a brown porter, but not as much as a stout. English brown and robust porters are excellent with grilled meat, gruyere cheese, and excellent with baked goods that include both chocolate and peanut butter. Goes well with marbled steaks.

Robust Porter: Key Characteristics		Notable Robust Porters
Attribute	Description	Founders Porter
ABV	5.1–6.6% — stronger than Brown Porter, but not a Stout	Double Decker
IBU (Bitterness)	25–40 — moderate to high; bitterness balances malt sweetness	Harpoon Porter
Color (SRM)	Very dark brown to black — often opaque with ruby highlights	Iron Belly
Body	Medium to full — smooth, sometimes creamy	Black Strap Molasses Porter
Carbonation	Moderately low to moderately high — supports aroma and texture	Founders Porter
Finish	Dry to medium-sweet — depends on malt bill and attenuation	Smuttynose Robust Porter

Taste: Malty | Complex | Roasty
Food Pairings: Smoked Brisket | Burnt Ends | Grilled Veggie | Espresso Desserts

Food Pairing Guide for Robust Porters

Robust Porter is a dark ale with backbone—perfect for those who love roast complexity without the full weight of a stout. It's a style that plays beautifully with barbecue, especially when you're working with smoked meats or rich sauces.

Cheese Pairings
- Smoked Cheddar or Gouda: Echoes the beer's smoky depth
- Blue Cheese (Stilton, Roquefort): Bold funk meets roasted malt
- Aged Parmesan or Gruyère: Nutty and salty, balanced by bitterness

Meat & Savory Dishes
- Grilled Steak or Lamb Chops: Charred crust matches the beer's roast
- Smoked Brisket or Pulled Pork: Deep, savory flavors enhanced by porter's intensity
- Beef Chili or Mole: Spicy, earthy dishes that play off cocoa and bitterness

Vegetables & Sides
- Grilled Mushrooms or Eggplant: Umami-rich and earthy
- Roasted Root Vegetables: Sweetness contrasts the beer's dryness
- Black Bean Burgers or Lentil Stew: Hearty and satisfying

Desserts
- Dark Chocolate Cake or Brownies: Cocoa-on-cocoa pairing that sings
- Molasses Cookies or Gingerbread: Spiced and sweet, perfect with roasted malt
- Espresso Ice Cream or Tiramisu: Coffee and cream meet porter's depth

Cowboy Sliders

A cowboy beef slider—typically loaded with smoky grilled beef, tangy barbecue sauce, crispy onions, and melty cheese—pairs brilliantly with a robust porter because the beer's roasty intensity, bitterness, and dark malt sweetness complements and elevate every layer of the slider. Crispy onions add texture and a hint of bitterness, which plays beautifully with the porter's hop edge.

Ingredients:
1 1/2 pounds ground round
1/2 tsp. kosher salt
1/4 tsp. freshly ground black pepper
1/4 tsp. granulated garlic
1/2 tsp. onion powder
1 Tbsp. Worcestershire sauce
1/2 cup barbecue sauce
1 (12 count) package Hawaiian rolls, cut in half horizontally, without separating individual rolls
2 cups shredded Cheddar cheese
6 slices bacon, cooked until crisp
1 jalapeno , thinly sliced, or more to taste
1/2 cup crispy fried onions

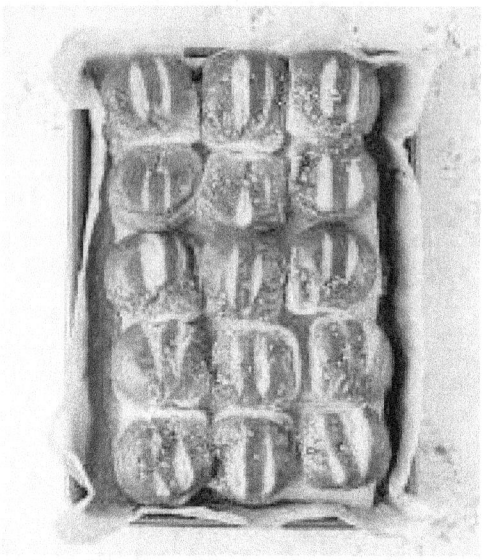

Instructions:
1. Preheat the oven to 350 ° F Heat a large skillet over medium-high heat. Add beef and cook while crumbling with a spoon until it is no longer pink, about 5 minutes.
2. Add salt, pepper, garlic powder, onion powder, and Worcestershire, and stir. Add barbecue sauce and stir until well combined. Bring a simmer and cook for 2 minutes. Remove from heat.
3. Place the bottom half of Hawaiian rolls on a small, rimmed baking sheet. Top with half of the shredded cheese. Top with meat mixture, bacon, jalapenos, crispy onions, and remaining cheese. Place the top half of the rolls on top and cover the pan with foil.
4. Bake in the preheated oven until the rolls are toasted and the cheese is melted and gooey, 15 to 20 minutes.

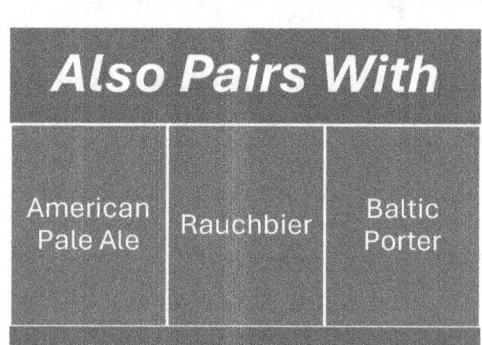

Also Pairs With: American Pale Ale | Rauchbier | Baltic Porter

Cowboy Slider Special Sauce

½ cup mayonnaise
2 Tbsp. BBQ sauce (smoky or spicy style)
1 Tbsp. ketchup
1 Tbsp. Dijon or spicy brown mustard
1 tsp. Worcestershire sauce
1 tsp. apple cider vinegar

1 tsp. honey or maple syrup
½ tsp. smoked paprika
¼ tsp. garlic powder
¼ tsp. onion powder
Pinch of cayenne or hot sauce (optional for heat)
Salt and black pepper to taste

Mix all the ingredients in a bowl until smooth and creamy. Add more BBQ sauce for smokiness, more vinegar for tang, or more honey for sweetness. Chill for 15–30 minutes to let the flavors meld. Serve on toasted slider buns, over patties, or as a dipping sauce.

Stouts

Stout is a dark, full-bodied ale known for its roasted malt character and creamy texture. With flavors ranging from coffee and chocolate to caramel and smoke, stouts are among the most complex and satisfying beer styles. Originally developed as a stronger version of porter, stouts have grown into a diverse family of beers enjoyed worldwide.

Flavor Profile Breakdown

Characteristic	Typical Range
Color	Deep brown to jet black
Aroma	Coffee, chocolate, caramel, toast
Body	Medium to full
Bitterness	Moderate to high (20–60 IBU)
ABV	4% – 12% depending on style

Styles of Stout by Region

Style	Flavor Profile	ABV Range
Dry Stout	Roasty, bitter, creamy	4–5%
Sweet Stout (Milk Stout)	Chocolatey, smooth, sweet (lactose added)	4–6%
Oatmeal Stout	Silky mouthfeel, nutty, mild roast	4.5–6%
American Stout	Bold roast, hoppy edge	5–7%
Imperial Stout	Intense malt, high alcohol, often barrel-aged	8–12%
Foreign Extra Stout	Stronger, export-style with rich roast	6–8%

Food Pairing Tips
- Match with Rich, Roasted Meats
- Echo Chocolate and Coffee Notes
- Balance with Salty and Umami-Rich Foods
- Contrast with Spicy Dishes

Awesome Food Pairings

Stout Style	Best Pairings
Dry Stout	Oysters, shepherd's pie, aged cheddar
Milk Stout	BBQ ribs, chocolate cake, glazed ham
Oatmeal Stout	Roast chicken, mushroom risotto, nutty desserts
American Stout	Burgers, spicy chili, smoked meats
Imperial Stout	Blue cheese, braised lamb, flourless chocolate torte

Dry Stout

Dry Stout is a very dark, roasty, bitter, creamy ale. It shares its history with porters, and the most common example is brewed by the Guinness brewery. It is the draught version of what is otherwise known as Irish stout. It goes well with grilled or smoked game, red meat, beef ribs and pit beef.

Dry Stout: Key Characteristics		Notable Dry Stout
Attribute	**Description**	Dangerous Man Dry Irish Stout
ABV	4.0–5.0% — low alcohol, highly sessionable2	Guinness Draught
IBU (Bitterness)	30–45 — firm bitterness, often from roasted grains	Murphy's Irish Stout
Color (SRM)	25–40 SRM — jet black to deep brown with ruby highlights	Beamish Irish Stout
Body	Medium-light to medium-full — creamy but not heavy	Black Cat Stout
Carbonation	Low to moderate — often served on nitrogen for a smooth mouthfeel	Dry Irish Stout
Finish	Dry, roasty, and clean — no lingering sweetness	Black House Nitro Stout

Taste: Burnt Toast | Some Bitterness |
Food Pairings: Grilled Meats | Barbecue | Chocolate Desserts | Shellfish | Pasta\Pizza

Food Pairing Guide for Dry Stouts

Dry Stout is perfect for those who want roast complexity without the heaviness of imperial stouts or milk stouts.

Cheese Pairings
- Sharp Cheddar or Irish Dubliner: Bold and tangy, balanced by roast
- Blue Cheese (Stilton, Gorgonzola): Funky and creamy, cut by bitterness
- Smoked Gouda or Brie: Rich and savory, enhanced by dry stout's depth

Meat & Savory Dishes
- Oysters or Mussels: Classic pairing—briny shellfish meets roasted malt
- Shepherd's Pie or Beef Stew: Hearty comfort food with earthy depth
- Grilled Sausages or black pudding: Rich and savory, especially with Irish-style stouts
- Smoked Brisket or BBQ Pulled Pork: Roast and smoke in perfect harmony

Vegetables & Sides
- Grilled Mushrooms or Eggplant: Umami-rich and earthy
- Roasted Root Vegetables: Sweetness contrasts the beer's dryness
- Colcannon or mashed potatoes: Creamy sides that match the mouthfeel

Desserts
- Chocolate Cake or Brownies: Bittersweet cocoa-on-cocoa pairing
- Coffee, ice cream or Tiramisu: Espresso and cream echo stout's flavor
- Molasses Cookies or Gingerbread: Spiced and dark, perfect with roast

Pepper Stout Beef

The beef roast, often slow-cooked with black pepper and stout, develops rich, caramelized, and smoky flavors. A dry stout—with its roasted barley, espresso bitterness, and dark chocolate notes—mirrors and amplifies those flavors, creating a seamless bridge between sip and bite. The black pepper adds heat and pungency, which is beautifully tempered by the dry stout's creamy mouthfeel and low residual sweetness. The bitter edge enhances the spice without overwhelming it, keeping the palate engaged. If the roast is braised in stout, the pairing becomes even more harmonious—you're drinking the same beer that built the sauce.

Ingredients:
4lb Chuck Roast
2 big bell peppers (sliced)
1 Big Red Onion (sliced)
3 Big Jalapenos (sliced, seeds and all)
6 garlic cloves (minced)
1/4 cup Worcestershire Sauce
1 - 12oz Bottle Guinness Extra Stout
Kosher Salt and Black Pepper

Instructions:
1. Heavily season Chuck Roast with Kosher Salt and Fresh black pepper and cook indirectly in the 245°-260° range. You can add smoked wood chips for more flavor.
2. Cook until the internal temperature reaches 165°.
3. Once the roast hits 165°, combine the remaining ingredients in a pan. Then, place the roast into the pan directly on top and cover tightly with foil.
4. Continue cooking the roast in a smoker or oven at 350° for 2.5-3 hours or until it is fork tender.
5. Once tender, shred meat and continue to cook uncovered until the liquid is reduced by half.
6. Serve meat on Texas Toast with or without cheese. Place some pepper jack or gorgonzola on top. Horseradish would be another good condiment.

Creamy Horseradish Sauce
½ cup sour cream
2 Tbsp. prepared horseradish (adjust to taste)
1 Tbsp. mayonnaise
1 tsp. Dijon mustard
1 tsp. white wine vinegar or lemon juice
¼ tsp. garlic powder
Salt and black pepper to taste
Optional: chopped chives or parsley for garnish

Mix all ingredients in a bowl until smooth and well combined. Add more horseradish for heat, more vinegar for tang, or more mayo for richness. Chill for 15–30 minutes to let the flavors meld. Serve cold or at room temperature with meats, sandwiches, or roasted potatoes.

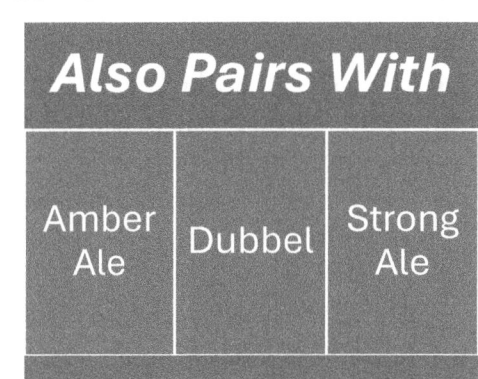

Also Pairs With

Amber Ale	Dubbel	Strong Ale

Sweet (Chocolate) Stout

Some of the best chocolate stouts on the market include real chocolate or its extracts to produce that unique flavor you enjoy. This is a high alcoholic beer. Notes prominent to the nose and tongue would be bourbon, vanilla, toasted malt, and barrel. Stout beer pairs well with rich food, like Kansas-style spareribs, macaroni and cheese, and mole sauce. It goes well with spicy BBQ beef, Memphis-style ribs or meats with vinegar-based tangy sauces.

Sweet Chocolate Stout: Key Characteristics		Notable Sweet Stouts
Attribute	Description	Belching Beaver Peanut Butter Milk Stout
ABV	4.0–6.0% — moderate strength, often leaning toward sessionable	Young's Double Chocolate Stout
IBU (Bitterness)	20–40 — low to moderate; bitterness is softened by sweetness	Left Hand Milk Stout
Color (SRM)	30–40 — deep brown to jet black, often opaque with tan head	Rogue Chocolate Stout
Body	Medium-full to full — creamy and smooth	Great Divide Chocolate
Carbonation	Low to moderate — enhances mouthfeel without sharpness	Coronado Barrel-Aged German Chocolate Cake
Finish	Sweet and lingering — chocolate and roast notes persist on the palate	

Taste: Malty | Sweet | Chocolaty | Caramel
Food Pairings: Barbecue | Cheese | Chocolate Desserts | Comfort Foods

Food Pairing Guide for Sweet Chocolate Stouts Sweet Chocolate Stout is a decadent, dessert-like beer style that blends the roasty depth of a stout with the creamy sweetness of lactose and the rich flavor of chocolate malts.

Cheese Pairings
- Triple-Crème Brie or Cambozola: Rich and creamy, balanced by roast and sweetness
- Smoked Gouda or Cheddar: Echoes the beer's depth and adds savory contrast
- Blue Cheese with Honey: Funky and sweet—perfect with chocolate stout's richness

Meat & Savory Dishes
- Pulled Pork Mac & Cheese: Smoky, creamy, and indulgent—mirrors the beer's body and sweetness
- Beef Chili with Cocoa or Mole: Spicy and earthy, enhanced by chocolate notes
- Grilled Steak with Coffee Rub: Roast-on-roast pairing with bold umami

Vegetables & Sides
- Roasted Root Vegetables: Sweet and earthy, great with malt depth
- Grilled Mushrooms or Eggplant: Umami-rich and smoky
- Sweet Potato Fries with Chipotle Aioli: Sweet, spicy, and creamy perfect match

Desserts
- Chocolate Lava Cake or Brownies: Cocoa-on-cocoa indulgence
- Tiramisu or Espresso Ice Cream: Coffee and cream echo stout's profile
- Peanut Butter Pie or S'mores: Sweet, nutty, and nostalgic

Pulled Pork Mac and Cheese

Pulled pork brings smoky, savory depth—often with sweet BBQ sauce or spice rub. Mac and cheese add creamy, salty richness. Sweet chocolate stout offers roasted malt flavors—dark chocolate, cocoa, and subtle caramel—that echo the BBQ sweetness and contrast the salt and smoke, creating a layered experience. The stout's roasted bitterness cuts through the fat of the cheese and pork, refreshing your palate between bites. The beer's chocolate and caramel sweetness enhance the comfort-food vibe of mac and cheese.

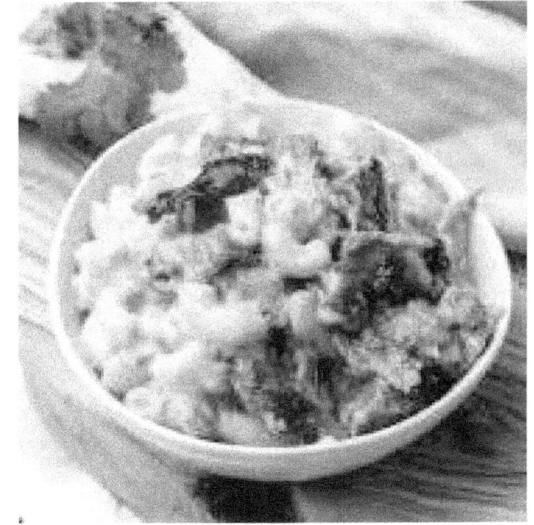

Ingredients:
16 ounces elbow noodle pasta
8 ounces pulled pork reheated
⅓ cup BBQ (homemade or your favorite one from the store)
4 ounces freshly shredded smoked Gouda
4 ounces freshly shredded medium cheddar
½ tsp. Morton kosher salt
½ tsp. freshly cracked black pepper
½ tsp. smoked paprika
½ cup thinly sliced green onions, divided
Panko for topping

Instructions:
1. Bring a large pot of salt water to boil. Add pasta and cook according to the package instructions until one minute less than al dente, about 10 minutes. Reserve ½ cup of the starchy pasta water and then drain the pasta and set it aside.
2. While the pasta is cooking, add the pulled pork to a medium bowl and pour BBQ sauce and warm for about 2 minutes. Add the Gouda and cheddar. And microwave until the cheese melts. Stir it often.
3. Drain the pasta when finished and add it to a large mixing bowl. Add heated meat and cheese and mix with a large spoon. If it's warm, serve topped with panko and sliced green onions. If not, or if reheating, place in a glass dish and heat in the oven for a few minutes until warm.

Mexican Street Corn (Elote)
4 ears of corn, husked
2 Tbsp. mayonnaise
2 Tbsp. sour cream or Mexican Crema
½ cup cotija cheese (crumbled)
1 tsp. chili powder (or Tajín for a citrusy kick)
1 Tbsp. fresh lime juice
1 Tbsp. chopped cilantro (optional)
Salt to taste | Lime wedges for serving

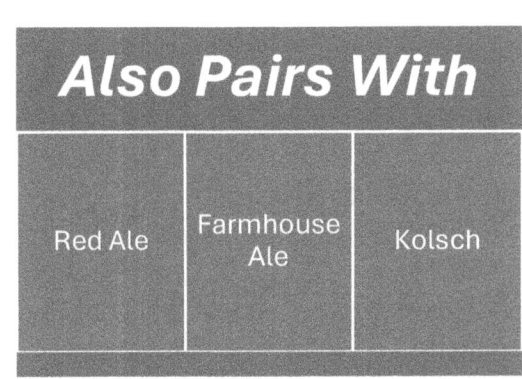

Also Pairs With

Red Ale	Farmhouse Ale	Kolsch

Grill corn over medium-high heat until charred in spots, turning occasionally (about 10 minutes). In a small bowl, combine mayo, sour cream, lime juice, and a pinch of salt. Brush the warm corn with the creamy sauce. Sprinkle generously with cotija cheese and chili powder. Top with chopped cilantro and serve with lime wedges for squeezing.

Oatmeal Stout

Oatmeal Stout is a sub-style of stout, the distinction being the inclusion of up to 20% oats by weight in the grist. Oatmeal stouts are often sweeter than dry stouts, but less sweet than sweet stouts or milk stouts. Hop bitterness varies with each brewer's interpretation of the style but is moderate, with an emphasis on bittering, rather than aroma hops. Pairs well with BBQ Brisket, Cheeseburger, Sharp cheddar, Dark chocolate cake, Tiramisu, and anything you had sauce too.

Oatmeal Stout: Key Characteristics		Notable Oatmeal Stouts
Attribute	Description	New Holland Dragons Milk Reserve Oatmeal Cookie
ABV	3.8–6.1% — moderate strength, often sessionable	Samuel Smith's Oatmeal Stout
IBU (Bitterness)	20–40 — balanced bitterness; enough to offset malt sweetness	Founders Breakfast Stout
Color (SRM)	22–40 SRM — dark brown to black, often opaque	Firestone Walker Velvet Merlin
Body	Medium-full to full — creamy, smooth, sometimes slick	Highland Black Mocha Stout
Carbonation	Medium — supports texture without sharpness	Naked Oat Stout
Finish	Medium-dry to medium-sweet — varies by interpretation	BrewDog

Taste: Coffee | Nutty | Earthy | Fruitiness | Roasty
Food Pairings: Beef or Pork BBQ | Root Veggies | Choc or Oatmeal Cookies | Chili

Food Pairing Guide for Oatmeal Stout
Oatmeal Stout is a silky, satisfying beer style that blends the roasty depth of a stout with the creamy smoothness of oats. It's a comfort beer with complexity—perfect for those who love rich malt character without overwhelming sweetness.

Cheese Pairings
- Aged Cheddar or Smoked Gouda: Sharp and savory, balanced by roast
- Brie or Camembert: Creamy and mild, echoing the beer's texture
- Blue Cheese with Honey: Funky and sweet—perfect with malt depth

Meat & Savory Dishes
- Beef Stew or Pot Roast: Hearty and slow-cooked, matched by the beer's richness
- Grilled Sausages or lamb chops: Charred and savory, enhanced by roasted malt
- Pulled Pork Mac & Cheese: Creamy, smoky, and indulgent—mirrors the beer's body

Vegetables & Sides
- Grilled Mushrooms or Eggplant: Umami-rich and earthy
- Roasted Root Vegetables: Sweetness complements malt
- Lentil Stew or Black Bean Chili: Hearty and satisfying

Desserts
- Chocolate Cake or Brownies: Cocoa-on-cocoa pairing that sings
- Oatmeal Cookies or Bread Pudding: Echoes the beer's grain and sweetness
- Coffee ice cream or Tiramisu: Creamy and roasty, a perfect match

Sticky Ribs

Sticky ribs often feature a glaze or BBQ sauce with brown sugar, molasses, or honey. Oatmeal stout brings roasted malt, cocoa, and subtle caramel notes that mirror and deepen the sweetness in the ribs. The beer's toasted grain and coffee flavors enhance the smoky char from the grill or smoker. Ribs are fatty and tender, and the stout's mild bitterness helps cleanse the palate between bites. Oats in the stout give it a silky, creamy body that pair beautifully with the sticky, saucy texture of the ribs.

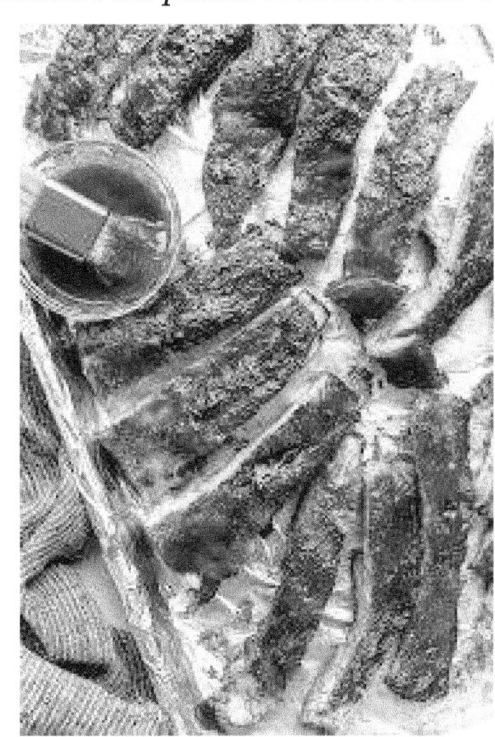

Ingredients:
1/4 cup light brown sugar
2 Tbsp. granulated sugar
1 tsp. chili powder
1 tsp. garlic powder
1 tsp. onion powder
1 tsp. paprika
Kosher salt and freshly ground black pepper
One 3-pound slab baby back ribs
2 cups BBQ sauce

Instructions:
1. Preheat the oven to 300 degrees F.
2. Combine the brown sugar, granulated sugar, chili powder, garlic powder, onion powder, paprika, 2 tsp. salt and a generous amount of freshly ground black pepper in a small.
3. Place the ribs on a piece of foil large enough to fold over and seal, then place on a baking sheet. Sprinkle the dry rub all over the top of the meaty side of the ribs. Wrap the foil around the ribs and seal tightly so that no juices can escape during baking. Bake until the meat is tender and can easily be pulled away from the bones with a fork, about 2 hours.
4. Heat the BBQ sauce in a small pan over medium heat until warm. Remove the ribs from the oven and open the foil pack. Remove the ribs from the foil and pour any juices that have accumulated into the BBQ sauce and mix to combine. Continue simmering the sauce until thickened, about 7 minutes.
5. Heat a grill or grill pan for cooking at medium-high heat.
6. Slice the ribs into 1-bone pieces. Brush all over with the BBQ sauce. Place the ribs on the grill and cook until grill marks appear, a few minutes on each side. Brush with more BBQ sauce and remove from the heat, then serve with the remaining BBQ sauce on the side.

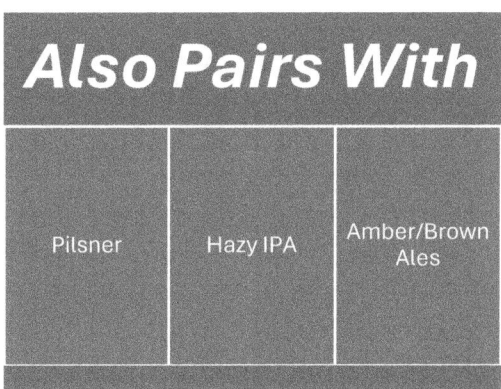

Imperial Stout

The American-style imperial stout is the strongest in alcohol and body of the stouts. Black in color, these beers typically have an extremely rich malty flavor and aroma with full, sweet malt character. Bitterness can come from roasted malts or hop additions. Goes well with smoked game birds, Memphis tangy BBQ sauce but can overpower many dishes.

Imperial Stout: Key Characteristics		Notable Imperial Stouts
Attribute	Description	North Coast Old Rasputin Imperial Stout
ABV	8–12% — high alcohol, warming and bold	Goose Island Bourbon County Stout
IBU (Bitterness)	50–90+ — assertive bitterness, often balancing rich malts	Founders KBS
Color (SRM)	30–40+ SRM — jet black to opaque brown, often with a tan or mocha head	Bell's Expedition Stout
Body	Full to very full — viscous, mouth-coating, luxurious	North Coast Old Rasputin
Carbonation	Moderate to low — enhances texture and aroma	Three Floyds Dark Lord
Finish	Long and complex — lingering roast, sweetness, and alcohol warmth	Prairie Bomb!

Taste: Balanced | Rich | Malty | Fruitiness | Barrel Aged Flavors
Food Pairings: Slow Cooked Meats | Cheeseburgers | Chili | Chocolate | Short Ribs

Food Pairing Guide for Imperial Stouts

Imperial Stout is the heavyweight champion of the stout family—bold, intense, and unapologetically complex.

Cheese Pairings
- Aged Gouda or Cheddar: Sharp and nutty, balanced by sweetness and roast
- Blue Cheese (Stilton, Roquefort): Funky and bold—perfect with dark fruit and bitterness
- Triple-Crème Brie or Camembert: Rich and creamy, softened by the beer's warmth

Meat & Savory Dishes
- Braised Short Ribs or Beef Stew: Deep, slow-cooked flavors match the beer's intensity
- Smoked Brisket or BBQ Ribs: Char and sweetness echo roasted malt and molasses
- Duck Breast or Venison: Gamey meats pair beautifully with dark fruit and cocoa notes

Vegetables & Sides
- Grilled Mushrooms or Eggplant: Earthy umami meets roasted malt
- Roasted Root Vegetables: Sweet and caramelized—great with molasses tones
- Black Bean Chili or Lentil Stew: Hearty and bold enough to match the beer

Desserts
- Chocolate Torte or Flourless Cake: Cocoa-on-cocoa indulgence
- Molasses Cookies or Gingerbread: Spiced and sweet—perfect with roast
- Cheesecake with Berry Compote: Creamy and tart, balanced by dark fruit and alcohol warmth

KC Burnt Ends

Burnt ends are the caramelized, smoky, fatty tips of brisket—packed with umami, bark, and BBQ glaze. Imperial stouts offer roasted malt flavors like espresso, dark chocolate, and charred grain, which mirror and enhance the smoky crust and deep beef flavor. KC-style burnt ends often feature a sweet, sticky BBQ sauce with molasses or brown sugar. The stout's bittersweet profile—with notes of cocoa, coffee, and sometimes dark fruit—balances the sweetness and adds complexity without overwhelming the palate. Burnt ends are rich, fatty, and bold, and imperial stouts are high-ABV, full-bodied, and intense—neither gets lost in the pairing.

Ingredients:
1 cup brown sugar
1 cup granulated sugar
1/2 cup salt
1/3 cup chili powder
1/4 cup paprika
6 Tbsp. black pepper
3 Tbsp. ground cumin
3 Tbsp. garlic powder
3 Tbsp. onion powder
1 Tbsp. cayenne pepper
One 10- to 12-pound whole, packer trim beef brisket or point

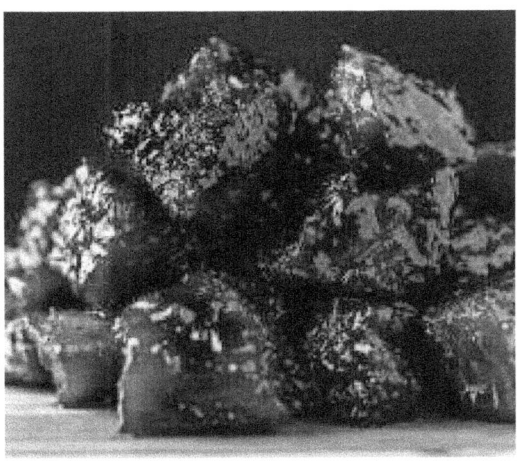

Instructions:
1. Sift the brown sugar, granulated sugar, salt, chili powder, paprika, black pepper, cumin, garlic powder, onion powder and cayenne pepper into a medium bowl and mix well. Set aside.
2. Trim all the hard fat from the brisket. Trim all the soft fat to 1/4 inch. Prepare a smoker or a grill, following the manufacturer's directions. Stabilize the temperature at 220 degrees F. Use a mild wood such as hickory or cherry for the smoke flavor. Generously cover all sides of the brisket with the rub and gently massage it in. Reserve the leftover rub. Smoke the meat until an instant-read thermometer registers 170 to 185 degrees F when inserted into the flat part of the brisket, about 1 hour per pound. For example, a 10-pound brisket may need to smoke for about 10 or more hours. Monitor the internal temperature.
3. Separate the point of the meat from the flat. At this time, you can slice the flat part off the brisket and eat. Trim the visible fat from the brisket point and coat it with the reserved rub. Return the meat to the smoker and continue cooking until the internal temperature of the brisket point reaches 200 degrees F. Remove the brisket from the smoker to a cutting board and let it sit for 10 to 20 minutes. Cut into chunks and transfer them to a serving platter. Serve it hot.

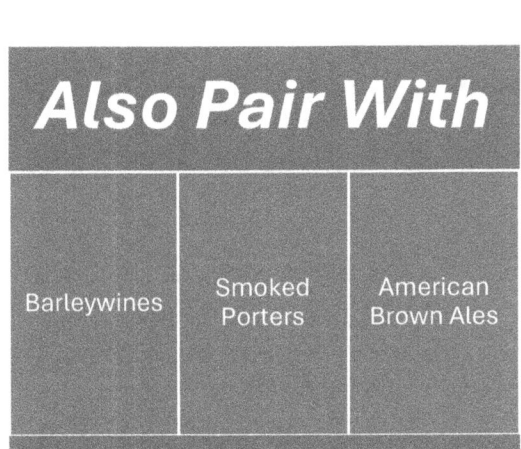

Foreign Stout

A Foreign Stout, also known as a Foreign Extra Stout (FES), was first brewed by Guinness in 1801 for export. It withstood long voyages, especially to destinations in Asia, Africa, and the Caribbean. To preserve the beer during these extended journeys, it was brewed with extra hops and had a higher alcohol content. Expect flavors of coffee, dark chocolate, and roasted grains. Some versions may have hints of dark cherries and a touch of buttery diacetyl. Foreign Stout is more heavily hopped than other Guinness stouts, resulting in a bitter taste. Typically, Foreign Stouts have an ABV (alcohol by volume) of around 7.5%. The extra hops served as a natural preservative for the long sea journeys.

Foreign Stout Key Characteristics		Notable Foreign Stouts
Attribute	**Description**	Guinness Foreign Extra Stout
ABV	6.3–8.0% — stronger than Dry Stout, warming but not overpowering	Foreign Extra Stout
IBU (Bitterness)	50–70 — firm bitterness, often from roasted grains and hops	Dolden Dark
Color (SRM)	30–40 SRM — very dark brown to black, often opaque	Nitro McCarthy Stout
Body	Medium-full to full — smooth, sometimes creamy	Sinebrychoff Porter
Carbonation	Moderate to moderately high — supports mouthfeel and aroma	
Finish	Can be dry (export versions) or sweet (tropical versions)	

Taste: Malty | Bittersweet | Roasty | Burnt notes
Food Pairings: Smoked Meats | Jerk Chicken |

Food Pairing Guide for Foreign Stouts

Foreign Stout—often called Foreign Extra Stout—is a bold, roasty, and moderately strong beer style that bridges the gap between Dry Stout and Imperial Stout.

Cheese Pairings
- Smoked Gouda or Aged Cheddar: Bold and savory, balanced by sweetness
- Blue Cheese with Fig Jam: Funky and fruity—perfect with dark fruit notes
- Brie or Camembert: Creamy and mild, softened by roast and sweetness

Meat & Savory Dishes
- Jerk Chicken or Spicy BBQ Ribs: Heat and char balanced by sweet roast
- Braised Short Ribs or Oxtail Stew: Deep, slow-cooked flavors match the beer's richness
- Grilled Lamb or Duck Breast: Gamey meats pair beautifully with molasses and cocoa

Vegetables & Sides
- Grilled Mushrooms or Eggplant: Earthy umami meets roasted malt
- Sweet Potato Fries or Plantains: Sweet and starchy—great with molasses tones
- Black Bean Chili or Lentil Stew: Hearty and bold enough to match the beer

Desserts
- Chocolate Cake or Brownies: Cocoa-on-cocoa indulgence
- Molasses Cookies or Gingerbread: Spiced and sweet—perfect with roast
- Rum Cake or Banana Bread: Tropical sweetness echoes the beer's origin

Crockpot Bourbon BBQ Meatballs

Bourbon BBQ sauce often includes molasses, brown sugar, and smoky bourbon—creating a sticky, sweet glaze. Foreign stouts feature roasted malt, molasses, and dark fruit notes (like raisin or plum), which echo and deepen the sauce's sweetness while adding complexity. The meatballs are fatty and savory, and the stout's roasty bitterness helps cut through that richness. The bourbon in the sauce brings warmth and vanilla, which is paired beautifully with the higher ABV and warming finish of a foreign stout.

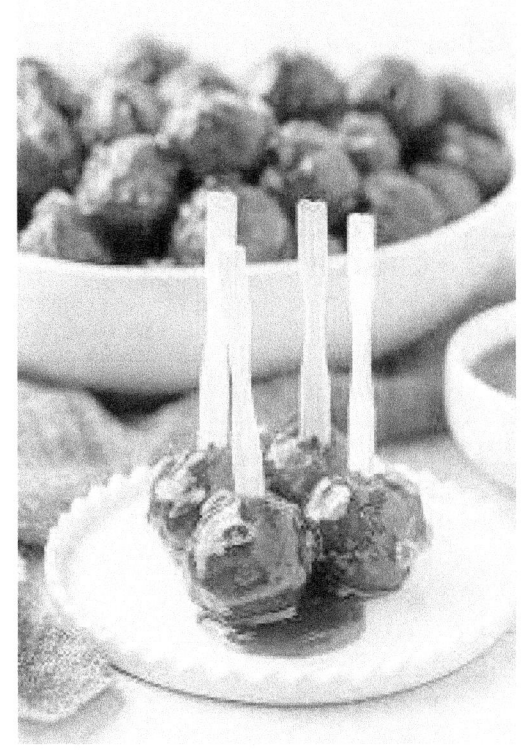

Ingredients:
32 oz bag fully cooked frozen meatballs *thawed*
2 cups bottled BBQ
3/4 cup bourbon
1/2 cup honey
1/3 cup molasses
1 Tbsp finely minced fresh garlic
1 Tbsp Worcestershire sauce
1/2 tsp cayenne pepper
fresh minced parsley

Instructions:
1. Add meatballs to the slow cooker. Set aside.
2. In a bowl, mix BBQ sauce, bourbon, honey, molasses, garlic, Worcestershire sauce, and cayenne pepper. Pour over the meatballs and stir to coat.
3. Cover and cook on LOW for 3-4 hours.
4. Stir before serving, then serve hot, sprinkled with minced fresh parsley if desired.

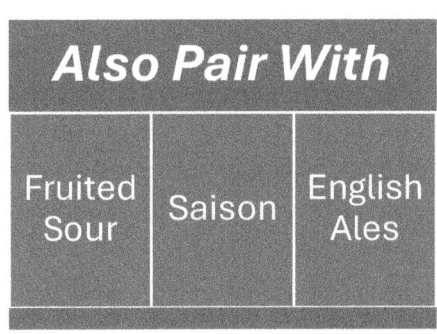

Also Pair With

Fruited Sour	Saison	English Ales

Cowboy Beans
1 lb. ground beef
6 slices thick-cut bacon, chopped
1 small onion, diced
2 cloves garlic, minced
1 (15 oz) can pinto beans, drained
1 (15 oz) can butter beans, drained
1 (15 oz) can black beans, drained
1 (15 oz) baked beans (with sauce)
½ cup ketchup
¼ cup brown sugar
2 Tbsp. molasses or maple syrup
1 Tbsp. yellow mustard
1 Tbsp. Worcestershire sauce
1 tsp. chili powder
Salt and pepper to taste

In a large skillet or Dutch oven, cook chopped bacon until crispy. Remove and set aside. In the same pan, cook the ground beef until browned. Drain excess fat. Add diced onion and garlic to the beef. Cook until softened (about 3–4 minutes). Stir in all the beans, ketchup, brown sugar, molasses, mustard, Worcestershire, chili powder, and cooked bacon. Mix well. Cover and simmer on low heat for 30–45 minutes, stirring occasionally. For a deeper flavor, bake uncovered at 350°F for 45 minutes.

Milkshake Stout

Milkshake Stout is a type of beer inspired by the flavors and characteristics of a milkshake. Milkshake stouts aim to replicate the creamy and indulgent qualities of a milkshake. Lactose is unfermentable by brewer's yeast, so it remains in the beer, adding sweetness and body. Chocolate and roasted malts contribute to the stout's flavor, providing notes of coffee, dark chocolate, and roasted grains. Expect a lightly sweet taste that mirrors the sweetness of milkshakes. The lactose adds a touch of creaminess. Some variations may include additional flavors like vanilla, fruit, or even spices.

Milkshake Stout: Key Characteristics		Notable Milkshake Stouts
Attribute	Description	Left Hand Nitro Peanut Butter Milk Stout
ABV	5.0–7.5% — moderate to strong; varies by brewer	Sweet Josie Brown Ale
IBU (Bitterness)	15–35 — low to moderate; bitterness is softened by sweetness	Milk Stout Nitro
Color (SRM)	30–40+ SRM — deep brown to black; may vary with adjuncts	Dragon's Milk Stout
Body	Full to very full — creamy, thick, and smooth	Coffee Snob Vanilla Latte Stout
Carbonation	Low to moderate — enhances mouthfeel without sharpness	Chocolate Coconut Cream Stout
Finish	Sweet and lingering — dessert-like with adjunct echoes	Imperial Bounty

Taste: Sweet | Malty | Coffee & Toffee Notes | Dessert-like | Creamy
Food Pairings: Chocolate or fruit Desserts | Barbecue with Sweet Glaze | Chili | Steak

Food Pairing Guide for Milkshake Stout

Milkshake Stout is a modern, indulgent twist on traditional stouts—designed to be dessert-like, creamy, and often bursting with adjunct flavors like vanilla, fruit purée, or chocolate.

Cheese Pairings
- Triple-Crème Brie or Camembert: Rich and buttery, echoing the beer's texture
- Mascarpone with Berries: Soft and sweet—perfect with fruit-infused stouts
- Blue Cheese with Honey or Fig Jam: Funky and sweet, balanced by roast

Meat & Savory Dishes
- Candied Bacon or Bacon-Wrapped Dates: Sweet-savory contrast that sings
- Pulled Pork with Sweet BBQ Sauce: Smoky and sticky—mirrors the beer's sweetness
- Spicy Sausage or Mole Chicken: Heat balanced by creamy sweetness

Vegetables & Sides
- Sweet Potato Fries with Marshmallow Dip: Sweet and salty indulgence
- Roasted Carrots or Beets: Earthy and sweet—great with malt depth
- Grilled Mushrooms with Balsamic Glaze: Umami meets sweetness

Desserts
- Chocolate Lava Cake or Brownies: Cocoa-on-cocoa decadence
- Strawberry Shortcake or Berry Tart: Fruit-forward stouts shine here
- Peanut Butter Pie or S'mores: Nostalgic and rich—perfect match

Jamaican Jerk Chicken

Jerk chicken is fiery, smoky, and spiced with allspice, Scotch bonnet peppers, and herbs. Milkshake stouts are sweet, creamy, and often infused with vanilla, chocolate, or fruit. The stout's lactose sweetness and smooth body cool the heat and soften the spice, creating a delicious contrast that keeps your palate engaged. Jerk chicken's grilled, charred exterior matches beautifully with the stout's roasted malt backbone—think cocoa, coffee, and toasted grain. If your milkshake stout includes fruit flavors (like strawberry, cherry, or banana), they add a tropical twist that plays off the Caribbean roots of jerk seasoning.

Ingredients
7 to 8 whole allspice*
3 Tbsp. of salt seasoning, such as Lawry's*
1 to 2 Scotch Bonnet peppers, quartered
1 bundle green onions, cut into 1-inch sections
1 sprig fresh thyme, leaves coarsely chopped
1 whole chicken, cleaned and quartered

Instructions:
1. Smash the allspice as finely as possible using a mortar and pestle. Put in a food processor and add the seasoning salt, peppers, green onions, thyme and 1/2 cup water. Blend the consistency of lumpy oatmeal and pour into a bowl.
2. Rub the chicken with the jerk seasoning and stuff the jerk seasoning between the skin and the meat. Place the chicken pieces into a storage pan and let marinade overnight (at least 12 hours).
3. Remove the excess seasoning from the chicken. Heat the grill to high heat (about 350 degrees F) and then place the chicken meat-side down first as to not let the chicken burn too quickly. Flip the chicken every 5 to 7 minutes until the skin has a nice brown color with grill marks, and then every 7 to 10 minutes on lower heat until cooked, around 40 minutes total or until the internal temperature of the chicken reaches 165 degrees F.
4. Chop each quarter into 4 to 5 pieces to get the real Jamaican jerk experience.

Authentic Jamaican Jerk Sauce (*Replace in Recipe)

4–6 scallions (green onions), chopped
1 small onion, chopped
3 cloves garlic
1–2 Scotch bonnet peppers (or habaneros), stemmed and seeded for less heat
1 Tbsp. fresh thyme (or 1 tsp. dried)
1 Tbsp. ground allspice
1 tsp. ground cinnamon
1 tsp. ground nutmeg
1 Tbsp. brown sugar
1/4 cup soy sauce
2 Tbsp. lime juice
2 Tbsp. white vinegar
2 Tbsp. vegetable oil
1/2 tsp. salt
1/2 tsp. black pepper
Optional: 1 Tbsp. grated fresh ginger

Also Pair With

Kolsch	Euro Pale Ale	Pilsner

Blend all ingredients in a food processor or blender until smooth. Add more lime juice for tang, more sugar for sweetness, or more pepper for heat. Use as a marinade or basting sauce. For best results, marinate meat for at least 4 hours or overnight.

American Stout

An American Stout is a bold and flavorful beer style that exhibit a deep, dark brown to black color. Expect flavors of roasted coffee, dark chocolate, and toasted malt. American hops contribute to the aroma and flavor, often with citrus or piney notes. American stouts typically have an ABV ranging from 5.7% to 8.9%. The bitterness level varies, falling between 35 and 60 IBU. American stouts are terrific companions to hearty foods.

American Stout: Key Characteristics		Notable American Stouts
Attribute	**Description**	Castle Danger George Hunter Stout
ABV	5.0–8.0% — moderate to strong; warming but not overwhelming	Shakespeare Stout by Rogue Ales
IBU (Bitterness)	35–75 — medium to high; bitterness from both hops and roasted grains	Obsidian Stout by Deschutes Brewery
Color (SRM)	30–40 SRM — jet black to deep brown; opaque with tan to mocha head	Black Cliffs by Boise Brewing
Body	Medium to full — smooth, sometimes creamy	Sierra Nevada Stout
Carbonation	Medium to high — supports aroma and texture	Bell's Kalamazoo Stout
Finish	Medium-dry to dry — often with lingering roast and hop bitterness	Great Lakes Edmund Fitzgerald

Taste: Bittersweet Choc | Coffee | Herbal
Food Pairings: Brisket | Burnt Ends | Most Smoked and Grilled Items | Dark Choc Desserts

Food Pairing Guide for American Stouts

American Stout is a bold, hop-forward evolution of traditional stouts—dark, roasty, and unapologetically American. It takes the rich malt backbone of English and Irish stouts and layers in assertive hop character, creating a beer that's both intense and balanced.

Cheese Pairings
- Smoked Cheddar or Gouda: Echoes the beer's smoky depth
- Aged Blue Cheese: Funky and bold—balanced by roast and bitterness
- Sharp Provolone or Asiago: Salty and intense, perfect with hop bite

Meat & Savory Dishes
- Grilled Steak or Lamb Chops: Charred crust matches roasted malt
- Spicy BBQ Ribs or Brisket: Sweet heat balanced by bitterness
- Blackened Chicken or Cajun Sausage: Spice and smoke meet hop and roast

Vegetables & Sides
- Grilled Portobello Mushrooms: Earthy umami plays off roasted malt
- Roasted Brussels Sprouts with Bacon: Bitter and salty—great with stout's edge
- Sweet Potato Fries with Chipotle Aioli: Sweet, spicy, and creamy contrast

Desserts
- Dark Chocolate Cake or Brownies: Cocoa-on-cocoa indulgence
- Espresso Ice Cream or Tiramisu: Coffee and cream echo stout's profile
- Molasses Cookies or Gingerbread: Spiced and sweet—perfect with roast

Smoked Baby Back Ribs

The ribs bring intense smoky, savory, and slightly sweet flavors from the rub and smoke. American stouts, with their roasted malt backbone, echo those smoky notes with hints of coffee, chocolate, and char. Ribs often have a glaze or sauce with brown sugar, molasses, or honey. The Stouts bitterness cuts through that sweetness, keeping the palate from getting overwhelmed. The carbonation in the stout helps cleanse the palate from the ribs' rich, fatty texture, making each bite feel fresh. Many American stouts have a smooth, velvety mouthfeel that complements the tender, juicy meat, enhancing the overall sensory experience.

Ingredients
2 Racks Pork Baby Back Ribs
4 Tbsp Yellow Mustard (For the binder)
8 Tbsp Rib Rub
6 Tbsp warmed Honey
4 Tbsp Butter
1/2 cup BBQ Sauce

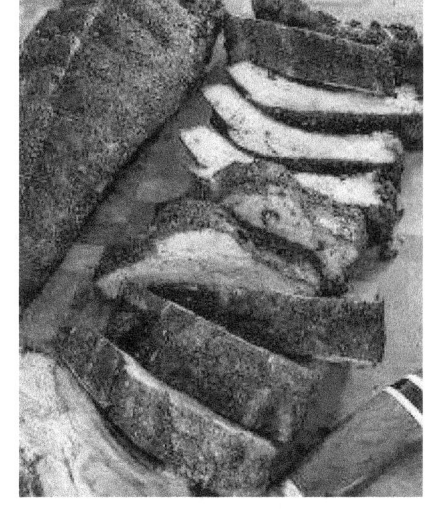

Instructions:
1. Rinse the ribs in cold water and pat them dry. Trim any excess fat or connective tissue. Remove the membrane from the bone side of the ribs. Apply a thin coating of yellow mustard evenly over the surface of the ribs. This binder helps the rub stick to the surface throughout the early part of the smoking process.
2. Now you can apply a generous coating of your favorite rub, covering all the sides and edges of the ribs.

3-2-1 Rib Method.
3. Preheat the smoker to 225°F. Once the smoker is at the proper temp, place the ribs on the grill, meat side UP. Smoke The Uncovered Ribs For 3 Hours.
4. Spritz their ribs every 30-45 minutes with a 50/50 mixture of apple cider vinegar and water.
5. After three hours, remove the ribs from the smoker and place each rack on a sheet of heavy-duty tin foil. Brush melted butter over the tops of the ribs and then add some melted honey. At this time, you can spritz the ribs for extra moisture. Cover both sides of the ribs with butter and melted honey. Now, wrap the ribs in foil.
6. Afterwards, the ribs are wrapped tightly in foil. Place the ribs back on the smoker with the meat side DOWN, keeping the temp at 225°F for 2 hours.
7. Remove the ribs from the foil and place them back on the grill with the meat side UP. Brush the ribs with your favorite BBQ sauce. Smoke the ribs for 1 more hour at 225°F. Check for doneness using a combination of the rib meat temperature (198-203 degrees), the pick-up test (should have a nice arch), and the amount of exposed bone. (1/4 to 1 ½ inches of exposed bone).
8. Let the ribs rest for 15 minutes. You can loosely wrap the ribs in foil or put a foil tent over them.
9. Cut the ribs with a sharp knife on a cutting board.

Also Pairs With

Robust Porter	Marzen	Double IPA

Lagers Beers

Lager is a type of beer brewed using bottom-fermenting yeast (Saccharomyces pastorianus) at cooler temperatures (typically 45–55°F / 7–13°C). After fermentation, lagers undergo a period of cold storage known as lagering, which smooths out flavors and creates a clean, crisp finish. The word "lager" comes from the German lager, meaning "to store."

History and Origin
The term "lager" comes from the German word lagern, meaning "to store"—a nod to the cold storage process used to mature the beer. Bottom-fermenting yeast (Saccharomyces pastorianus) was key to lager's development. Unlike ale yeast, it ferments at cooler temperatures and settles at the bottom of the vessel. The earliest lagers were brewed in Bohemia (modern-day Czech Republic) and Germany, where brewers stored beer in cool caves or cellars during the summer.

Key Characteristics
Fermentation: Bottom-fermented at cool temperatures
Maturation: Cold storage for weeks or months
Taste: Clean, smooth, less fruity than ales
ABV Range: Typically, 4–7%, depending on style

Lagers are beloved for their drinkability and versatility. Whether you're sipping a crisp pilsner or a rich Dunkel, there's a lager for every palate.

Common Lager Styles

Style	Color	Flavor Profile	ABV Range
Pale Lager / Pilsner	Light gold	Crisp, hoppy, refreshing	4.5-5.5
Helles	Pale gold	Malty, smooth, less bitter	4.8-5.4
Dunkel	Dark brown	Malty, bready, caramel notes	4.5-6.0
Schwarzbier	Black	Roasty, smooth, light-bodied	4.4-5.4

Awesome Food Pairings
Pale Lager: Grilled chicken, sushi, pretzels
Helles: German Fare, Grilled Meats, Seafood, Vegetarian Dishes, Spicy Foods
Dunkel: Pork schnitzel, sausages, roast pork or beef, Barbecue, Root Veggies, Bread Pudding
Schwarzbier: Smoked sausage, Grilled pork chops, Roast beef, Pulled pork, brisket, ribs with smoky or sweet sauces

LAGER BEER & FOOD PAIRINGS

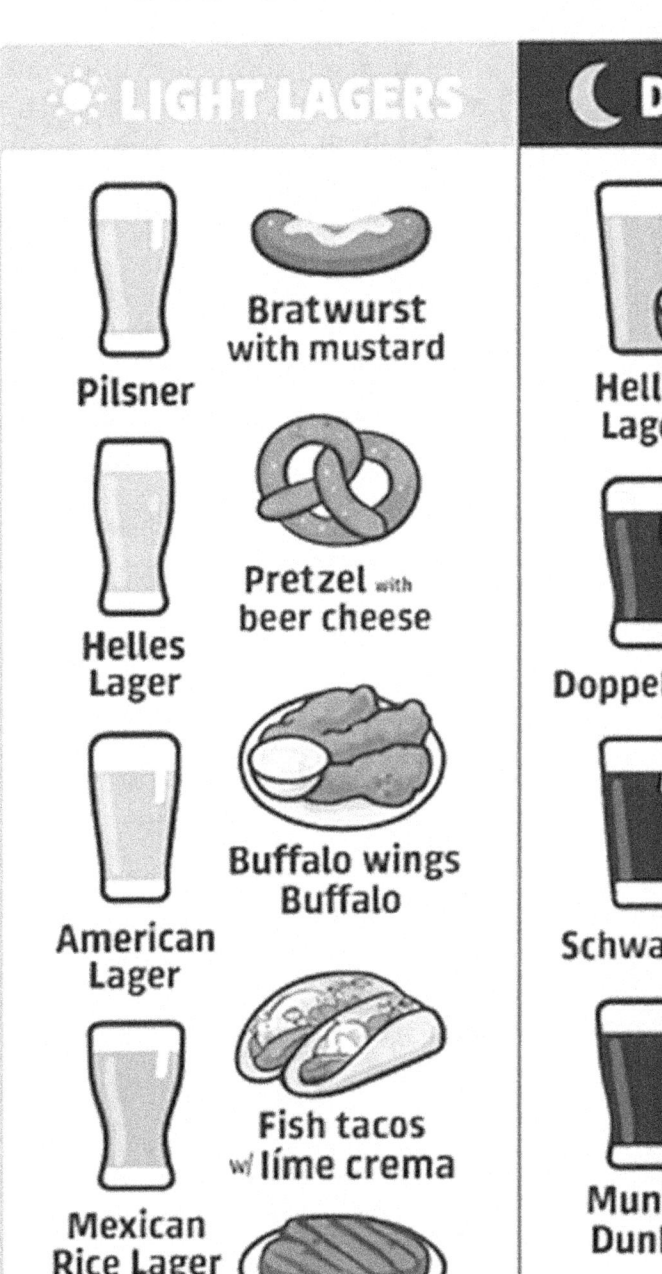
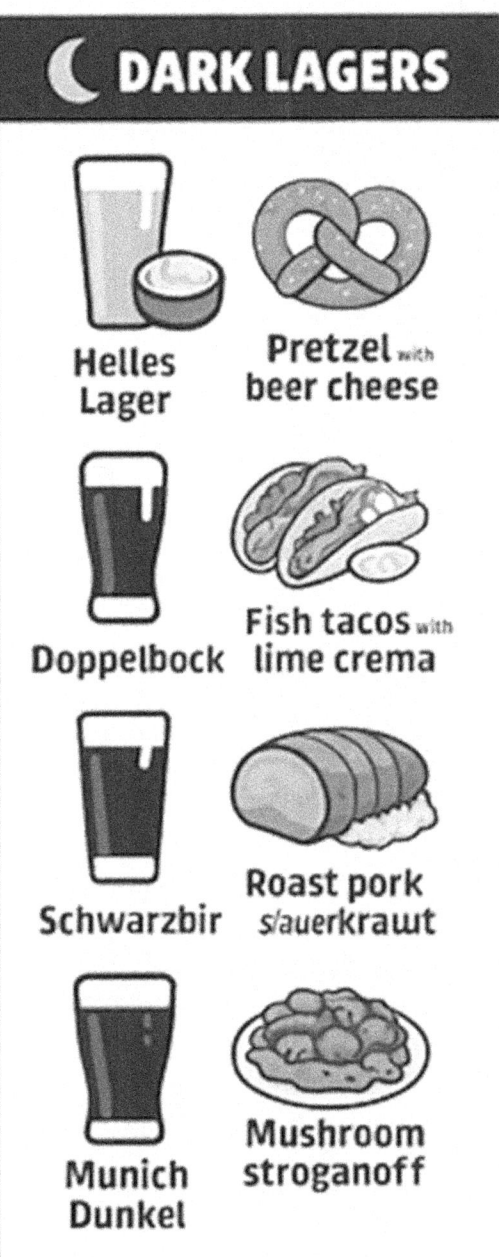

Pale Lagers

Pale Lagers are crisp, clean, and highly refreshing beers that emphasize balance and drinkability. Brewed with pale malts and bottom-fermenting yeast at cool temperatures, they showcase a smooth malt sweetness, subtle hop bitterness, and brilliant clarity.

Pale Lager Characteristics
Appearance: Pale golden color with brilliant clarity
Flavor: Crisp, clean, and refreshing with mild malt sweetness and subtle hop bitterness
Aroma: Light floral or herbal hop notes, sometimes with faint grain or biscuit undertones
Body: Light to medium, with high carbonation for a refreshing mouthfeel
ABV: Typically ranges from 4% to 6%, making it easy-drinking and sessionable
Fermentation: Cold-fermented using bottom-fermenting yeast for a smooth, clean finish

Pale Lager Styles by Region

Region	Style/Name	Key Characteristics	Notable Examples
Germany	Pilsner, Helles, Dortmunder Export	Crisp, dry, noble hops; Helles is maltier and softer	Warsteiner, Bitburger, Paulaner Helles
Czech Republic	Czech Pilsner (Bohemian)	Rich malt, floral Saaz hops, smooth bitterness	Pilsner Urquell
United States	American Pale Lager	Light body, mild hops, often brewed with corn or rice	Budweiser, Coors Banquet
Mexico	Mexican Lager	Refreshing, mild bitterness, often served with lime	Corona Extra, Modelo Especial
Japan	Japanese Pale Lager	Clean, dry, subtle malt and hops	Asahi Super Dry, Sapporo Premium
Netherlands	International Pale Lager	Balanced, smooth, mild bitterness	Heineken
Denmark	Dortmunder-style Export	Slightly stronger, balanced malt and hop profile	Carlsberg

Food Pairing Tips
- Pale lagers are delicate and clean, so pair them with foods that won't overpower their flavor.
- Their carbonation and dry finish cut through salty, greasy, or spicy dishes.
- Pale lagers pair beautifully with citrus, herbs, and vinegar-based dishes.
- Pale lagers are perfect with simple, nostalgic foods—think backyard BBQ or ballpark snacks.

Pale Lager Styles & Food Pairings

Pale Lager Style	Flavor Profile	Best Food Pairings
German Pilsner	Crisp, bitter, floral noble hops	Bratwurst, schnitzel, pretzels, grilled white fish
Czech Pilsner	Smooth, malty, Saaz hops, soft bitterness	Roast chicken, creamy cheeses, potato pancakes
American Pale Lager	Light, mild, often adjuncts (corn/rice)	Burgers, hot dogs, nachos, fried chicken
Mexican Lager	Light, refreshing, often served with lime	Tacos, ceviche, elote (grilled corn), tortilla chips
Japanese Pale Lager	Clean, dry, subtle malt and hops	Sushi, tempura, yakitori, miso soup
International Lager	Balanced, mild bitterness, smooth finish	Pizza, pasta with light sauces, grilled vegetables

Pale Lager

Pale lager is a very pale -to- golden -colored lager beer with a well- attenuated body and a varying degree of noble hop bitterness. Light beers go great when paired with poultry, fruits, salads, and appetizers. Pilsners go great with poultry, seafood and smaller plates. Some of the barbeque meals that can work correctly with the light lagers are fried fish, Buffalo wings, and any poultry.

Pale Lager: Key Characteristics		Notable Pale Lager
Attribute	**Description**	Pilsner Urquell
ABV	4.0–6.0% — low to moderate; ideal for session drinking	Weihenstephaner Original
IBU (Bitterness)	10–30 — mild to moderate; bitterness varies by sub-style	Bitburger Premium Pils
Color (SRM)	2–6 SRM — pale straw to light gold; crystal clear appearance	Modelo Especial
Body	Light to medium-light — crisp and easy-drinking	Stella Artois
Carbonation	High — adds to the refreshing mouthfeel	
Finish	Clean and dry — minimal lingering flavors; very quaffable	

Taste: Malty | Citrusy | Hoppy | Grassy | Floral | Sweetness
Food Pairing: Grilled Chicken | Fish Tacos | Fresh Salads | Sushi | Spicy Dishes

Food Pairing Guide for Pale Lagers
Pale Lager is the ultimate crowd-pleaser—simple in appearance but refined in execution. Whether you're exploring regional variations or pairing it with barbecue sides, it's a versatile style that plays well with almost any dish.

Cheese Pairings
- Mild Cheddar or Monterey Jack: Soft and creamy, balanced by crispness
- Mozzarella or Burrata: Fresh and milky—great with lager's subtle malt
- Swiss or Havarti: Nutty and mellow, echoing the beer's smoothness

Meat & Savory Dishes
- Grilled Bratwurst or Hot Dogs: Classic combo—salt, smoke, and refreshment
- Fried Chicken or Schnitzel: Crunchy and rich, cut by carbonation
- Fish Tacos or Shrimp Po'boys: Briny and spicy—lager cools and complements

Spicy & Global Cuisine
- Thai Curry or Pad Thai: Lager's lightness cools heat and balances sweetness
- Buffalo Wings or Jalapeno Poppers: Crisp finish tames spice and salt
- Indian Samosas or Chaat: Refreshing contrast to bold spices

Vegetables & Sides
- French Fries or Onion Rings: Salty and crispy—perfect with carbonation
- Grilled Corn or Zucchini: Sweet and smoky—echoes malt notes
- Coleslaw or Potato Salad: Creamy sides balanced by dry finish

Desserts
- Lemon Bars or Fruit Tarts: Bright and tangy—great with lager's clean profile
- Shortbread Cookies or Pound Cake: Buttery and simple—echoes malt sweetness
- Pretzels with Chocolate Dip: Sweet-salty contrast that pops

Chicken in White Wine Sauce

Chicken in white wine sauce is paired wonderfully with a pale lager because the chicken is typically poached or sautéed, with a sauce made from white wine, butter, herbs, and sometimes cream. Pale lagers are light-bodied and mildly malty, so they don't overpower the dish—they let the nuanced flavors of the sauce shine. The white wine sauce brings a touch of acidity and brightness. Pale lagers, with their dry finish and subtle carbonation, mirror that brightness and refresh the palate, especially between bites of buttery sauce. Herbs like thyme, parsley, or tarragon in the sauce pair well with gentle floral or herbal hop notes in a pale lager.

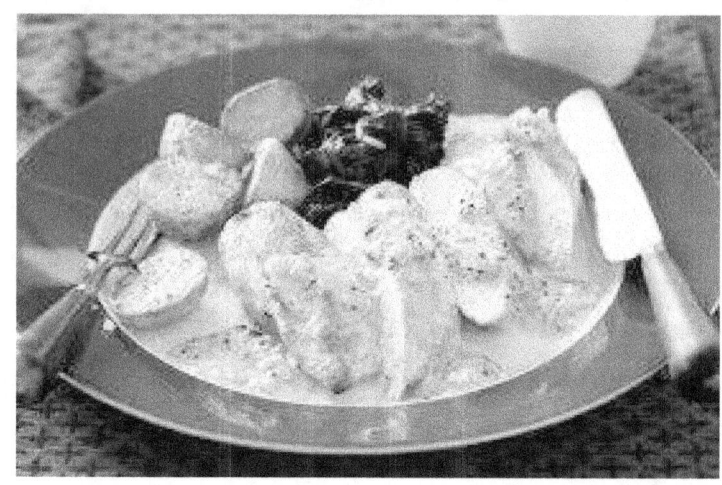

Ingredients:
3 Tbsp. all-purpose flour
4 thin-sliced chicken breasts
1/4-1/2 tsp. garlic powder
kosher salt & black pepper
1 Tbsp. olive oil
3 Tbsp. butter, divided
1/2 cup chicken broth
1/2 cup dry white wine
1/4 tsp. dried thyme | fresh herbs optional garnish

Instructions:
1. Place the flour in a small bowl or plate. Sprinkle the chicken breasts evenly on both sides with garlic powder and a small amount of salt and pepper. Warm olive oil and 1 Tbsp. of the butter in a large skillet over medium-high heat.
2. Lightly dredge each chicken breast in the flour. Shake gently to remove any excess, then place each piece in the hot pan. Cook for 1-2 minutes per side, until browned on the outside but not fully cooked through. Remove the chicken pieces and set aside.
3. Add broth and wine to the pan, bring to a simmer, and let it bubble for 1-2 minutes, scraping the bottom to remove any browned bits. Add the remaining 2 Tbsp. butter and thyme. Simmer for another 1-2 minutes, while the butter melts.
4. Return the chicken to the pan, lower the heat to medium-low, and simmer for another 3-4 minutes, until the sauce thickens slightly, and the chicken is cooked through. Garnish with fresh herbs.

Oven-Roasted Vegetables
4 cups mixed vegetables, chopped (e.g., carrots, zucchini, onion, broccoli, cauliflower, sweet potatoes)
2–3 Tbsp. olive oil
1 tsp. kosher salt
½ tsp. black pepper
1 tsp. garlic powder or minced garlic
1 tsp. dried herbs (thyme, rosemary, oregano, or Italian seasoning)

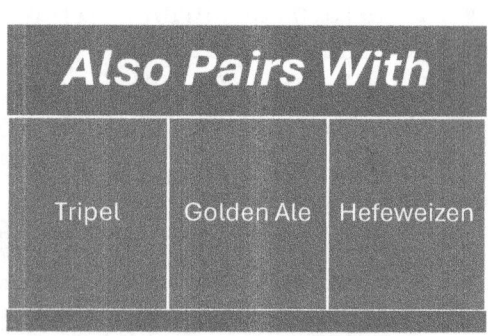

Also Pairs With		
Tripel	Golden Ale	Hefeweizen

Set oven to 425°F. Line a baking sheet with parchment paper or foil. Wash and chop the vegetables into uniform bite-sized pieces for even cooking. Toss the veggies in a large bowl with olive oil, salt, pepper, garlic, and herbs. Add vinegar or lemon juice if using. Spread in a single layer on the baking sheet. Roast for 25–35 minutes, flipping halfway, until golden and tender with crispy edges.

Light Lager

These lighter flavored beers go very well with lighter BBQ foods. Some of them have a refreshing balance of floral fruit hops, like pilsner, and bready malt. While others have a hint of sweetness from a toasted caramel malt flavor. Complements lemongrass, ginger, garlic, cilantro, and similar flavors; add depth to light dishes such as spring rolls and salads. Goes great with Southern BBQ and lighter fare like chicken and seafood.

Light Lager: Key Characteristics		Notable Light Lager
Attribute	**Description**	Bud Light
ABV	2.5–5.0% — low alcohol; ideal for casual, all-day sipping	Coors Light
IBU (Bitterness)	8–12 — very low; just enough to balance sweetness	Miller Lite
Color (SRM)	2–4 SRM — pale straw to light gold; crystal clear appearance	Michelob Ultra
Body	Very light — dry, crisp, and highly carbonated	Corona Light
Calories	Typically, 90–110 per 12 oz; designed for low-calorie appeal	Amstel Light
Finish	Clean and dry — no lingering malt or hop flavors	Bud Light

Taste: Cereal | Clean | Very Little Flavors : High Carbonation | Dry Finish
Food Pairing: Grilled Chicken | Fish | Sushi | Light Fare | Spicy Wings or Nachos

Food Pairing Guide for Light Lagers
Light Lager is a no-frills refresher. Light Lager is the ultimate easy-drinker—crisp, clean, and designed for maximum refreshment with minimal complexity.

Cheese Pairings
- Mild Cheddar or Colby: Soft and creamy, balanced by crispness
- Mozzarella or Provolone: Fresh and milky—great with lager's subtle malt
- Queso Fresco or Monterey Jack: Light and salty, perfect with carbonation

Meat & Savory Dishes
- Grilled Hot Dogs or Bratwurst: Classic combo—salt, smoke, and refreshment
- Fried Chicken or Chicken Tenders: Crunchy and rich, cut by carbonation
- Fish Tacos or Shrimp Po'boys: Briny and spicy—lager cools and complements

Spicy & Global Cuisine
- Buffalo Wings to jalapeno Poppers: Crisp finish tames spice and salt
- Thai Curry or Pad Thai: Lager's lightness cools heat and balances sweetness
- Mexican Street Corn or Tacos al Pastor: Sweet, spicy, and savory—perfect match

Vegetables & Sides
- French Fries or Onion Rings: Salty and crispy—perfect with carbonation
- Grilled Corn or Zucchini: Sweet and smoky—echoes malt notes
- Coleslaw or Potato Salad: Creamy sides balanced by dry finish

Desserts
- Lemon Bars or Fruit Tarts: Bright and tangy—great with lager's clean profile
- Shortbread Cookies or Pound Cake: Buttery and simple—echoes malt sweetness
- Pretzels with Chocolate Dip: Sweet-salty contrast that pops

Green Chile Stew

New Mexico green chili stew pairs beautifully with a light lager because the beer's crisp, clean profile complements the stew's spicy, earthy, and savory depth without competing for attention. Green chili stew packs a gentle to moderate heat from roasted Hatch chiles. Light lagers—low in bitterness and high in carbonation—cool the palate, making the spice more enjoyable and less overwhelming. The stew's base of slow-cooked pork or beef, potatoes, and onions deliver hearty, umami-rich flavors. A light lager's dry finish and subtle malt backbone cut through the richness, keeping each bite feeling fresh.

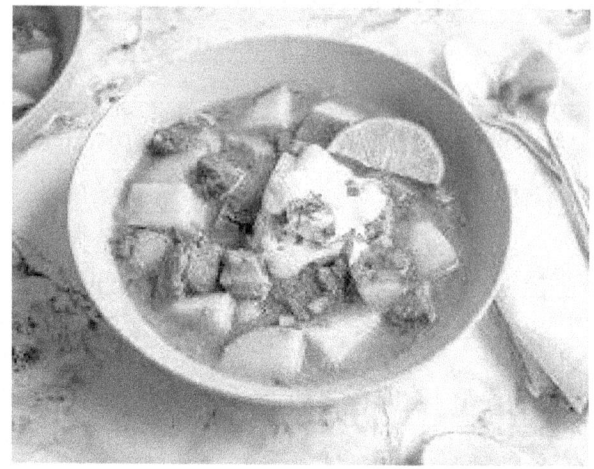

3 lbs. Boston Pork Butt, cut into 1 1/2 " cubes
2 tbsp vegetable oil
2 large onions, peeled and chopped
2 cloves garlic, peeled and minced
2 qts Free range chicken stock
18 Hatch chiles, roasted, peeled, seeded, and chopped (approx. 1 1/2 cups)
6 small tomatoes, peeled, seeded and chopped
6 med potatoes, peeled and diced
1/2 tsp each toasted Mexican oregano, toasted ground cumin, & salt to taste
1 bunch cilantro, fresh
1 jar crema Mexicana* Optional as this makes the soup thick. Most New Mexicans surveyed, omit.

In a large skillet, brown pork over medium-high heat for about 10 minutes. Transfer the pork to a large stockpot. Add oil to the skillet. Add onions and cook over medium heat until softened, about 7 minutes. Reduce heat, add garlic and sauté for 1 minute. Transfer the onions and garlic to the stockpot. Add one-quart stock to skillet and deglaze it. Add this stock, the remaining stock, chiles, tomatoes, potatoes, oregano and cumin to the stockpot. Salt to taste. Simmer on low heat for 1 1/2 hours, until pork is very tender. Ladle into bowls, garnish with cilantro leaves. Stir crema Mexicana into the soup for a creamy consistency.

Green Chile–Friendly Cornbread
1 cup yellow cornmeal
1 cup all-purpose flour
1 tbsp baking powder
½ tsp baking soda
½ tsp salt
2 tbsp sugar
1 cup buttermilk
2 eggs
¼ cup each melted butter, creamed corn & shredded cheddar or pepper jack
1–2 tbsp chopped roasted green chiles or jalapenos (for a flavor echo)

Preheat oven to 400°F. Butter a cast-iron skillet or 8x8 baking dish. Mix dry ingredients: In a large bowl, whisk together cornmeal, flour, baking powder, baking soda, salt, and sugar. In another bowl, whisk buttermilk, eggs, melted butter, and creamed corn. Stir wet into dry until just combined. Fold in cheese and chiles, if using. Pour into prepared pan and bake for 20–25 minutes until golden and a toothpick comes out clean.

Also Pairs With		
Mexican Lager	Fruited Gose	Euro Pale Ale

Euro Pale Lager

Euro Pale Lagers are pale gold and exhibit excellent head retention. Expect hops with a hint of graininess. These beers are bitter, with a full body and the taste of toasted malt and spicy hops. They are brewed with an all-malt base and noble hop varieties.

Euro Pale Lager: Key Characteristics		Notable Euro Pale Lagers
Attribute	**Description**	Grolsch Premium Lager
ABV	4.0–6.0% — moderate strength; ideal for casual sipping	Heineken
IBU (Bitterness)	18–25 — moderate; enough to balance malt sweetness	Stella Artois
Color (SRM)	2–6 SRM — pale straw to light gold; brilliant clarity	Peroni Nastro Azzurro
Body	Light to medium — smooth and refreshing	Harp Lager
Carbonation	Medium to high — enhances crispness and drinkability	Bitburger Premium Pils
Finish	Clean and slightly sweet — with a touch of hop bitterness	

Taste: Crisp, Balanced, Biscuity, Earthy
Food Pairings: Grilled Sausages | Barbecue | Roasted Chicken | Seafood

Food Pairing Guide for Euro Pale Lagers

Euro Pale Lager is a refined refresher—perfect for barbecue menus when you're pairing with lighter meat or sides.

Cheese Pairings
- Emmental or Gruyère: Nutty and mellow—echoes malt sweetness
- Young Gouda or Havarti: Creamy and mild, balanced by carbonation
- Brie with Apple Slices: Soft and buttery, lifted by a crisp finish

Meat & Savory Dishes
- Roast Chicken or Pork Loin: Simple and savory—perfect with malt depth
- Bratwurst or Weisswurst: Classic Bavarian pairing with herbal hops
- Schnitzel or Fish & Chips: Fried and crispy—cut by carbonation

Vegetables & Sides
- German Potato Salad or Spaetzle: Rich and starchy—balanced by a dry finish
- Grilled Asparagus or Zucchini: Earthy and fresh—echoes hop character
- Sauerkraut or Pickled Veggies: Tangy and sharp—softened by malt

Spicy & Global Cuisine
- Thai Basil Chicken or Pad See Ew: Sweet-savory heat cooled by lager
- Tacos al Pastor or Carnitas: Pork and spice balanced by crispness
- Indian Butter Chicken or Samosas: Creamy and spiced—lifted by carbonation

Desserts
- Apple Strudel or Pear Tart: Fruity and flaky—great with malt sweetness
- Shortbread Cookies or Pound Cake: Buttery and simple—echoes biscuit notes
- Pretzels with Chocolate Dip: Sweet-salty contrast that pops

Carolina Pulled-Pork Sandwiches

Carolina pulled pork is famous for its vinegar-forward BBQ sauce, which is tangy, sharp, and acidic. Euro pale lagers have a gentle malt sweetness (think honeyed bread or biscuit) that softens the acidity and brings balance to the bite. The pork is slow-cooked, tender, and fatty, often with a smoky edge. Euro lagers are clean and crisp, with moderate carbonation that cuts through the richness and refreshes the palate. The sandwich layers flavors—meat, sauce, slaw, bun. Euro pale lagers offer herbal or floral hop notes and a smooth, dry finish that complement without competing, letting the sandwich shine.

Ingredients:

For dry rub
3 Tbsp. coarsely ground black pepper
3 Tbsp. (packed) dark brown sugar
3 Tbsp. paprika
2 Tbsp. coarse salt
1 tsp. cayenne pepper
2 untrimmed boneless pork shoulder halves (also known as Boston butt; about 6 pounds total)
1 pint of creamy coleslaw

For mop
1 cup of apple cider vinegar
1/2 cup of water
2 Tbsp. Worcestershire sauce
1 Tbsp. coarsely ground black pepper
1 Tbsp. coarse salt
2 tsp. of vegetable oil

Instructions:

Make dry rub:
1. Mix the first 5 ingredients in a small bowl to blend.
2. Place the pork, fat side up, on the work surface. Cut each piece lengthwise in half. Place it on a large baking sheet. Sprinkle dry rub all over pork; press into pork. Cover with plastic; refrigerate at least 2 hours. (Can be made 1 day ahead. Keep chilled.)

Make mop:
1. Mix the first 6 ingredients in a medium bowl. Cover and refrigerate.
2. Following manufacturer's instructions and using lump charcoal and 1/2 cup drained wood chips for smokers or 1 cup for barbecue, start a fire and bring the temperature of the smoker or barbecue to 225°F to 250°F. Place the pork on the rack in the smoker or barbecue. Cover; cook until meat thermometer inserted into center of pork registers 165°F., turning pork and brushing with cold mop every 45 minutes, about 6 hours total. Add more charcoal as needed to maintain 225°F to 250°F temperature and more drained wood chips (1/2 cup for a smoker or 1 cup for a barbecue with each addition) to maintain smoke level.
3. Transfer the pork to a clean rimmed baking sheet. Let it stand until it's cool enough to handle. Shred into bite-size pieces. Mound on platter. Pour any juice from the sheets over the pork. (Can be made 1 day ahead. Transfer the pork and any juices to the baking dish. Cover with foil, chill. Before continuing, rewarm the pork, covered, in a 350°F oven about 30 minutes.)
4. Divide the pork among the bottoms of buns. Drizzle lightly with barbecue sauce. Top with coleslaw. Cover with the tops of buns.

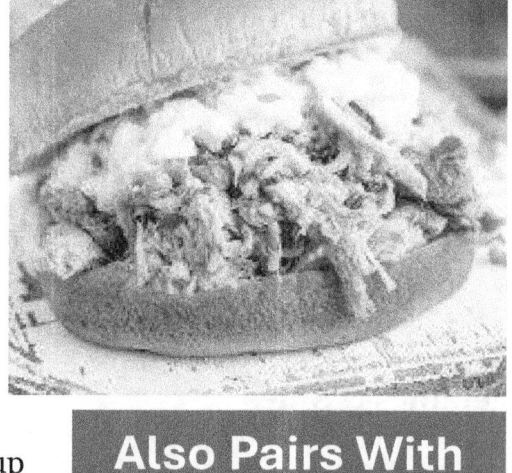

Also Pairs With

| Cider Ale | Vienna Lager | Cream Ale |

Pilsner

A drier beer with a hint of bitterness helps balance buttery flavors, especially in seafood. Some Pilsners have some floral hops flavors like Lagers, and it goes well with chicken, beef, port, and duck. Works well with salmon, tuna & other high-fat, oily fish and with marbled meats; bitterness offers a pleasing contrast with sweet reductions and sauces. Go grill beer for anything. It does well with chicken, beef, pork, brats, salmon, and duck — all in barbeque especially anything skewered with veggies.

Pilsner: Key Characteristics		Notable Pilsners
Attribute	Description	Brooklyn Pilsner
ABV	4.0–5.3% — moderate strength; highly sessionable	Slow Pour Pils
IBU (Bitterness)	30–40+ — noticeable but balanced; varies by sub-style	Pivo Pils
Color (SRM)	3–7 SRM — pale straw to light gold; brilliant clarity	Prima Pils
Body	Light to medium — crisp and clean	Beck's
Carbonation	Medium to high — enhances mouthfeel and aroma	Bitburger Premium Pils
Finish	Dry and refreshing — with lingering hop bitterness or malt sweetness depending on style	Oskar Blues Mama's Little

Taste: Crisp | Grainy | Grassy | Bready | Herbal
Food Pairings: Brats | Barbecue | Seafood | Spicy Dishes | Vietnamese Food

Food Pairing Guide for Pilsner
Pilsner is the gold standard of refreshment—simple in ingredients, but masterful in execution.

Cheese Pairings
- Goat Cheese or Feta: Tangy and salty—balanced by pilsner's crispness
- Gruyère or Emmental: Nutty and mellow—echoes malt sweetness
- Fresh Mozzarella or Burrata: Creamy and delicate—lifted by carbonation

Meat & Savory Dishes
- Grilled Sausages or Bratwurst: Classic pairing—herbs and hops in harmony
- Roast Chicken or Turkey: Light and savory—perfect with pilsner's clean finish
- Fish & Chips or Fried Shrimp: Crunchy and rich—cut by carbonation and bitterness

Spicy & Global Cuisine
- Thai Green Curry or Pad Thai: Sweet heat cooled by crisp lager
- Mexican Street Tacos or Elote: Spice and salt balanced by dry finish
- Indian Samosas or Tandoori Chicken: Bold spices softened by malt and bubbles

Vegetables & Sides
- Grilled Asparagus or Zucchini: Earthy and fresh—echoes hop character
- Potato Salad or Spaetzle: Creamy and starchy—balanced by carbonation
- Pickled Veggies or Kimchi: Tangy and sharp—softened by malt

Desserts
- Lemon Tart or Apple Strudel: Bright and fruity—great with pilsner's clean profile
- Shortbread Cookies or Pound Cake: Buttery and simple—echoes biscuit notes
- Pretzels with Chocolate Dip: Sweet-salty contrast that pops

Crispy Beer Batter Fish

The fish's crunchy, golden batter is rich and slightly oily. Pilsners are highly carbonated and dry, which means they cut through the fat, cleanse the palate, and keep each bite feeling light and fresh. Pilsners have a light malt backbone—think crackers or bread crust—that mirrors the flavor of the batter. This creates a flavor echo that ties the dish and drink together without overwhelming the delicate fish. Pilsners often feature herbal or floral hop notes, especially in Czech or German styles. These subtle hops add complexity and lift the mild flavor of white fish, like cod or haddock, without clashing.

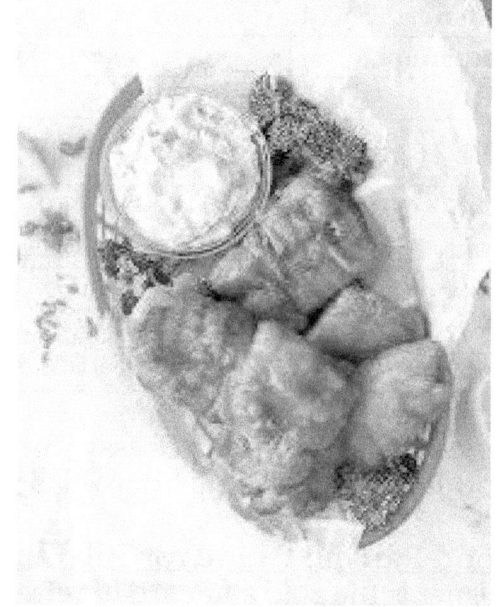

Ingredients:
2 lbs. white fish, like cod or tilapia or Your Catch of the Day
1 tsp of salt
1/2 tsp black pepper
1 cup all-purpose flour
1 tbsp garlic powder
1 tbsp paprika
2 tsp seasoned salt
1 large egg, lightly beaten
1 1/3 cups of beer
Canola oil for frying

Instructions:
1. Add oil to a large, heavy-bottomed pot or deep fryer until it's about 2 to 3 inches deep. Heat oil to 375 degrees F.
2. Meanwhile, cut the fish into stick shapes, about 1 inch wide and 3 inches long. Pat dry with paper towels and season with salt and pepper.
3. Whisk together the flour, garlic powder, paprika and seasoned salt. Stir in the lightly beaten egg, then gradually whisk in the beer until the batter forms and is no longer lumpy.
4. Quickly dip the fish, one piece at a time, into the batter, then place in the hot oil. Cook for 3 to 4 minutes, or until the fish is a nice golden brown. Drain on a wire rack and enjoy while hot!

Classic Tartar Sauce
½ cup mayonnaise
2 Tbsp. finely chopped dill pickles or cornichons
1 Tbsp. fresh lemon juice
1 Tbsp. finely chopped capers
1 tsp. Dijon mustard
1 tsp. pickle juice
1 Tbsp. finely chopped fresh parsley or dill
½ tsp. garlic powder, or minced shallots
Salt and black pepper to taste

Mix all ingredients in a bowl until well combined. Add more lemon juice for brightness, more pickles for crunch, or mustard for zing. Chill for 30 minutes to let the flavors meld.

Also Pairs With		
Helles Lager	Light Lager	Lime Gose

Czech Pilsner

The Czech Pilsner was originally brewed in the town of Pilsen (Plzeň) in what is now the Czech Republic. Czech Pilsners are pale gold in color and brilliantly clear. Aroma: Expect hops with a hint of graininess. These beers are bitter, with a full body and the taste of toasted malt and spicy hops. Floor-malted barley slightly caramelized, along with Saaz (Žatec) hops. The long, rounded finish leaves you refreshed.

Czech Pilsner: Key Characteristics		Notable Czech Pilsner
Attribute	**Description**	Pilsner Urquell
ABV	4.2–5.8% — moderate strength; highly sessionable	Budweiser Budvar Original
IBU (Bitterness)	30–45 — firm but smooth; never harsh	Staropramen
Color (SRM)	3–6 SRM — pale gold to deep gold; brilliant clarity	Znojemské Pivo
Body	Medium — fuller than German Pils; soft and rounded mouthfeel	Březnický Ležák
Carbonation	Light to moderate — supports drinkability without sharpness	
Finish	Long and balanced — can lean toward malt or hops, but always smooth	

Taste: Balanced | Biscuity | Toasty | Crisp | Spicy | Clean
Food Pairings: Roast Chicken | Pork | Vietnamese Food | Tacos

Food Pairing Guide For Czech Pilsners

Czech Pilsner—also known as Bohemian Pilsner—is a style that balances bready malt richness with floral, spicy noble hops, all wrapped in a smooth, rounded finish.

Cheese Pairings
- Aged Gouda or Gruyère: Nutty and rich—balanced by hop bitterness
- Fresh Goat Cheese or Feta: Tangy and salty—lifted by crisp carbonation
- Czech Olomoucké Tvarůžky (if available): Pungent and funky—tempered by malt sweetness

Meat & Savory Dishes
- Roast Pork with Caraway or Garlic: Classic Czech pairing—echoes malt and spice
- Grilled Sausages or Kielbasa: Smoky and savory—perfect with herbal hops
- Schnitzel or Chicken Cutlets: Crispy and rich—cut by carbonation and bitterness

Vegetables & Sides
- Braised Cabbage or Sauerkraut: Tangy and earthy—softened by malt
- Potato Pancakes or Dumplings: Starchy and hearty—balanced by a dry finish
- Grilled Mushrooms or Asparagus: Umami and herbal—mirrors hop character

Spicy & Global Cuisine
- Vietnamese Bánh Mi or Thai Basil Chicken: Bright herbs and spice cooled by crisp lager
- Mexican Street Tacos or Elote: Salt, spice, and char—perfect with pilsner's snap
- Indian Pakoras or Butter Chicken: Creamy and spiced—lifted by carbonation

Desserts
- Apple Strudel or Pear Tart: Fruity and flaky—echoes malt sweetness
- Shortbread Cookies or Almond Cake: Buttery and simple—pairs with biscuit notes
- Pretzels with Caramel Dip

Pork Cabbage Rolls

Cabbage rolls often feature braised or fermented cabbage, which brings a slightly sour, earthy edge. Czech pilsners—especially those brewed with Saaz hops—offer a spicy, herbal bitterness that cuts through the tang and refreshes the palate. The pulled pork filling is tender, fatty, and deeply savory. Czech pilsners have a dry, clean finish and moderate carbonation, which cleanses the palate and balances the richness of the meat without overwhelming it. Czech pilsners are more malt-forward than their German cousins, with flavors of fresh bread, biscuit, and honey. These malt notes complement the sweetness in the pork and any tomato-based sauce, creating a cozy, cohesive flavor profile.

Ingredients:
head of cabbage, leaves removed
1-2 lbs. pork butt or shoulder, fat removed, and cut into 4 chunks
1 white onion, sliced
2 Tbsp paprika
2 Tbsp Italian seasoning
1 tsp salt and pepper
2 large carrots, chopped finely
1 cup of water
fresh parsley

For Sauce
1 6 oz can tomato paste
1/2 cup unsweetened almond milk
1 Tbsp Italian seasoning
1 cup of broth from the crockpot

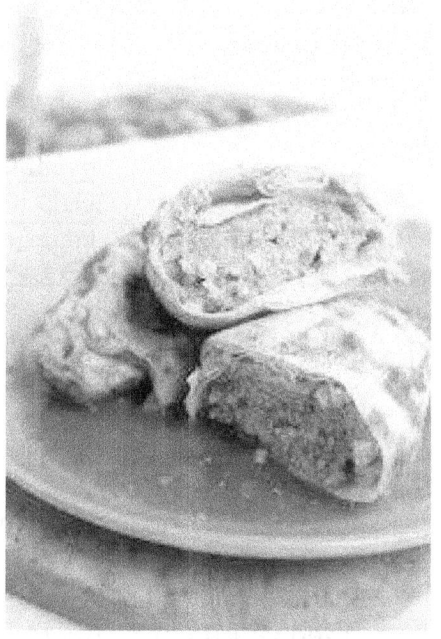

Instructions:
1. Stick your cut pork shoulder or butt into your crock pot with the diced onion, salt and pepper, and 1 cup water
2. Cook on low for about 6-8 hours. One hour before the meat is done, take out and shred with 2 forks. Return to crock pot and add in finely chopped carrot, paprika and Italian seasoning.
3. Blanch your cabbage leaves by steaming them for approx. 3 minutes then sticking them in freezing water or an ice bath.
4. Take your meat and place it on your leaf. Roll it up and put it in a baking dish, seam side down.
5. Pour a little of the juice from the crockpot into the bottom of the baking dish and stick in a 375° oven for 8-10 min.
6. While the rolls are cooking, make your sauce by adding in tomato paste, unsweetened almond milk, Italian seasoning, and broth from the crockpot. Stir and simmer until the rolls are done.
7. Top the rolls with the sauce and garnish with fresh parsley.

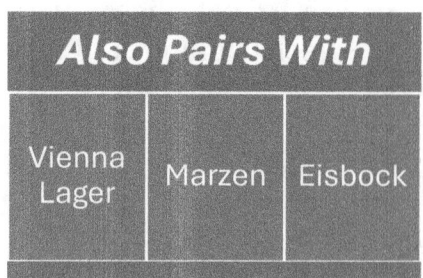

Also Pairs With

| Vienna Lager | Marzen | Eisbock |

German Pilsner

German Pilsners are golden-colored and exhibit excellent head retention. Expect a floral hop aroma. These beers are bitter, with a moderately malty backbone. Hop Bitterness: Perception of hop bitterness is medium to high. Noble type hop aroma and flavor are moderate and obvious. German Pilsners are distinctly different from Bohemian-style pilsners. They are lighter in color and body and have a lower perceived hop bitterness.

German Pilsner: Key Characteristics		Notable German Pilsner
Attribute	Description	Prima Pils
ABV	4.6–5.3% — moderate strength; ideal for session drinking	Bitburger Premium Pils
IBU (Bitterness)	25–50 — medium to high; clean, lingering bitterness	Rothaus Tannenzäpfle Pils
Color (SRM)	3–4 SRM — pale straw to light gold; brilliant clarity	Jever Pilsener
Body	Low to medium-low — crisp and dry	Warsteiner Premium Verum
Carbonation	Medium to high — enhances mouthfeel and aroma	Krombacher Pils
Finish	Dry to medium-dry — with a clean, bitter aftertaste	Beck's Pilsner

Taste: Bready | Floral | Herbal | Spicy | Crisp | Dry
Food Pairings: Grille Fish | Roast Chicken | Thai or Vietnamese | Indian Food | Mexican

Food Pairing Guide for German Pilsners

German Pilsner—often simply called "Pils"—is a crisp, hop-forward lager that highlights precision, balance, and refreshment.

Cheese Pairings
- Emmental or Gruyère: Nutty and mellow—echoes malt sweetness
- Fresh Goat Cheese or Feta: Tangy and salty—lifted by carbonation
- Camembert or Brie: Creamy and soft—balanced by crisp bitterness

Meat & Savory Dishes
- Bratwurst or Weisswurst: Classic Bavarian pairing—herbs and hops in harmony
- Roast Chicken or Pork Schnitzel: Crispy and savory—cut by carbonation
- Grilled Fish or Seafood Skewers: Light and briny—enhanced by pilsner's snap

Spicy & Global Cuisine
- Thai Basil Chicken or Vietnamese Spring Rolls: Bright herbs and spice cooled by crisp lager
- Indian Pakoras or Butter Chicken: Creamy and spiced—lifted by carbonation
- Mexican Street Tacos or Elote: Salt, spice, and char—perfect with pilsner's dry finish

Vegetables & Sides
- Grilled Asparagus or Zucchini: Earthy and fresh—echoes hop character
- German Potato Salad or Spaetzle: Rich and starchy—balanced by dry finish
- Pickled Veggies or Sauerkraut: Tangy and sharp—softened by malt

Desserts
- Apple Strudel or Pear Tart: Fruity and flaky—great with malt sweetness
- Shortbread Cookies or Almond Cake: Buttery and simple—echoes biscuit notes
- Pretzels with Caramel Dip: Sweet-salty contrast that pops

Carne Asada Street Tacos

Carne asada is grilled beef, often marinated with citrus, garlic, and spices, then seared to perfection. German pilsners have a snappy bitterness from noble hops that cuts through the smoky richness and stresses the seasoning. Street tacos are typically topped with onions, cilantro, lime, and salsa. The beer's herbal and floral hop notes echo the fresh herbs and citrus, creating a flavor bridge that ties everything together. If your tacos include spicy salsa or jalapenos, the pilsner's high carbonation and dry finish help cool the heat and refresh the palate between bites.

Ingredients:
2 Tbsp. vegetable oil
3 lbs. flank steak, or you can use skirt steak
1 onion chopped
2 fresh limes plus extra for toppings
1 bundle of cilantro
1 tsp. salt
1 tsp. pepper
½ stick butter
16 mini corn tortillas
Couple handfuls of cabbage

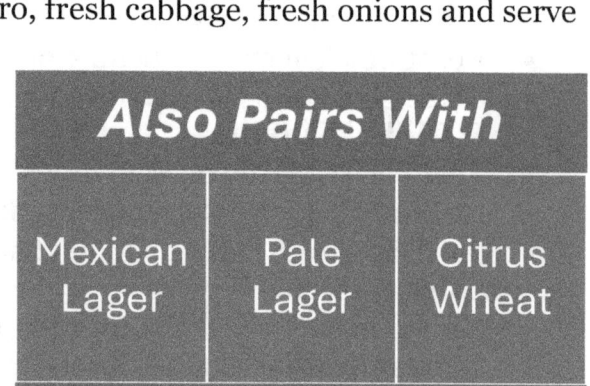

Instructions:
1. Thinly slice the steak. Then chop into bite site pieces. In a skillet, brown the steak in the oil. Add half the onions to the skillet and cook until soft. Save the rest of the onions.
2. Meanwhile, season with salt and pepper. Squeeze the juice of two fresh limes over the meat and onion mixture. Continue cooking until the meat is cooked through.
3. While the steak is cooking, melt the butter in another skillet or I used an electric skillet.
4. Fry the mini corn tortillas in the melted butter for 1 minute until they are soft. Allow them to cool slightly. You will need 2 mini corn tortillas per taco.
5. Spoon the meat mixture onto the tortillas. Top with cilantro, fresh cabbage, fresh onions and serve with lime.

Easy Refried Beans
1 (15 oz) can pinto beans (or black beans), drained and rinsed
2 Tbsp. olive oil or butter
2 cloves garlic, minced
¼ cup finely chopped onion
½ tsp. ground cumin
¼ tsp. chili powder
Salt to taste
¼ cup water, vegetable broth, or bean liquid

Also Pairs With		
Mexican Lager	Pale Lager	Citrus Wheat

In a skillet over medium heat, warm oil or butter. Add garlic (and onion if using) and sauté until fragrant and soft—about 2 minutes. Stir in the beans, cumin, chili powder, and a pinch of salt. Cook for 2–3 minutes to warm through. Add water or broth and mash beans with a potato masher or fork until it is mostly smooth, leaving some texture. Simmer for 5–7 minutes, stirring often, until thickened to your liking. Put some in your taco or eat on the side.

American Lager

American lager is a beer style that was initially modeled on the European pale lager. American lagers are characterized by lighter bodies, little to no bitterness, and low ABV. Contrary to their German styles which uses only barley, American lager uses wheat and rye, making it easier to drink. Offers the perfect contrast to Thai, Pan-Asian, Latino Fusion, Mexican, Peruvian, and other spicy cuisines. Pairs with extremely sweet or spicy barbecue.

American Lager: Key Characteristics		Notable American Lagers
Attribute	**Description**	Foster's Lager
ABV	4.2–5.3% — low to moderate; ideal for casual sipping2	Samuel Adams Boston Lager
IBU (Bitterness)	8–18 — very low; just enough to balance sweetness2	Brooklyn Lager
Color (SRM)	2–4 SRM — pale straw to light gold; crystal clear2	Sierra Nevada Summerfest
Body	Low to medium-low — light and crisp	Narragansett Lager
Carbonation	High — adds sprightliness and a refreshing bite	California Lounge Chair
Finish	Dry and clean — no lingering malt or hop flavors	Money Cat

Taste: Crisp | Clean | Balanced | Cracker Notes | Floral | Herbal | Light Body
Food Pairings: Hot Dogs | Burgers | Fried Chicken | Grilled Corn | Spicy Wings

Food Pairing Guide for American Lager
American Lager is the quintessential easy-drinking beer—light, crisp, and designed for mass appeal.

Cheese Pairings
- American Cheese or Mild Cheddar: Classic combo—simple and creamy
- Monterey Jack or Colby: Soft and buttery—balanced by crispness
- Queso Dip or Cheese Curds: Salty and rich—cut by carbonation

Meat & Savory Dishes
- Hot Dogs or Burgers: Backyard staples—lager refreshes and complements
- BBQ Pulled Pork or Ribs: Sweet and smoky—lager cools and balances
- Fried Chicken or Chicken Wings: Crunchy and fatty—cut by carbonation

Spicy & Global Cuisine
- Buffalo Wings or Jalapeno Poppers: Heat and salt cooled by crisp lager
- Tacos or Nachos: Bold flavors softened by clean finish
- Korean Fried Chicken or Thai Street Food: Sweet-spicy contrast that pops

Vegetables & Sides
- French Fries or Onion Rings: Salty and crispy—perfect with bubbles
- Coleslaw or Potato Salad: Creamy and tangy—balanced by dryness
- Grilled Corn or Baked Beans: Sweet and earthy—echoes malt notes

Desserts
- Apple Pie or Peach Cobbler: Fruity and flaky—great with subtle malt
- Vanilla Ice Cream or Root Beer Float: Creamy and nostalgic—lifted by carbonation
- Pretzels with Chocolate Dip: Sweet-salty contrast that sings

Grilled Chicken Caesar Salad

Pairing a Grilled Chicken Caesar Salad with an American Lager is all about balance, refreshment, and subtle enhancement. Creamy Caesar dressing has bold flavors—garlic, anchovy, Parmesan, and lemon—that can overwhelm delicate beers. But American lagers are crisp and clean, offering a refreshing contrast without competing. Grilled chicken adds a smoky, savory layer. The mild malt backbone of a lager complements this without adding heaviness. Romaine lettuce and croutons bring crunch and texture. The carbonation in the lager helps cleanse the palate between bites, keeping each forkful fresh.

Ingredients:
For the Grilled Chicken Marinade
½ of a lemon, juiced
2 Tbsp. olive oil
1 Tbsp. Dijon mustard
1 tsp. minced garlic
1 Tbsp. fresh minced rosemary or 1 tsp. dried
¾ tsp. kosher salt
freshly ground black pepper to taste
1-pound boneless, skinless chicken breasts

For the Caesar Salad
1 head romaine, chopped
½ cup shredded Parmesan
freshly ground black pepper, to taste
1 cup Caesar Salad Dressing, or more as needed
Garlic croutons

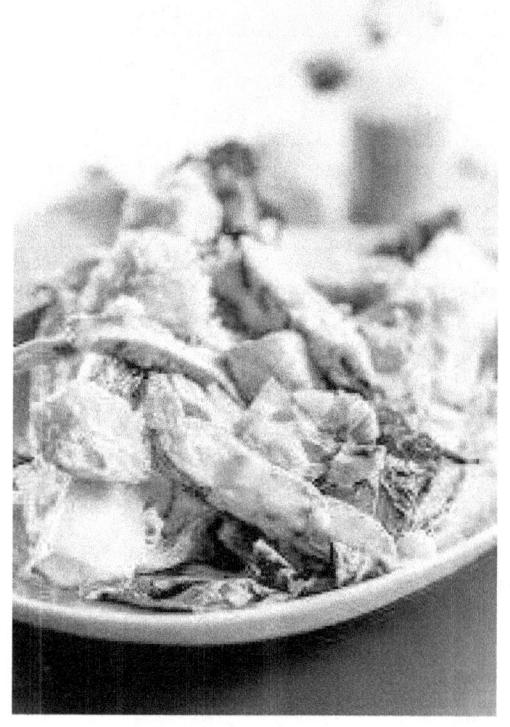

Instructions:
Grilled Chicken
1. Combine the lemon juice, olive oil, Dijon, garlic, rosemary, salt, and pepper in a small bowl. Whisk it well to combine.
2. Place the chicken in a zippered plastic storage bag. Pour the marinade over the top. Press out as much air as you can and seal the bag. Use your hands to move the chicken around in the bag until it is well coated with marinade. Refrigerate for at least an hour or for up to 8 hours.
3. Grill the chicken on your outdoor or stovetop grill for 4 to 5 minutes per side until the internal temperature reads 165 degrees F when checked with an instant-read thermometer. If we use thicker pieces of chicken, the cooking time will increase.
4. Transfer grilled chicken to a cutting board and slice into small strips (3-inches). Set aside while you prepare the remaining ingredients.

Also Pairs With

Helles Lager	Belgian Witbier	Blonde Ale

Assemble the Salad
Chop romaine and toss with about half of the Caesar dressing and half of the shredded Parmesan. Season with pepper, to taste. Top with sliced chicken. Sprinkle with the remaining Parmesan. Top the salad with the Croutons and serve with remaining dressing on the side.

Dortmunder

Dortmunder beer is a pale, well-hopped lager that ranges in color from golden to light amber. It has aromas of sweet malt and a mild hop flavor. The beer offers a medium-bodied mouthfeel and a moderately dry finish. The Dortmunder lager was originally made for 19th-century German industrial workers. High levels of sulfate in the region's water gave the beer a distinct sulfur flavor that balanced with the bitterness from the hops. Named after its city of origin, Dortmund, this lager was never less than 5% ABV—light enough to quench a coal miner's thirst, yet hearty enough to reward a long day of manual labor.

Dortmunder Export: Key Characteristics		Notable Dortmunder
Attribute	**Description**	DAB Original
ABV	5.0–6.0% — slightly stronger than a Helles or Pils	Great Lakes Dortmunder Gold
IBU (Bitterness)	20–30 — moderate; clean and balanced bitterness	Ayinger Jahrhundert Bier
Color (SRM)	4–6 SRM — pale gold to deep straw; brilliant clarity	Berghoff DortWunder Lager
Body	Medium — fuller than a Pils, lighter than a Bock	Three Floyds Jinx Proof
Carbonation	Medium to high — crisp and refreshing	
Finish	Clean and smooth — with a subtle malt sweetness and dry hop edge	

Taste: Balanced | Biscuity | Earthy | Smooth | Slightly Sweer
Food Pairings: Pulled Pork | Sauerkraut Street Tacos | Spicy Foods|

Food Pairing Guide for Dortmunder
Dortmunder-style beer—also known as Dortmunder Export—is a classic German pale lager that strikes a perfect balance between malt richness and hop bitterness.

Cheese Pairings
- Aged Gouda or Gruyère: Nutty and rich—echoes malt depth
- Fontina or Havarti: Creamy and mild—balanced by carbonation
- Smoked Cheddar: Bold and savory—lifted by herbal hops

Meat & Savory Dishes
- Grilled Bratwurst or Kielbasa: Smoky and spiced—perfect with malt and hops
- Roast Chicken or Pork Loin: Savory and juicy—balanced by a dry finish
- Pulled Pork Cabbage Rolls: Earthy and tangy—complemented by malt sweetness

Vegetables & Sides
- German Potato Salad or Spaetzle: Rich and starchy—cut by carbonation
- Grilled Mushrooms or Asparagus: Umami and herbal—mirrors hop character
- Braised Cabbage or Sauerkraut: Tangy and earthy—softened by malt

Spicy & Global Cuisine
- Thai Basil Chicken or Vietnamese Bánh Mi: Bright herbs and spice cooled by crisp lager
- Mexican Street Tacos or Elote: Salt, spice, and char—balanced by malt and hops
- Indian Butter Chicken or Samosas: Creamy and spiced—lifted by carbonation

Desserts
- Apple Strudel or Pear Tart: Fruity and flaky—echoes malt sweetness
- Shortbread Cookies or Almond Cake: Buttery and simple—pairs with biscuit notes
- Pretzels with Caramel Dip

Smoked Pork Tenderloin

Smoked pork tenderloin has a deep, savory flavor with hints of char and wood. Dortmunder lagers offer a bready, honeyed malt profile that echoes the caramelized edges of the pork and adds a touch of sweetness to balance the smoke. Pork tenderloin is lean and tender, so it benefits from a beer that's not too heavy. Dortmunder's medium body and dry finish keep the pairing light and refreshing, enhancing the meat's texture without adding weight. If the pork is seasoned with garlic, rosemary, or pepper, the beer's herbal hop character creates a flavor bridge, tying the dish and drinking together. The moderate bitterness in Dortmunder helps cut through the smoky richness, cleansing the palate and preparing you for the next bite.

Ingredients:
2 1-pound pork tenderloins
3 Tbsp. Favorite Rub
½ cup Favorite BBQ Sauce (Fruity, Boozy Sauces Rock)

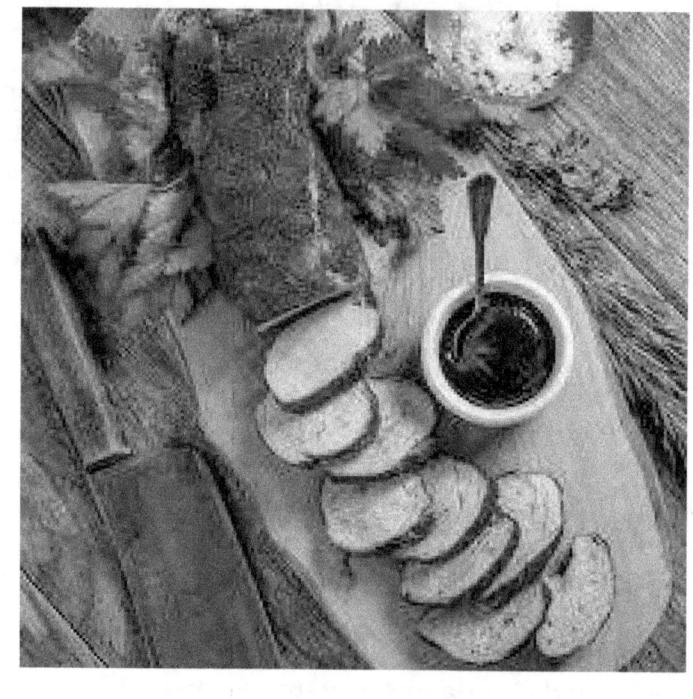

Instructions:
1. Remove your pork tenderloins from the package and use a sharp knife to remove any excess fat and silver skin.
2. Preheat your smoker to 225 degrees F.
3. Season the tenderloins on all sides with the sweet rub. Place the tenderloins on the grill, close the lid, and smoke until the internal temperature of the tenderloins reaches 135 degrees F.
4. Baste on all sides with BBQ Sauce. Cook until the internal temperature of the tenderloin reaches 145 degrees F, and the sauce tightens up.
5. Remove the pork tenderloin from the grill. Slice against the grain into 1/2-inch medallions. Serve immediately.

Gingered Cranberry Sauce
12 oz fresh or frozen cranberries
¾ cup sugar
½ cup water
¼ cup orange juice or apple cider
1–2 tsp. fresh grated ginger
Zest of 1 orange
Pinch of salt

Also Pairs With

Vienna Lager	Cider Ale	Belgian Dubbel

In a medium saucepan, combine water, orange juice, sugar, ginger, and salt. Bring to boil. Stir in the cranberries and reduce the heat to medium. Simmer for 10–15 minutes, stirring occasionally, until berries burst and sauce thickens. Stir in orange zest if using. Taste and adjust sweetness or ginger level. Let cool to room temperature—sauce will thicken as it cools. Serve warm or refrigerate until ready to use. Keeps well for up to a week.

California Common- Steam Beer

The California Common, also known as Steam Beer, is brewed with lager yeast but fermented at ale fermentation temperatures. This method dates to the late 1800s in California, when refrigeration was a great luxury. Brewers had to improvise to cool the beer down, so shallow fermenters were used. In a way, the lager yeast was trained to ferment quicker at warmer temperatures. Some mild fruitiness along with an herbal yet assertive hop bitterness is also typical.

California Common: Key Characteristics		Notable Steam Beer
Attribute	**Description**	Anchor Steam Beer
ABV	4.5–5.5% — moderate strength; highly sessionable	Steam Donkey
IBU (Bitterness)	30–45 — firm bitterness; clean and lingering	California Commo
Color (SRM)	10–14 SRM — medium amber to light copper; clear	Common Sense
Body	Medium — smooth and grainy with a dry edge	Steam Punk
Carbonation	Medium to medium-high — supports crispness and aroma	California Dreamin'
Finish	Fairly dry and crisp — with lingering hop bitterness and grainy malt flavor	

Taste: Caramel | Earthy | Toffee | Woody | Clean | Fruity
Food Pairings: BBQ Chicken| | Pork chops | Grilled foods | Smoked Foods | Roasted Veggies

Food Pairing Guide for California Common Steam Beer California Common is a uniquely American hybrid style that blends lager yeast with ale fermentation temperatures, creating a beer that's toasty, balanced, and full of rustic charm.

Cheese Pairings
- Smoked Gouda or Aged Cheddar: Rich and sharp—echoes malt depth
- Fontina or Havarti: Creamy and mild—balanced by bitterness
- Blue Cheese or Gorgonzola: Bold and funky—tempered by earthy hops

Meat & Savory Dishes
- Grilled Tri-Tip or Flank Steak: Charred and juicy—perfect with toasty malt
- BBQ Pulled Pork or Brisket: Sweet and smoky—balanced by hop bitterness
- Roast Chicken or Duck: Savory and rich—lifted by dry finish

Vegetables & Sides
- Roasted Root Veggies or Mushrooms: Earthy and caramelized—mirrors malt character
- Grilled Corn or Zucchini: Sweet and smoky—echoes toasty notes
- Baked Beans or Mac & Cheese: Rich and hearty—cut by carbonation

Spicy & Global Cuisine
- Korean BBQ or Bulgogi: Sweet heat and char—balanced by malt and hops
- Carnitas Tacos or Enchiladas: Bold and savory—lifted by dry finish
- Indian Butter Chicken or Rogan Josh: Creamy and spiced—tempered by bitterness

Desserts
- Apple Crisp or Bread Pudding: Toasty and fruity—echoes malt and esters
- Caramel Flan or Butterscotch Bars: Sweet and creamy—balanced by earthy hops
- Chocolate Chip Cookies or Brownies: Rich and chewy—cut by carbonation

Santa Maria Grilled Tri-Tip Beef

Tri-tip is grilled over red oak, giving it a smoky, caramelized crust. California Common has a toasty, biscuit-like malt backbone that echoes the char and enhances the meat's savory depth. The traditional rub includes garlic, black pepper, salt, and sometimes rosemary or paprika. Steam beer's Northern Brewer hops offer woody, earthy bitterness that mirrors the spice and adds a subtle contrast. Tri-tip is juicy and beefy, with a medium-fat content that benefits from a beer that cleanses the palate. California Common's dry finish and moderate carbonation keep the pairing light and refreshing, even with bold flavors.

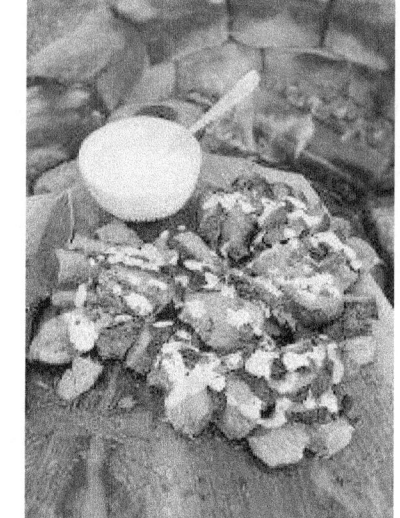

Ingredients:
2 tsp. each salt, freshly ground black pepper
2 tsp. garlic powder
1 ½ tsp. paprika
1 tsp. onion powder
1 tsp. dried rosemary
¼ tsp. cayenne pepper
1 (2 1/2 pound) beef tri-tip roast
⅓ cup red wine vinegar
⅓ cup vegetable oil
4 cloves crushed garlic
½ tsp. Dijon mustard

Instructions:
1. Stir salt, black pepper, garlic powder, paprika, onion powder, rosemary, and cayenne pepper together in a bowl.
2. Place the tri-tip in a glass baking dish and coat on all sides with the spice mixture. Cover the dish with plastic wrap and refrigerate for 4 hours.
3. Combine vinegar, vegetable oil, crushed garlic, and Dijon mustard in a sealable container. Cover the container and shake until the ingredients are blended.
4. Remove the tri-tip from the refrigerator. Let it sit uncovered at room temperature for 30 minutes.
5. Preheat an outdoor grill for high heat; lightly oil the grates.
6. Place the tri-tip on the preheated grill and brush with the vinegar mixture. Cook for 4 minutes, flip, and baste. Flip and baste every 4 minutes until the tri-tip firms up and is reddish-pink and juicy in the center, 25 to 30 minutes total. An instant-read thermometer inserted into the center should read 130° F.

Avocado Crema
1 ripe avocado
½ cup sour cream or Greek yogurt
1 Tbsp. fresh lime juice
1 small garlic clove (minced or grated)
Salt to taste

Also Pairs With		
West Coast IPA	Scotch Ale	Hoppy Pale Ale

Blend all ingredients in a food processor or blender until smooth and creamy. Add more lime for tang, salt for balance, or sour cream for silkiness. Chill for 15–30 minutes to let the flavors meld.

Dark Lagers

Dark lagers are a rich and versatile beer style that combines the smooth drinkability of lagers with the deep, roasted flavors of darker malts. Here's a quick guide to their key characteristics and ideal food pairings:

Dark Lager Characteristics
- **Color:** Deep amber to dark brown, sometimes black
- **Flavor Profile:** Toasted bread, caramel, cocoa, coffee, and subtle nuttiness, Low to moderate bitterness, Clean finish typical of lagers, without the fruity esters found in ales
- **Body:** Medium, with smooth carbonation
- **Aroma:** Roasted malt, mild chocolate, and hints of dark bread or cookie dough
- **ABV:** Typically ranges from 4.5% to 6%, depending on the style (e.g., Dunkel, Schwarzbier, Czech Dark Lager)

Dark Lager by Region

Region	Style	Flavor Profile	Notable Examples
Germany	Dunkel, Schwarzbier	Dunkel: malty, bready, caramel; Schwarzbier: crisp, roasty, subtle chocolate	Ayinger Altbairisch Dunkel, Köstritzer Schwarzbier2
Czech Republic	Czech Dark Lager (Tmavé)	Smooth, rich malt, mild roast, balanced bitterness	Bohemia Regent Dark, U Fleků Tmavý Ležák
United States	American Dark Lager	Clean, mild roast, sometimes adjuncts like corn	Yuengling Dark Lager, craft variants
Mexico	Mexican Dark Lager	Light-bodied, mild caramel, smooth finish	Negra Modelo, Victoria
Austria	Dunkle Lager	Toasty, nutty, slightly sweet	

Food Pairing Tips for Dark Lagers
- Match with Roasted and Grilled Meats
- Complement Earthy and Spiced Dishes
- Echo with Chocolate and Caramel Desserts

Food Pairings Tips for Dark Lager

Dish	Why It Works
Grilled Meats (steak, pork ribs)	The charred edges match the beer's roasted malt notes
Bratwurst with caramelized onions	Classic German pairing—malty beer complements savory sausage
Shepherd's Pie or Meatloaf	Comfort food meets comforting beer; rich flavors balance beautifully
Mushroom Stroganoff or Fried Rice	Earthy mushrooms echo the beer's nutty, toasted profile
BBQ Burritos or Tacos with Black Beans	Smoky and spicy elements play well with the beer's depth
Dark Chocolate Desserts	Cocoa notes in the beer enhance chocolate-based sweets like brownies or mousse

Dark Lager

These beers have toasty, nutty, or lightly roasted malt flavor that compliments the similar flavors produced by your grill or smoker. They also often have a hint of caramel flavor that will bring a little sweetness to the mix. This type of combination will allow your beer to pair with any type of meat. try to go with one that falls in the 5 to 6% ABV range so it does not fall short or overpower your food. Dark lager works wonderfully with a variety of seafood, especially salmon.

Dark Lager: Key Characteristics		Notable Dark Lager
Attribute	Description	New Belgium 1554 Dark Ale
ABV	4.5–6.0% — moderate strength; varies by substyle	Jack's Abby Copper Legend
IBU (Bitterness)	18–30 — low to moderate; bitterness is clean and balanced	Heineken Dark
Color (SRM)	18–30 SRM — deep amber to dark brown; often clear with ruby highlights	Spaten Oktoberfest
Body	Medium — smooth and rounded	Hofbrau Oktoberfestbier
Carbonation	Medium to high — enhances drinkability	Great Lakes Eliot Ness
Finish	Clean and dry to slightly sweet — depends on malt and yeast profile	

Taste: Malty | Roasty | Sweet | Earthy | Chocolate | Nutty | Some Bitterness
Food Pairings: Roast Beef or Pork | BBQ Ribs | Smoked Chicken | Mac & Cheese | Root Veggies

Food Pairing Guide For Dark Lager
Dark Lager is a beautifully balanced style that combines the clean, crisp profile of a lager with the rich, toasty flavors of darker malts.

Cheese Pairings
- Smoked Gouda or Aged Cheddar: Bold and nutty—echoes malt depth
- Gruyère or Fontina: Creamy and mellow—balanced by roastiness
- Blue Cheese or Gorgonzola: Funky and sharp—tempered by malt sweetness

Meat & Savory Dishes
- Grilled Sausages or Bratwurst: Smoky and spiced—perfect with toasty malt
- Roast Beef or Pork Shoulder: Rich and savory—lifted by a clean finish
- BBQ Ribs or Smoked Chicken: Sweet and smoky—balanced by subtle bitterness

Vegetables & Sides
- Roasted Root Veggies or Mushrooms: Earthy and caramelized—mirrors malt character
- Braised Cabbage or Sauerkraut: Tangy and rich—softened by malt
- Mac & Cheese or Potato Gratin: Creamy and hearty—cut by carbonation

Spicy & Global Cuisine
- Korean Bulgogi or BBQ: Sweet heat and char—balanced by roast and fizz
- Carnitas Tacos or Mole Sauce: Deep flavors and spice—echoed by malt complexity
- Indian Rogan Josh or Dal Makhani: Spiced and creamy—lifted by dry finish

Desserts
- Chocolate Cake or Brownies: Rich and fudgy—mirrored by cocoa notes
- Bread Pudding or Sticky Toffee: Toasty and sweet—echoes caramel malt
- Nutty Tarts or Pecan Pie: Sweet and earthy—perfect with a nutty roast

Savory Smoked Sausage and Potatoes

Smoked sausage brings bold, meaty flavors with hints of spice and char. Dark lagers—like Munich Dunkel or Schwarzbier—offer toasty, bready malt notes that echo the caramelized edges of the sausage and enhance its richness. Roasted or pan-fried potatoes have a starchy, earthy base and often pick up crispy, golden bits. The beer's subtle cocoa, coffee, or nutty undertones complement the potatoes' texture and flavor, adding depth without heaviness. Sausage is fatty and juicy, and potatoes can be buttery or oily. Dark lagers have moderate carbonation and a clean finish, which cut through the richness and refresh the palate between bites. If the sausage includes pepper, garlic, or paprika, the beer's low-to-moderate bitterness and herbal hop notes provide a gentle contrast that keeps the flavors lively.

Ingredients:
1 small onion, finely diced
1 carrot, finely diced
1 lb. smoked beef sausage
6 medium potatoes, peeled and cubed
1 Tbsp olive oil
3 c reduced-sodium chicken broth
1/4 tsp garlic powder
1/4 tsp celery seed
2 Tbsp parsley flakes
3/4 tsp salt
1/4 tsp black pepper
1/3 c all-purpose flour

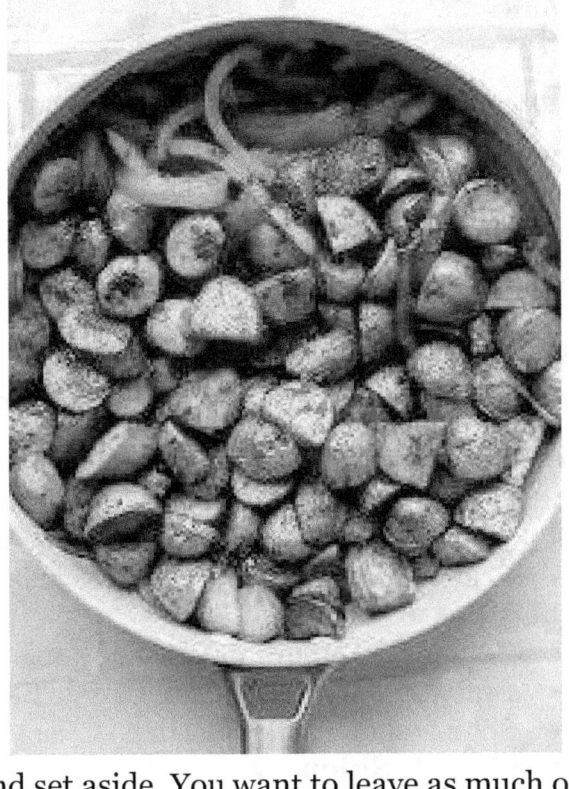

Instructions:
1. Preheat oven to 350°F. Finely dice the onion and carrot and set aside. You can use a food processor for this.
2. Cut sausage about 1/2 inch - 3/4-inch slices. Set aside. Peel and cube the potatoes. Set aside.
3. Heat a large oven-safe pot. Add olive oil and brown the sausage.
4. Remove the sausage from the pot with a slotted spoon and set aside. You want to leave as much oil as possible in the pot.
5. Add the diced carrot and onion to the pot and cook for just a minute.
6. Add the sausage back.
7. Add the potatoes.
8. Add the garlic powder, celery seed, parsley, salt, and pepper. Give it a good mix.
9. Then add the flour and mix well.

Also Pairs With

Munich	Dunkelweizen	Belgian Pale Ale

Helles

Helles is a malt accented lager beer that balances a pleasant malt sweetness and body with floral Noble hops and restrained bitterness. The German word hell can be translated as "bright", "light", or "pale". Malty flavors go well with beer, seafood, pork, brats, slow roasted meats, and sauced chicken.

Helles Lager: Key Characteristics		Notable Helles
Attribute	**Description**	Spaten Lager
ABV	4.7–5.4% — moderate strength; ideal for session drinking	Weihenstephaner Original
IBU (Bitterness)	16–22 — low to moderate; bitterness is clean and restrained	Spaten Premium Lager
Color (SRM)	3–5 SRM — pale gold to bright straw; brilliant clarity	Hacker-Pschorr Münchner Gold
Body	Medium-light to medium — smooth and rounded	Paulaner Original
Carbonation	Medium — supports crispness without sharpness	Ayinger Lager Hell
Finish	Clean and slightly malty — with a soft, dry edge that invites another sip	

Taste: Malty | Bready | Balanced | Med Body | Low Bitterness | Sessionable
Food Pairings: Seafood | Salads | Grilled items | Roast Chicken | German Potato Salad

Food Pairing Guide for Helles
Helles is a classic German lager style that embodies balance, subtlety, and drinkability.

Cheese Pairings
- Emmental or Havarti: Mild and creamy—echoes malt sweetness
- Young Gouda or Fontina: Buttery and smooth—balanced by carbonation
- Brie with Apple Slices: Soft and fruity—lifted by a crisp finish

Meat & Savory Dishes
- Roast Chicken or Pork Loin: Simple and savory—perfect with malt depth
- Bratwurst or Weisswurst: Classic Bavarian pairing—herbs and hops in harmony
- Schnitzel or Chicken Cutlets: Crispy and rich—cut by carbonation

Vegetables & Sides
- German Potato Salad or Spaetzle: Starchy and hearty—balanced by dry finish
- Grilled Asparagus or Zucchini: Earthy and fresh—mirrors hop character
- Braised Cabbage or Sauerkraut: Tangy and rich—softened by malt

Spicy & Global Cuisine
- Thai Basil Chicken or Pad See Ew: Sweet-savory heat cooled by lager
- Tacos al Pastor or Carnitas: Pork and spice balanced by malt and fizz
- Indian Butter Chicken or Samosas: Creamy and spiced—lifted by carbonation

Desserts
- Apple Strudel or Pear Tart: Fruity and flaky—echoes malt sweetness
- Shortbread Cookies or Pound Cake: Buttery and simple—pairs with biscuit notes
- Pretzels with Chocolate Dip: Sweet-salty contrast that pops

Chicken Sausage and Vegetable Foil Packet Dinner

Chicken sausage is lighter and less fatty than pork, often seasoned with herbs, garlic, or fennel. Helles lagers have a bready, honeyed malt backbone that complements the mild savoriness of the sausage without overpowering it. Roasted or sautéed vegetables—like zucchini, bell peppers, or onions—bring earthy, sweet, and slightly caramelized notes. The beer's clean, crisp finish and moderate carbonation help lift and refresh these flavors, keeping the dish light and vibrant. If the sausage or veggies include thyme, rosemary, or pepper, the Helles's gentle floral or herbal hop character creates a flavor bridge, enhancing the aromatic elements of the dish.

Ingredients:
1 4 pack al fresco all-natural sundried tomato chicken sausage, thinly sliced
1-pound green beans, trimmed
1 red pepper, cored and thinly sliced
1 yellow bell pepper, cored and thinly sliced
1 small red onion
3 Tbsp. olive oil
2 cloves garlic, grated
1 Tbsp. fresh thyme leaves
1 tsp. dried oregano
1 tsp. dried basil
1 tsp. kosher salt
1 small zucchini, trimmed, cut lengthwise and cut into half-moons
1 small yellow summer squashed, trimmed, cut lengthwise and cut into half-moons
1 tsp. crushed red pepper flakes, optional

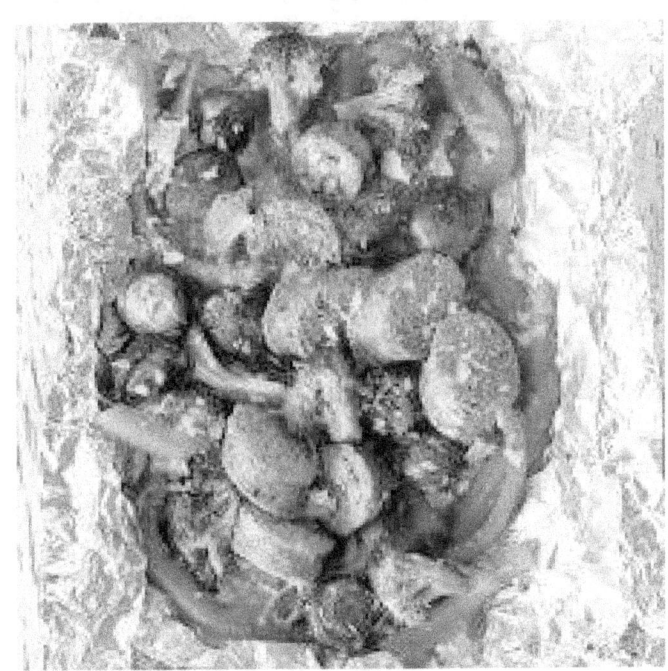

Instructions:
1. Preheat your grill to medium-high heat.
2. In a large bowl, add all ingredients and toss to combine and equally coat in oil and seasoning.
3. Lay out 4 16-inch-long pieces of foil and divide the mixture equally and put into the middle of each piece of foil. Wrap up the foil so that there are no holes. If you have super thin foil or there is too much to adequately close the pouch, tear off another piece of foil and double-wrap your packet.
4. If cooking on the grill, add the packets to the grill and cook for about 20 minutes, flipping the packet halfway through cooking. Remove one packet and check to see if the vegetables are cooked to your desired doneness. If not, continue cooking until you reach your desired level of vegetable doneness.
5. If cooking in the oven, add your packets to a large baking sheet and cook at 425 degrees for about 20 minutes or until everything is fully cooked in the packet.

Also Pairs With

| Cream Ale | Gose | English Ale |

German Pilsner

On the heavier end for lagers, German Lagers feature bready, caramelly, or toasty flavors with dark malts that cut through the fat of the meat and complement flavors nicely. Natural for any type of sausage, smoked or grilled.

German Lager: Key Characteristics		Notable German Lagers
Attribute	**Description**	St Pauli Girl
Fermentation	Cold fermentation with Saccharomyces Pastorious (lager yeast)	Weihenstephaner Original
Maturation	Lagered (stored cold) for weeks to months for smoothness and clarity	Bitburger Premium Pils
ABV Range	Typically, 4.5–6.5%, depending on substyle	Augustiner Bräustuben Helles
IBU Range	16–50+ — bitterness varies widely by style	Spaten Oktoberfestbier
Color Range	2–30 SRM — pale straw to deep brown	
Body	Light to full — varies by malt bill and style	
Finish	Always clean — can be dry, malty, or bitter depending on the variant	

Taste: Crisp | Floral | Grassy | Biscuity | Malt-Forward
Food Pairings: Brats | Roast Chicken | Fish & Chips | Tri-tip | Duck

Food Pairing Guide for German Pilsner
German Lager isn't just one style—it's a family of precision-brewed beers that range from pale and crisp to dark and malty.

Cheese Pairings
- Emmental or Gruyère: Nutty and mellow—balanced by hop bitterness
- Goat Cheese or Feta: Tangy and salty—lifted by crisp carbonation
- Camembert or Brie: Creamy and soft—cut by dry finish

Meat & Savory Dishes
- Bratwurst or Weisswurst: Classic Bavarian pairing—herbs and hops in harmony
- Roast Chicken or Schnitzel: Crispy and savory—cut by carbonation
- Grilled Fish or Seafood Skewers: Light and briny—enhanced by pilsner's snap

Vegetables & Sides
- Grilled Asparagus or Zucchini: Earthy and fresh—mirrors hop character
- German Potato Salad or Spaetzle: Rich and starchy—balanced by dry finish
- Pickled Veggies or Sauerkraut: Tangy and sharp—softened by malt

Spicy & Global Cuisine
- Thai Basil Chicken or Vietnamese Spring Rolls: Bright herbs and spice cooled by crisp lager
- Indian Pakoras or Butter Chicken: Creamy and spiced—lifted by carbonation
- Mexican Street Tacos or Elote: Salt, spice, and char—perfect with pilsner's dry finish

Desserts
- Apple Strudel or Pear Tart: Fruity and flaky—great with malt sweetness
- Shortbread Cookies or Almond Cake: Buttery and simple—echoes biscuit notes
- Pretzels with Caramel Dip: Sweet-salty contrast that pops

Flat Iron Steak

Flat iron steak is well-marbled and flavorful, often grilled to develop a caramelized crust. German pilsners—known for their noble hop bitterness—cut through the umami and char, keeping the palate fresh and lively. The steak is often seasoned with salt, pepper, garlic, or herbs. Pilsners brewed with Hallertau or Tettnang hops offer floral and herbal notes that mirror and enhance the seasoning. Flat iron steak has a juicy, tender texture that can feel heavy. German pilsners have a light body and dry finish, which cleanses the palate and prepares you for the next bite.

Ingredients:
1 (2 pound) flat iron steak
2 ½ Tbsp. olive oil
2 cloves garlic, minced
1 tsp. chopped fresh parsley
¼ tsp. chopped fresh rosemary
½ tsp. chopped fresh chives
¼ cup Cabernet Sauvignon (or other dry red wine)
½ tsp. salt
¾ tsp. ground black pepper
¼ tsp. dry mustard powder

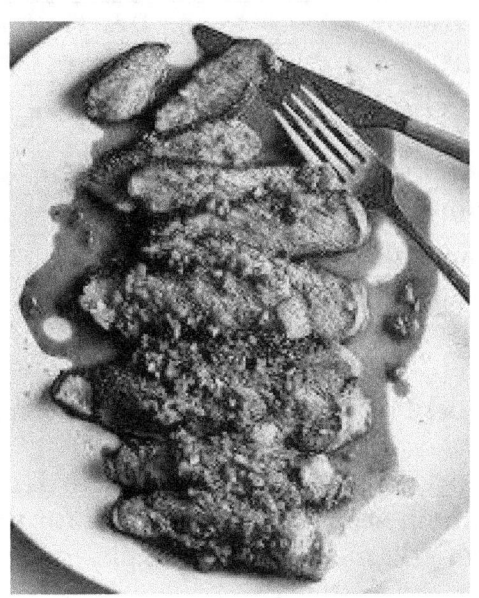

Instructions:
1. Place the steak inside a large resealable bag. Stir olive oil, garlic, parsley, rosemary, chives, red wine, salt, pepper, and mustard powder together in a small bowl.
2. Pour the marinade over the steak in the bag. Press out as much air as you can and seal the bag. Marinate in the refrigerator for 2 to 3 hours.
3. Heat a nonstick skillet over medium-high heat. Place the steak in the hot skillet and discard any remaining marinade; sear and cook the steak for 3 to 4 minutes on each side for medium rare, or to your desired doneness. An instant-read thermometer inserted into the center should read 130°F for medium rare. Allow me to rest for about 5 minutes.

Red Wine Sauce for Steak
1 Tbsp. olive oil or butter
1 small shallot, finely minced
1 clove garlic, minced
¾ cup dry red wine (Cabernet, Merlot, or Pinot Noir)
½ cup beef broth
1 tsp. fresh thyme
1 Tbsp. cold butter (for finishing)
Salt and black pepper to taste

Also Pairs With

Robust Porter	American Brown Ale	Black IPA

In a skillet over medium heat, warm olive oil or butter. Add shallots and garlic, cooking until soft and fragrant (about 2–3 minutes). Pour in the red wine and scrape up any browned bits from the pan. Simmer for 3–5 minutes until reduced by half. Stir in the beef broth and thyme. Simmer another 5–7 minutes until sauce thickens slightly. Remove from the heat and whisk in cold butter for a glossy finish. Season with salt and pepper to taste.

Munich\Dunkel

Munich, with its 1,000 years of brewing tradition in Bavaria. Monks in monasteries were the first brewmasters, and churches used beer as an incentive for attendance. The famous Purity Law of 1516 ensured that beer could only be made from barley, hops, water, and yeast, guaranteeing high-quality brews.

Munich | Dunkel: Key Characteristics		Notable Munich's
Attribute	Description	Paulaner Munich Lager
ABV	5.8-6.3% moderate strength; sessionable yet satisfying	Spaten Premium Lager
IBU (Bitterness)	18–25 — low to moderate; bitterness is subtle and clean	Ayinger Altbairisch Dunkel
Color (SRM)	6–9 SRM — amber to deep reddish-brown; brilliant clarity	Hofbräu Dunkel
Body	Medium — smooth and rounded with a soft mouthfeel	Spaten Oktoberfestbier
Carbonation	Medium — supports drinkability without sharpness	Löwenbräu Original
Finish	Rich, toasty, slightly sweet, brewed for festivals	

Taste: Bready | Toast | Clean | Medium Body | Low Bitterness
Food Pairings: Stews | Game | Chocolate Desserts | Grilled Chicken | Roasted Pork

Food Pairing Guide for Munich Dunkel Beers

Munich-style beers are known for their malt-forward character, clean fermentation, and sessionable strength, making them staples in beer halls and festivals across Munich.

Cheese Pairings
- Smoked Gouda or Aged Cheddar: Bold and nutty—echoes malt depth
- Gruyère or Alpine-style: Creamy and earthy—balanced by roastiness
- Blue Cheese or Gorgonzola: Funky and sharp—tempered by malt sweetness

Meat & Savory Dishes
- Roast Pork or Beef: Rich and savory—lifted by clean finish
- Bratwurst or Kielbasa: Smoky and spiced—perfect with toasty malt
- Sauerbraten or Meatloaf: Deeply flavored and hearty—mirrored by malt complexity
- Pulled Pork Cabbage Rolls: Tangy and earthy—softened by caramel malt

Vegetables & Sides
- Braised Cabbage or Sauerkraut: Tangy and earthy—balanced by malt
- Roasted Root Vegetables or Mushrooms: Umami and caramelized—mirrors malt character
- German Potato Salad or Spaetzle: Starchy and comforting—cut by carbonation

Spicy & Global Cuisine
- Carnitas Tacos or Mole Sauce: Deep flavors and spice—enhanced by roast and fizz
- Indian Rogan Josh or Dal Makhani: Spiced and creamy—lifted by dry finish
- Korean BBQ or Bulgogi: Sweet heat and char—balanced by malt and hops

Desserts
- Chocolate Cake or Brownies: Rich and fudgy—mirrored by cocoa notes
- Bread Pudding or Sticky Toffee: Toasty and sweet—echoes caramel malt
- Nutty Tarts or Pecan Pie: Sweet and earthy—perfect with a nutty roast

Caramelized Pork Ribs

Pork ribs glazed with caramelized sauces (like honey, brown sugar, or molasses) develop deep, sweet-savory crusts. Munich Dunkel's bready, biscuit-like malt and hints of caramel and cocoa mirror those flavors, creating a seamless flavored bridge. If the ribs are smoked or spiced with garlic, paprika, or pepper, the beer's roasty undertones and gentle herbal hops add depth without overpowering. The beer's low bitterness lets the ribs shine while still providing contrast. Pork ribs are rich and fatty, especially when slow-cooked or grilled. Munich Dunkel's medium body and crisp carbonation help cut through the richness, keeping each bite satisfying and refreshing.

Ingredients:
1/2 Cup granulated sugar
1 cup of water
3 tbsp. fish sauce
1/4 cup finely chopped Lemongrass or lemongrass paste
6 cloves garlic
2 tbsp lime juice
1 tbsp minced fresh ginger root
1 tbsp packed brown sugar
1 tsp five-spice powder
4 lb. pork back ribs
1 tbsp peanut or vegetable oil

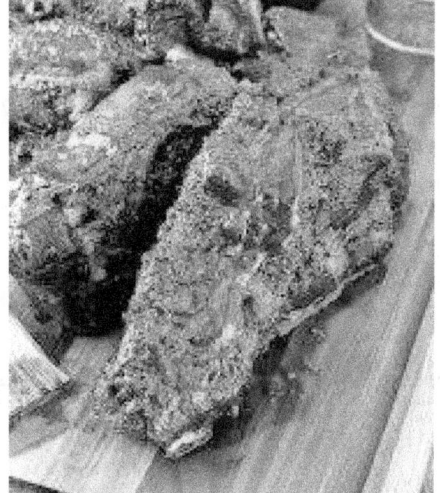

Instructions:
Caramel Sauce
1. In a medium, heavy-bottomed saucepan, over high heat, stir granulated sugar with 1/2 cup water until the sugar dissolves. Bring to a boil, reduce heat to medium and cool, without stirring, for about 10 minutes or until deep golden brown. Immediately remove from the heat. Caramel may darken still - don't worry, it can get quite dark.
2. Carefully pour in the rest of the water and fish sauce (mixture will bubble up). Return the pot to low heat and cook, stirring, to dissolve any hardened caramel.
3. Stir in lemongrass, garlic, lime juice, ginger, brown sugar, and five-spice powder. Simmer over low heat for 10 minutes to blend the flavors. (Sauce can be covered and chilled up to several days ahead).

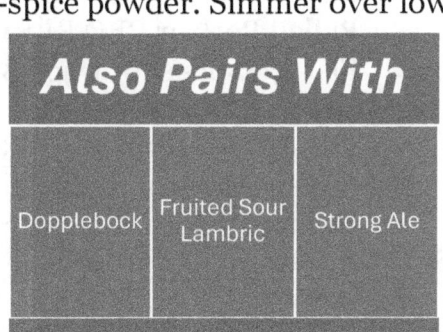

Ribs
In Oven
1. Preheat oven to 425F. Slice ribs between bones. Place it in a large pot with enough water to cover and bring it to a boil. Reduce heat and simmer, covered, for 50 to 60 minutes until meat is fork-tender. Drain. Let stand until it's cool enough to handle.
2. In a bowl, toss the ribs with half of the caramel sauce until evenly coated. Arrange in a single layer on a shallow parchment-lined baking dish. Bake ribs in a preheated oven, turning once or twice, for 30 minutes or until well browned and most of the sauce has evaporated.

In Smoker
1. Preheat the smoker to 225. Use the 3:2:1 method for ribs. For the final 1 stage, Slice the ribs between bones. Toss with Carmel sauce, reserving some. Place all ribs on a wire rack or directly on the smoker grate. Turn ribs over and baste ribs every 15 minutes with remaining Carmel sauce.

Schwarzbier

Schwarzbier, meaning "black beer" in German. Schwarzbier has an opaque, black color with hints of chocolate or coffee flavors. It is like stout because it is made from roasted malt, which gives it its dark hue. Schwarzbiers are made using a cool fermentation method, classifying them as lagers. The alcohol content typically ranges from 4.4% to 5.4% ABV.

Schwarzbier: Key Characteristics		Notable Schwarzbier's
Attribute	**Description**	Kostritzer Schwarzbier
ABV	4.4–5.4% — moderate strength; easy-drinking and sessionable	Sprecher Black Bavarian
IBU (Bitterness)	20–30 — low to moderate; bitterness is clean and balanced	Samuel Adams Black Lager
Color (SRM)	25–40 SRM — deep brown to black; often with ruby highlights	New Belgium 1554 Black Lager
Body	Light to medium — surprisingly smooth and crisp for a dark beer	
Carbonation	Medium — supports drinkability and aroma	
Finish	Dry and clean — with subtle roast lingering gently on the palate	

Taste: Malty | Roasty | Sweet | Earthy | Coffee | Light Floral
Food Pairings: Grilled Pork | Root Vegetables |

Food Pairing Guide For Schwarzbier

Despite its deep color, Schwarzbier is light-bodied, crisp, and refreshingly smooth, making it one of the most approachable dark beer styles out there.

Cheese Pairings
- Smoked Gouda or Aged Cheddar: Bold and nutty—echoes roast
- Gruyère or Alpine-style: Creamy and earthy—balanced by a crisp finish
- Blue Cheese or Gorgonzola: Funky and sharp—tempered by malt sweetness

Meat & Savory Dishes
- Grilled Lamb or Brisket: Charred and juicy—mirrored by roasty malt
- Smoked Sausages or Kielbasa: Savory and spiced—lifted by carbonation
- Pulled Pork or BBQ Ribs: Sweet and smoky—balanced by a dry finish
- Flat Iron Steak or Duck Breast: Rich and flavorful—cut by crisp roast

Vegetables & Sides
- Roasted Mushrooms or Root Veggies: Earthy and caramelized—echoes malt character
- Braised Cabbage or Sauerkraut: Tangy and rich—softened by malt
- German Potato Salad or Spaetzle: Hearty and starchy—balanced by fizz

Spicy & Global Cuisine
- Carnitas Tacos or Mole Sauce: Deep flavors and spice—enhanced by roast and fizz
- Indian Rogan Josh or Dal Makhani: Spiced and creamy—lifted by dry finish
- Korean Bulgogi or BBQ: Sweet heat and char—balanced by malt and hops

Desserts
- Chocolate Cake or Brownies: Rich and fudgy—mirrored by cocoa notes
- Bread Pudding or Sticky Toffee: Toasty and sweet—echoes caramel malt
- Nutty Tarts or Pecan Pie: Sweet and earthy—perfect with a nutty roast

Taco Chicken Enchiladas

Chicken enchiladas often feature seasoned meat with chili, cumin, garlic, and paprika. Schwarzbier's subtle cocoa and coffee notes add a layer of depth that complements the spices without clashing. Melted cheese and enchilada sauce bring richness and tang, which can coat the palate. Schwarzbier's light body and dry finish help cut through the fat, keeping each bite fresh and balanced. The toasted tortilla and caramelized edges of the enchiladas echo the bready, toasty malt, creating a flavor bridge that ties the dish and drink together. Schwarzbier's gentle hop bitterness and cooling carbonation help temper the heat from chili peppers and salsa, making the spice more enjoyable.

Ingredients:
4 whole medium boneless, skinless chicken breast halves
3 Tbsp. Taco Seasoning
2 cups Enchilada Sauce (see Below)
12 corn tortillas
1-2 cups of Monterrey Jack Cheese shredded

Instructions:
1. Place the chicken breasts in the slow cooker and sprinkle 2 Tbsp. of the taco seasoning over the top. Cook on low for 4 hours or until the chicken is tender and shreds easily. Shred the chicken and stir in the remaining taco seasoning and ¼ C of water. Return cover and cook an additional 10 minutes.
2. Spread ½ C of enchilada sauce onto the bottom of a 9x13 pan.
3. Heat tortillas until pliable and place about ¼ C of the chicken in the middle of each tortilla with about 2 Tbsp. of the cheese. Roll and arrange in the 9x13 pan. Repeat until all the chicken and tortillas are used.
4. Pour the remaining enchilada sauce over the top of the enchiladas and top with the remaining cheese. Cover pans with foil and bake 375 degrees for 20 minutes, remove foil and bake an additional 10-15 minutes or until enchilada sauce is bubbling and cheese is well melted.
5. Serve with sour cream, lettuce, and tomato.

Homemade Enchilada Sauce
2 Tbsp. vegetable oil
2 Tbsp. all-purpose flour
2 Tbsp. chili powder
1 tsp. ground cumin
½ tsp. garlic powder
½ tsp. onion powder
¼ tsp. dried oregano
¼ tsp. salt (or to taste)
Pinch of cinnamon (optional for warmth)
2 Tbsp. tomato paste
2 cups of chicken or vegetable broth
Optional: ½ tsp. smoked paprika or a splash of apple cider vinegar for depth

Also Pairs With

Mexican-Style Lager	American Wheat Ale	Cream Ale

In a medium saucepan, heat the oil over medium heat. Whisk in the flour and cook for 1 minute to form a light roux. Stir in chili powder, cumin, garlic powder, onion powder, oregano, salt, and cinnamon. Cook for 30 seconds to bloom the spices. Whisk in tomato paste, then slowly add broth while whisking to avoid lumps. Bring to a gentle boil, then reduce heat and simmer for 10–15 minutes until thickened.

Ambers Beers

Amber beers are a broad category of brews known for their reddish-gold to deep copper color and balanced flavor profile. They sit comfortably between pale ales and dark beers, offering a satisfying mix of toasted malt sweetness and moderate hop bitterness. Amber beers get their color and flavor from roasted crystal malts, which also contribute to their rich mouthfeel and subtle sweetness.

Origins & History
- Early versions were part of the English bitter and pale ale family, often served from casks at cellar temperature.
- The term "amber" comes from the beer's distinct reddish-golden hue, created by using roasted or kilned malts.
- Pioneering breweries like New Belgium, North Coast, and Bell's reimagined traditional styles with American hops, adding citrusy and piney notes while preserving the caramel malt backbone.

Key Characteristics
- **Color**: Golden red to deep amber (10–17 SRM)
- **Flavor**: Caramel, biscuit, toffee, sometimes light chocolate, or fruit
- **Aroma**: Malty and nutty with subtle hop notes
- **Body**: Medium, smooth, and slightly creamy
- **ABV**: Typically, 4.5% to 6.0%
- **Bitterness**: Moderate (25–45 IBU)

Style	Flavor Profile	Color	ABV Range
Amber Ale	Toasty, moderate hop bitterness, Carmel	Copper to Redish Brown	4.5-6.0
Vienna Lager	Toasty, balanced, slightly sweet	Amber	4.7-5.5
Bock / Doppelbock	Rich, strong, sweet malt	Deep amber to brown	6.3-7.9

Food Pairings
Amber Ale: Smoked pork ribs, Sausages and bratwurst, Pepperoni pizza, Sharp cheddar or Gouda, Chocolate cheesecake
Vienna Lager: Grilled chicken, pork chops, burgers, bratwurst, Roast turkey, duck, or beef, enchiladas, Flan
Bock: Braised meats, aged cheeses, chocolate desserts

Their malt-forward profile complements caramelized flavors and balances spicy or salty foods. Amber beers are perfect for those who love the crispness of lagers but crave a little more depth and malt character.

AMBER BEERS
BEER & FOOD PAIRINGS

Beer			
Amber Ale	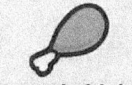 roasted chicken	burgers	cheddar
Irish Red Ale	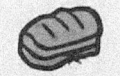 corned beef	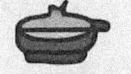 shepherd's pie	roasted pork
Amber Lager	BBQ ribs	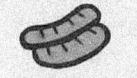 grilled sausage	pretzels
Rauchbier (Smoked Lager)	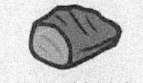 smoked brisket	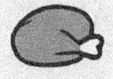 bacon	gouda
Märzen (Lager)	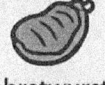 bratwurst	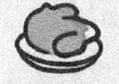 roast turkey	*potato salad*
Vienna	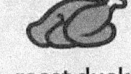 roast duck	sausage	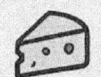 aged cheddar
Maibock/ Helles Bock	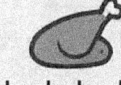 lamb shank	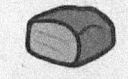 roasted beef	blue cheese
Doppelbock	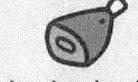 lamb schank	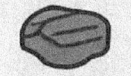 roasted beef	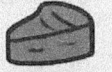 grilled steak
Eisbock	 chocolate cake	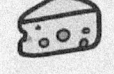 aged cheese	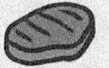 grilled steak

Amber Ales

Amber ales are known for their rich copper to deep amber color, toasty malt backbone, and moderate hop bitterness. Originating in the U.S. craft beer movement, this style has become a staple for those who enjoy flavorful yet approachable beers. It's a versatile choice that pairs well with a wide range of foods and suits any occasion.

Flavor Profile Breakdown
Color: Copper to reddish-brown
Body: Medium, smooth mouthfeel
Aroma: Toasted bread, caramel, light citrus, or pine
Taste: Balanced malt sweetness (caramel, toffee) with moderate hop bitterness
Finish: Clean, slightly dry, or lingering malt

Amber Ale Style by Region
- **American Amber Ale**: More hop-forward, often with citrus or pine notes
- **English Amber Ale**: Milder hops, more biscuit and toffee malt character
- **Red Ale**: Often used interchangeably, though some red ales lean sweeter or maltier

Food Pairing Tips for Amber Ales
- Match with Grilled and Roasted Meats
- Balance with Spicy and Zesty Dishes
- Echo Earthy and Sweet Flavors
- Enhance Caramel-Based Desserts

Awesome Food Pairings

American Amber Ale	Grilled burgers with cheddar and caramelized onions, BBQ pulled pork sandwiches, Sweet potato fries, Spicy tacos with chipotle crema
British Amber Ale / Bitter	Roast chicken with herbs, Bangers and mash, Shepherd's pie, Stilton, or aged cheddar
Irish Red Ale	Corned beef and cabbage, Meatloaf with tomato glaze, Gouda or Dubliner cheese, Bread pudding with whiskey sauce

Amber Ale

Amber ale is an American term used to describe a variety of beers that are brewed with a proportion of amber malt and sometimes crystal malt to produce an amber color ranging from light copper to light brown. They are slow-fermenting and are considered richer than pale ale, with a medium body. Complements rich, aromatic, spicy and smoked foods such as chili, BBQ ribs, grilled chicken, and beef steaks like a T-bone and burgers.

Amber Ale: Key Characteristics		Notable Amber Ales
Attribute	Description	Fat Tire Amber Ale
ABV	4.5–6.0% — moderate strength; sessionable yet flavorful	Alaskan Amber
IBU (Bitterness)	25–45 — balanced; noticeable but not overpowering	Boont Amber Ale
Color (SRM)	10–17 SRM — deep amber to reddish copper; clear with off-white head	Red Seal Ale
Body	Medium to medium-full — smooth and rounded	Amber Ale
Carbonation	Moderate — supports drinkability and aroma	Hop Head Red
Finish	Balanced and clean — with lingering malt sweetness or hop bitterness depending on the variant	

Taste: Malty | Caramel | Toasty | Earthy | Herbal
Food Pairings: Grilled Meats | BBQ | Pizza | Mexican Cuisine | Lamb

Food Pairing Guide for Amber Ale

Amber Ale is known for its gorgeous copper hue, caramel malt backbone, and moderate hop bitterness, making it a versatile and approachable choice for both casual drinkers and craft beer enthusiasts.

Cheese Pairings
- Aged Cheddar or Smoked Gouda: Bold and nutty—mirrors malt depth
- Monterey Jack or Colby: Mild and creamy—balanced by hop bitterness
- Blue Cheese or Stilton: Funky and sharp—tempered by caramel sweetness

Meat & Savory Dishes
- Grilled Burgers or Steaks: Charred and juicy—echoes toasty malt
- BBQ Ribs or Pulled Pork: Sweet and smoky—balanced by hops
- Roast Chicken or Turkey: Savory and herbaceous—lifted by carbonation

Vegetables & Sides
- Roasted Root Vegetables or Mushrooms: Earthy and caramelized—mirrored by malt
- Sweet Potato Fries or Mac & Cheese: Rich and starchy—cut by bitterness
- Grilled Corn or Zucchini: Sweet and smoky—enhanced by toasty notes

Spicy & Global Cuisine
- Buffalo Wings or Spicy Tacos: Heat and char—cooled by malt and fizz
- Indian Tikka Masala or Butter Chicken: Creamy and spiced—balanced by hops
- Thai Peanut Noodles or Pad Thai: Sweet-savory spice—lifted by carbonation

Desserts
- Pecan Pie or Carrot Cake: Nutty and spiced—echoes caramel malt
- Chocolate Chip Cookies or Brownies: Rich and chewy—mirrored by roast
- Apple Crisp or Bread Pudding: Toasty and fruity—balanced by bitterness

Blackened Salmon

Blackened salmon is coated in a bold spice rub—often with paprika, cayenne, garlic, and herbs—then seared to create a smoky, flavorful crust. Amber ale's toasty malt and caramel notes echo the browning and spice, creating a flavor bridge that enhances the dish without overpowering it. Salmon is a fatty, flavorful fish, and blackening intensifies its richness. Amber ale's moderate hop bitterness and carbonation help cut through the fat, keeping the palate refreshed and the flavors lively. The herbal and smoky elements of the blackened rub pair well with amber ale's subtle roast and malt complexity, adding layers of flavor without clashing.

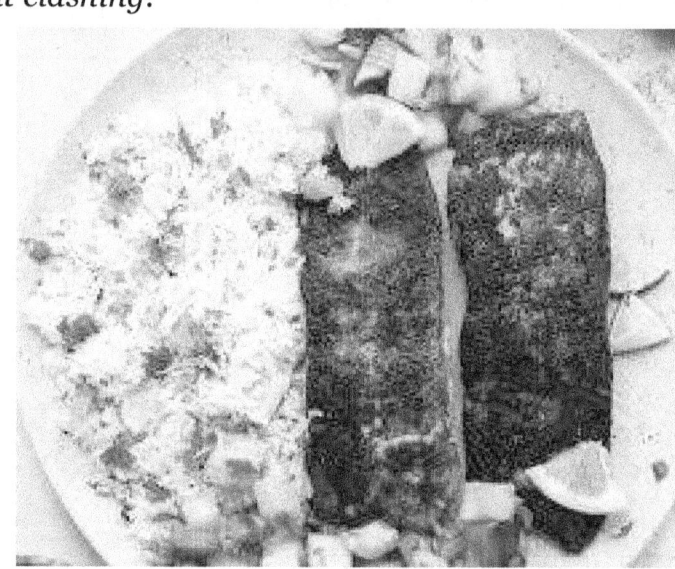

Ingredients:
2 tsp. packed brown sugar
1 1/2 tsp. kosher salt
1 tsp. paprika
1 tsp. garlic powder
1 tsp. dried oregano
1/2 tsp. freshly ground black pepper
1/2 tsp. onion powder
1/2 tsp. dried thyme
1/4 tsp. cayenne pepper
5 Tbsp. butter, divided
4 salmon fillets, skin on
Lime wedges, for serving

Instructions:
1. In a small bowl, whisk together the sugar and spices. In a microwave-safe bowl, melt 3 Tbsp. of butter. Brush butter on top of fillets and coat with seasonings.
2. In a large skillet over medium heat, melt the remaining 2 Tbsp. butter. Add salmon, skin side up, and cook for 3 minutes, then flip and cook 2 to 3 minutes more or until it flakes easily with a fork. Serve with limes.

Cilantro Lemon Rice
1 cup long-grain white rice (or basmati)
2 cups of water or vegetable broth
1 Tbsp. olive oil or butter
½ tsp. salt
Zest of 1 lemon
2 Tbsp. fresh lemon juice
¼ cup chopped fresh cilantro
Optional: pinch of garlic powder or minced garlic

Also Pairs With		
Farmhouse Ale	Golden Strong Ale	English ESB

In a saucepan, bring the water (or broth), rice, oil, and salt to a boil. Reduce heat to low, cover, and simmer for 15–18 minutes until rice is tender and liquid is absorbed. Remove from the heat and let sit covered for 5 minutes. Fluff with a fork. Stir in lemon zest, lemon juice, and cilantro. Mix gently to combine.

Irish Red Ales

Red is just a descriptor for a caramelly, full-bodied pale ale, often highly hopped. Red ales must possess a range of "mediums": medium or slightly fuller body; medium levels of the fruity aromas and flavors common in IPA; medium hop bitterness and flavor; medium to full malt character. Delicious with nuts, game meats and root vegetables, chicken, burgers, and spicy barbecue.

Irish Red Ale: Key Characteristics		Notable Irish Red Ales
Attribute	Description	Smithwick's Irish Red Ale
ABV	4.0–6.0% — moderate strength; highly sessionable[2]	Murphy's Irish Red
IBU (Bitterness)	20–28 — low to moderate; just enough to balance malt sweetness	Kilkenny Irish Cream Ale
Color (SRM)	11–18 SRM — copper-red to reddish-brown; clear with creamy off-white head	O'Hara's Irish Red
Body	Medium — smooth and rounded mouthfeel	Harp Red Lager
Carbonation	Moderate — supports drinkability and aroma	
Finish	Clean and mildly sweet to dry — varies by recipe	

Taste: Crisp, Clean, Caramel, Balanced
Food Pairings: Cabbage | Corned Beef | Roasted Meats | Grilled Sausage

Food Pairing Guide for Irish Red Ales

Irish Red Ale is a smooth, malt-forward ale with a distinctive reddish hue, known for its approachability, subtle sweetness, and clean finish.

Cheese Pairings
- Aged Cheddar or Red Leicester: Sharp and nutty—mirrored by malt depth
- Smoked Gouda or Irish Porter Cheese: Bold and creamy—balanced by roast
- Brie or Camembert: Soft and buttery—cut by carbonation

Meat & Savory Dishes
- Corned Beef or Shepherd's Pie: Rich and savory—echoed by caramel malt
- Roast Lamb or Pork Loin: Earthy and herbaceous—lifted by a clean finish
- Grilled Sausages or Meatloaf: Smoky and spiced—balanced by malt sweetness

Vegetables & Sides
- Roasted Root Vegetables or Mushrooms: Earthy and caramelized—mirrored by malt
- Colcannon or Mashed Potatoes: Creamy and starchy—cut by carbonation
- Braised Cabbage or Leeks: Sweet and savory—enhanced by toasty notes

Spicy & Global Cuisine
- Beef Tacos or Enchiladas: Spiced and cheesy—tempered by malt and fizz
- Indian Butter Chicken or Rogan Josh: Creamy and aromatic—lifted by a dry finish
- Thai Peanut Noodles or Satay: Sweet-savory spice—balanced by malt depth

Desserts
- Carrot Cake or Bread Pudding: Spiced and toasty—echoes caramel malt
- Chocolate Chip Cookies or Brownies: Rich and chewy—mirrored by roast
- Apple Crisp or Sticky Toffee Pudding: Fruity and sweet—perfect with nutty malt

Sausage Mushroom Pizza

Sausage adds bold, spiced, and fatty flavors. Mushrooms bring deep umami and earthiness. Cheese and tomato sauce layer tang and creaminess. This creates a complex, hearty flavor profile that benefits from a beer that can both complement and cleanse. Toasty caramel malts echo the browned sausage and crust. Mild bitterness cuts through the fat without overpowering. A clean finish refreshes the palate between bites. Subtle earthy notes mirror the mushrooms' depth. The ale's sweetness balances the salt and spice. Its effervescence lifts the richness of cheese and meat.

Ingredients:
1 Tbsp. olive oil
4 oz bulk Italian sausage
1 cup sliced mushrooms (3 oz)
3 cloves garlic, finely chopped
1 prepared Pizza Crust
1/2 cup tomato sauce (from an 8-oz can)
1/3 cup thinly sliced red onion
1 1/2 cups shredded mozzarella cheese (6 oz)
2 Tbsp. thinly sliced fresh basil leaves

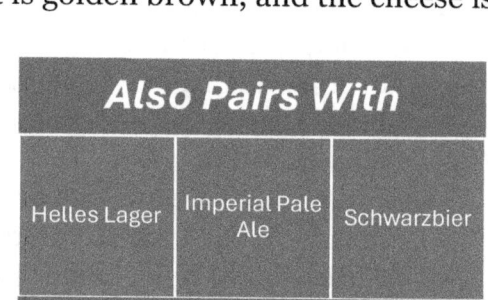

Instructions:
1. Spray a 15x10-inch or larger dark or nonstick cookie sheet with cooking spray. Heat oven to 400°F (425°F for all other pan types). In a 10-inch skillet, heat oil over medium heat. Add sausage, and cook 3 to 5 minutes, stirring occasionally, until no longer pink. Using a slotted spoon, transfer the pasta to a small bowl.
2. Add mushrooms to drippings in skillet; cook 3 to 5 minutes, stirring frequently, until softened and browned. Stir in garlic; remove from heat.
3. Spread tomato sauce evenly over the dough. Top with the mushroom mixture. Top with sausage, red onion, and cheese. Bake for 5 to 9 minutes or until the crust is golden brown, and the cheese is melted.
4. Top with basil.

Cheesy Garlic Bread
1 loaf French bread or Italian bread (halved lengthwise)
½ cup unsalted butter, softened
3–4 cloves garlic, minced
2 Tbsp. chopped fresh parsley (or 1 tsp dried)
1½ cups shredded mozzarella cheese
¼ cup grated Parmesan cheese
Optional: pinch of red pepper flakes or Italian seasoning

Also Pairs With		
Helles Lager	Imperial Pale Ale	Schwarzbier

Set to 400°F. Line a baking sheet with foil or parchment. Mix softened butter with garlic, parsley, and optional seasonings. Slather garlic butter over bread halves. Sprinkle evenly with mozzarella and Parmesan. Place on baking sheet and bake for 10–12 minutes until cheese is melted and bubbly. For extra crispiness, broil for 1–2 minutes at the end—watch closely!

Amber Lager

Amber lagers are a medium-bodied lager with a toasty or caramel-like malt character. Hop bitterness can range from extremely low to medium-high. Brewers may use decoction mash and dry hopping to achieve advanced flavors. Lager is beer that has been brewed and conditioned at low temperatures. Amber pale also complements jerk chicken and pulled pork. The flowery and light aroma will also make the barbeque experience exciting.

Amber Lager: Key Characteristics		Notable Amber Lagers
Attribute	Description	Great Lakes Eliot Ness
ABV	4.8–5.4% — moderate strength; sessionable and smooth	Negra Modelo
IBU (Bitterness)	18–30 — low to moderate; bitterness balances malt sweetness	Samuel Adams Boston Lager
Color (SRM)	10–17 SRM — amber to deep red; clear with off-white head	Devil's Backbone Vienna Lager
Body	Medium — rounded and smooth with a touch of malt weight	Ayinger Oktober Fest-Märzen
Carbonation	Medium — supports crispness and aroma	Jack's Abby Copper Legend
Finish	Clean and slightly malty — often with lingering caramel or toast	Brooklyn Lager

Taste: Crisp | Clean | Caramel | Balanced | Biscuit | Moderate Bitterness
Food Pairings: BBQ| Grilled Vegetables | Smoked Ribs |Roast Duck | Mac & Cheese

Food Pairing Guide for Amber Lagers
Amber Lager is a malt-forward, medium-bodied lager that offers a beautiful balance between toasty sweetness and clean drinkability.

Hearty & Savory Dishes
- Grilled sausages: Their caramel malt complements the char and spice.
- Smoked pork ribs: The beer's sweetness balances smoky, savory notes.
- Roast duck: Cuts through the fat while enhancing the roasted flavors.

Cheesy Comforts
- Fried cheese curds or mozzarella sticks: Crisp carbonation and malt sweetness play beautifully with melty textures.
- Mac & cheese: The beer's body stands up to creamy richness.

Earthy & Spiced Fare
- Mushroom risotto or goulash: Umami and spice are mellowed by the lager's smooth finish.
- Pupusas with cheese or pork: Roasted malt flavors echo the richness of the filling.

Grilled & Roasted Vegetables
- Charred peppers, onions, or zucchini: The toasty malt notes enhance caramelization.

Sweet & Savory Fusion
- BBQ dishes with sweet sauces: The beer's malt backbone complements the glaze.
- Savory pies or empanadas: Especially with spiced meat or mushroom fillings.

Beer Braised Chicken with Carrots and Red Potatoes

The caramel malt in the amber lager complements the roasted notes of the vegetables and the golden skin of the chicken. The beer's subtle bitterness cuts through the richness of the braise, keeping the dish from feeling heavy. The effervescence lifts the palate, making each bite feel fresh and satisfying. If the dish is cooked with amber lager, pairing it with the same beer enhances the continuity of flavor.

Ingredients:
4 (1-1/2 lb.) bone-in chicken thighs
Salt and pepper to taste
1 Tbsp. olive oil
2 Tbsp. of butter, divided
1 medium onion, finely chopped
1 lb. fresh baby carrots
1-1/2 lbs. red potatoes, cut into quarters
2 cloves garlic, minced
2 sprigs fresh rosemary
3 sprigs fresh thyme
1 (12 oz) bottle light beer
1/2 cup of chicken broth
2 Tbsp. of white whole wheat flour
Salt and pepper to taste

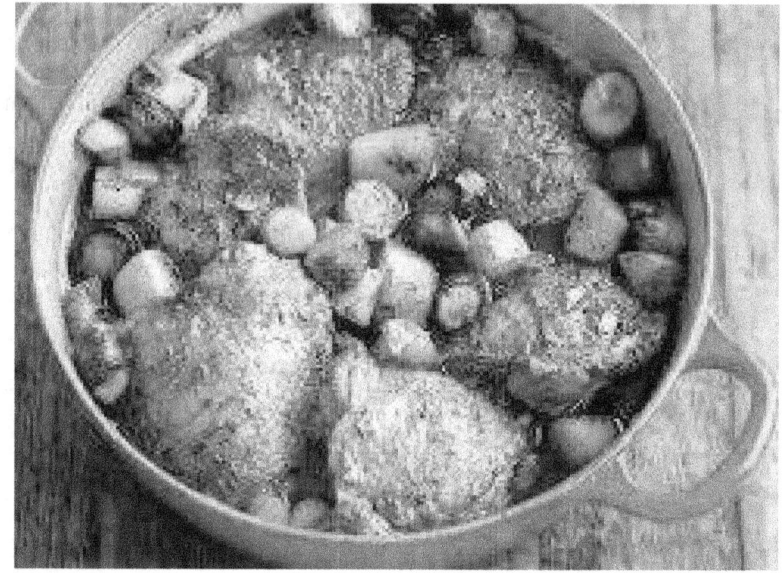

Instructions:
1. Season chicken thighs on both sides with salt and pepper. In a Dutch oven or large oven-safe saucepan over medium-high heat, sear chicken in oil and 1 Tbsp. butter on both sides 2-3 minutes until golden. Transfer the chicken to a plate and set aside.
2. Add the remaining Tbsp. butter to same skillet and then add onion, baby carrots, and potatoes. Sauté in butter 5-10 minutes until lightly golden. Add garlic and sauté 1 additional minute.
3. Nestle chicken back into pan and arrange herbs around it. Pour the beer and broth into the pan and bring to a low simmer. Cover the pan and place in a 350F oven. Bake chicken 40-45 minutes until the chicken is tender-apart and vegetables are tender.
4. Remove the chicken and vegetables and place them on a cutting board momentarily. Discard herb sprigs. Whisk flour with a little water and add the remaining liquids in pan. Bring to a simmer over medium heat, stirring occasionally until the sauce is slightly thickened.
5. Season the sauce with salt and pepper to taste and toss the vegetables and chicken back into the pan until coated in sauce.

Also Pairs With

Blonde Ale	Helles Lager	Oktoberfest

Rauchbier (Smoked Lager)

Smoked beer is a type of beer with a distinctive smoke flavor imparted by using malted barley dried over an open flame. It goes well with low and slow smoked meats. Best with ribs if you can find it in a store. Whether you're pairing it with smoked meat or exploring its regional variations.

Rauchbier: Key Characteristics		Notable Rauchbier
Attribute	Description	Aecht Schlenkerla Rauchbier Marzen
ABV	4.8–6.5% — moderate strength; varies by substyle (e.g., Märzen, Bock)	Aecht Schlenkerla Rauchbier Urbock
IBU (Bitterness)	20–30 — low to moderate; bitterness is clean and balanced	Spezial Rauchbier Lager
Color (SRM)	12–30 SRM — amber to dark brown; often clear with ruby highlights	Alaskan Smoked Porter
Body	Medium — smooth and rounded, sometimes creamy	Live Oak Rauchbier
Carbonation	Moderate — supports drinkability and aroma	Jack's Abby Smoke & Dagger
Finish	Dry to slightly sweet — with lingering smoke and malt complexity	

Taste: Malty | Smoky | Toasty | Smooth | Carmel
Food Pairings: Smoked Meats | Grilled Foods | Dark Chocolate Desserts | Pork Belly | Sausage

Food Pairing Guide for Rauchbier

Rauchbier — "smoke beer" is brewed with malt dried over an open flame, typically beechwood, which infuses the beer with aromatic phenols reminiscent of campfire, smoked meats, or even bacon.

Meaty & Smoky Classics
- Smoked sausages -the char and spice harmonize with Rauchbier's malt.
- Smoked ham, bacon, or porchetta: Fat and salt mellow the beer's intensity.
- Barbecue - Rauchbier mirrors grilled notes and balances spicy sauces.

Cheese Pairings
- Smoked cheeses (Rauchkäse): Mirror the beer's smoky malt.
- Aged Gouda or sharp cheddar: cut through the smoke with tang and texture.
- Blue cheese or ash-coated chèvre: Pierces the smoky haze with sharp, funky contrast.

Hearty German Comfort Foods
- *Schlenkerla beer cheese soup*
- *Sauerbraten* (pot roast)
- *Kartoffelsuppe* (potato soup)

Savory Snacks & Boards
- Charcuterie boards: Focus on savory items, skip the fruit, add pickles, olives, and caramelized onions.
- Bacon-wrapped bites: Smoky on smoky is a win.

Surprising Pairings
- Chinese food: The umami and sweet-savory sauces play well with Rauchbier's depth.
- Spicy dishes: The malt backbone balances heat while enhancing flavor complexity.

BBQ Dry Rub Ribs

Rauchbier (literally "smoke beer") is brewed with malts dried over open flames, giving it a rich, campfire-like aroma. Dry rub ribs, especially when smoked or grilled, carry deep charred flavors and spice. Together, they amplify each other's smokiness without clashing—like two instruments playing the same melody in harmony. Dry rubs often include paprika, cumin, garlic, and brown sugar. Rauchbier's toasty malt sweetness balances the heat and spice, while its earthy undertones echo the rub's complexity. The smoky aroma of the beer primes your palate for the ribs.

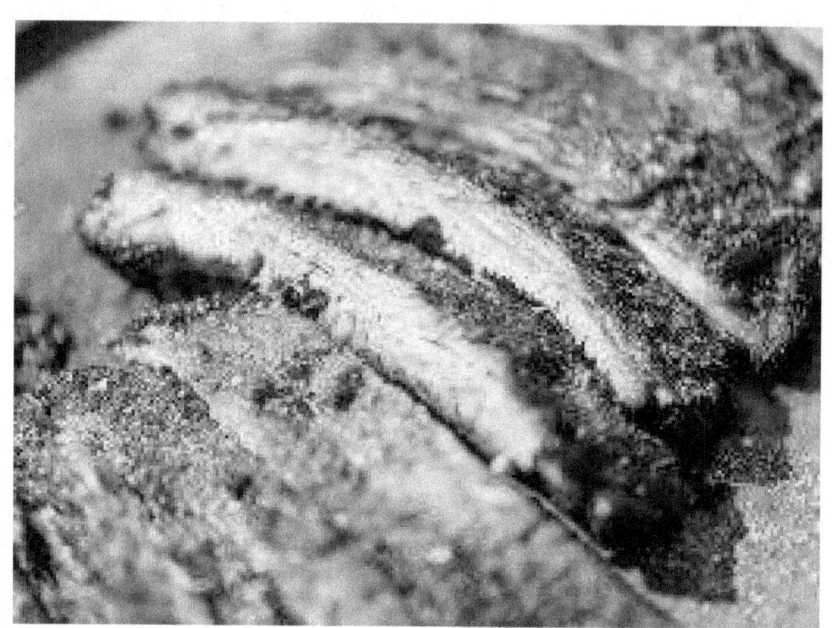

Ingredients
2 racks Pork ribs

For the dry rub/seasoning:
2 tbsp soft brown sugar
1 tsp paprika
2 tsp salt
1 tsp black pepper
1 tsp garlic powder
1 tsp onion powder
½ tsp mild Chilli Powder
1 tsp dried oregano

For the mop:
1 tbsp of the rub
1/2 cup chicken stock
1/4 cup Apple Cider Vinegar

Instructions
1. Preheat your BBQ or smoker to 250F and set the BBQ up for indirect cooking.
2. Whilst the BBQ is preheating, prepare the ribs and make the rub. Take the ribs out of the fridge an hour before you want to cook. Remove the membrane from the inside of the ribs.
3. Now make the rub, place all the rub ingredients in a bowl, and mix until fully combined.
4. Pat the ribs dry with some kitchen roll and sprinkle over 1 tbsp of the rub over each rack of ribs (2 tbsp in total). We don't want too much seasoning at this stage as we want the flavor of the smoke to penetrate the rib, creating a lovely bark.
5. Once the BBQ is up to temperature, then place a pan in the BBQ underneath where the ribs will be placed and pour in some water or weak chicken stock.
6. Add the ribs to the BBQ, close the lid, and leave them to smoke for 2 hours. While the ribs are cooking, make the mop. Add all the mop ingredients to a bowl and mix until combined.
7. After 2 hours, remove the ribs from the BBQ, mop them once and wrap them in foil tightly, then place them back on the BBQ for a further 1-2 hours, checking on them after 1 hour).
8. Take the ribs off and allow them to rest for 20 minutes before serving.
9. When you're ready to serve, mop the ribs and then sprinkle on the remaining dry rub.

Also Pairs With

Quadrupel	American IPA	Rauchbier

Marzen (Lager)

The beer style is characterized by a deep gold-copper hue, brilliant clarity, and a persistent head. On the nose, the beer gives off a distinct aroma of caramel and toasted malt, the Vienna or Munich variety. The malt gives off a delicate sweetness, perfectly balancing the moderate bitterness from the hops, nor overshadowing the other. And as all lagers should, it finishes crisp and clean on the palate. Caramelization of malts complements that of char-grilled and seared meats or hearty, spicy Mexican dishes, spicy barbecued chicken, sausage, and pork.

Märzen: Key Characteristics		Notable Marzen
Attribute	**Description**	Paulaner Oktoberfest Märzen
ABV	5.1–6.0% — moderate strength; warming but sessionable	Spaten Oktoberfestbier
IBU (Bitterness)	18–24 — low to moderate; bitterness is clean and balanced	Hacker-Pschorr Original Oktoberfest
Color (SRM)	8–14 SRM — deep gold to amber; brilliant clarity	Weihenstephaner Festbier
Body	Medium — smooth and rounded with a soft mouthfeel	Sierra Nevada Oktoberfest
Carbonation	Moderate — supports drinkability and aroma	Jack's Abby Copper Legend
Finish	Clean and slightly malty — with lingering toast & caramel notes	Great Lakes Oktoberfest

Taste: Toasty | Carmel | Toffee | Floral Malt-forward
Food Pairings: Mac & Cheese | Barbecue | Roasted Poultry | Sauerkraut

Food Pairing Guide for Marzen Lager

Märzen is a traditional German lager originally brewed in March ("März" in German) and stored in cool caves to be enjoyed during fall festivals—most famously Oktoberfest.

Classic German Pairings
- Bratwurst or Weisswurst: The beer's maltiness complements the savory sausage.
- Soft pretzels with mustard or cheese dip: Salt and carbs meet smooth malt.
- Sauerkraut or red cabbage: The beer's sweetness balances the tang.

Cheese Matches
- Emmental or Gruyère: Their mild nuttiness echoes Marzen's malt.
- Aged cheddar: Sharpness contrasts the beer's smooth body.
- Beer cheese dip: Especially if made with Marzen itself.

Roasted & Grilled Meats
- Roast chicken or turkey: Especially with herbs or gravy.
- Grilled pork chops: Sweet malt balances smoky edges.
- BBQ pulled pork: The beer's body stands up to bold flavors.

Hearty Comfort Foods
- Mac & cheese: Creamy richness meets malty depth.
- Shepherd's pie: Earthy and savory with a touch of sweetness.
- Mushroom risotto: Umami and malt are a natural match.

Sweet Pairings
- Apple strudel: Cinnamon and fruit play off the malt.
- Bread pudding: Especially with caramel or bourbon sauce.

Bourbon Brown Sugar Smoked Pork Loin

This pairing screams fall comfort—smoky meats, amber beer, and cozy flavors that feel right at home during Oktoberfest or a fall harvest dinner. Bourbon adds warmth, vanilla, and oak notes. Brown sugar brings caramelized sweetness and a glossy glaze. Smoked pork loin delivers deep umami and charred richness. Toasty caramel malts echo the brown sugar glaze. The caramel malt in Märzen mirrors the bourbon and sugar glaze. Its smooth texture enhances the pork's tenderness. The lager's crispness keeps the pairing from feeling heavy or cloying.

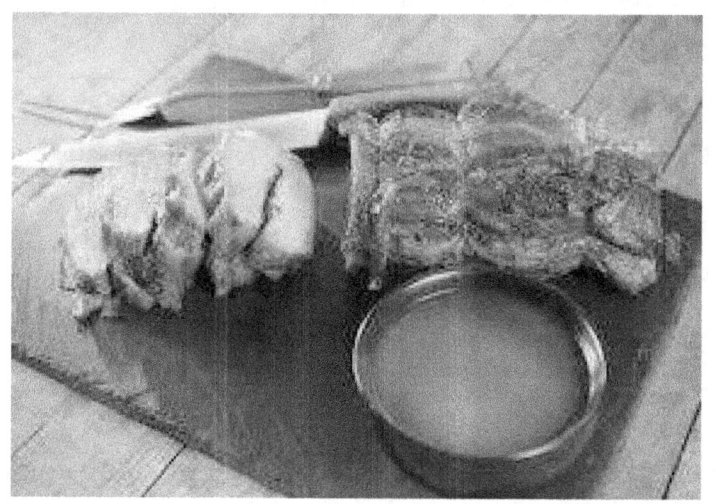

Ingredients:
For the pork:
1 center-cut piece of pork loin (2½ to 3 pounds)
3 Tbsp. Tennessee whiskey
2 Tbsp. of your favorite barbecue rub
3 Tbsp. Dijon mustard
½ cup firmly packed brown sugar
4 slices bacon

For the glaze:
3 Tbsp. salted butter
3 Tbsp. brown sugar
3 Tbsp. Dijon mustard
3 Tbsp. Tennessee whiskey
Barbecue sauce (optional), for serving

Instructions:

1. Butterfly the pork loin, opening the roast up as you would a book. Sprinkle the inside of the roast with 1 Tbsp. of the whiskey and let it marinate for 5 minutes. Sprinkle a third of the rub over the inside of the roast. Spread the mustard on top with a spatula, then sprinkle the brown sugar on top of the mustard. Sprinkle the remaining 2 Tbsp. of whiskey on top of the brown sugar. Fold the roast back together (like closing a book) and sprinkle the remaining rub over the outside.
2. Cut four 12-inch pieces of butcher's string. Place a slice of bacon across the strings and set the roast on top of the bacon. Tie each piece of string together around the roast so that they hold the slices of bacon against it. Set the pork roast aside.
3. Make the glaze: Combine the butter, brown sugar, mustard, and whiskey in a saucepan and boil until syrupy, 4 to 6 minutes. Set the glaze aside.
4. Ready smoker to 225 degrees. When ready to cook, place the pork roast on the hot grate, over the drip pan and away from the heat, and cover the grill. Cook the roast until cooked through, 1 to 1½ hours. To test for doneness, insert an instant-read meat thermometer into the side of the roast: The internal temperature should be about 160°F. Start basting the roast with some of the glaze after 30 minutes and continue basting every 15 minutes.
5. Transfer the cooked roast to a cutting board and let it rest for 5 minutes, then remove and discard the strings. Slice the roast crosswise and drizzle any remaining glaze over it. If you like, serve barbecue sauce alongside.

Also Pairs With

Scotch Ale	Robust Porter	Dunkelweizen

Vienna

Vienna Lager is a beer named after the city in which it originated. It is brewed using a three-step decoction boiling process. The malt bill typically includes Munich, Pilsner, Vienna, and dextrin malts, with wheat occasionally added. The color of Vienna Lager reliably falls between pale amber and medium amber, often exhibiting a reddish hue. Noble hops are used subtly, resulting in a beer with a crisp quality, a toasty flavor, and some residual caramel-like sweetness.

Vienna Lager: Key Characteristics		Notable Vienna
Attribute	**Description**	Dos Equis Ambar
ABV	4.7–5.5% — moderate strength; smooth and sessionable	Samuel Adams Boston Lager
IBU (Bitterness)	18–30 — balanced; enough to offset malt sweetness	Devils Backbone Vienna Lager
Color (SRM)	9–15 SRM — copper to amber; brilliant clarity with reddish hue	Sierra Nevada Vienna Style Lager
Body	Medium-light to medium — smooth and slightly creamy	Schell's FireBrick
Carbonation	Moderate — enhances drinkability and aroma	
Finish	Fairly dry and crisp — with lingering toast and hop bitterness	

Taste: Malty | Crisp | Toasty | Hop Bitterness | Floral | Spicy
Food Pairings: Barbecue Chicken | Brisket | Carmel Desserts | Roast Pork | Latin Dishes | Pretzels

Food Pairing Guide for Vienna

Vienna is a beautifully balanced amber lager that highlights toasty malt character, a crisp finish, and subtle hop bitterness.

Roasted & Grilled Meats
- Roast pork or pork tenderloin: The beer's malt sweetness complements the meat's natural richness.
- Grilled chicken thighs: Smoky char meets smooth malt.
- Beef tacos or carne asada: Especially with mild spice and citrus.

Cheese Pairings
- Havarti or Gouda: Their mild sweetness echoes the beer's malt.
- Swiss or Emmental: Nutty and smooth, perfect with Vienna's toasty notes.
- Queso Oaxaca or mild cheddar: Great for Mexican-style Vienna lagers.

Latin-Inspired Dishes
- Tamales: Especially pork or chicken, with mole or red sauce.
- Enchiladas: Mildly spiced with red chili or mole.
- Chiles rellenos: The beer's crispness cuts through the richness.

Comfort Foods
- Shepherd's pie: Earthy and savory with a touch of sweetness.
- Mushroom stroganoff: Umami and malt are a natural match.
- Grilled bratwurst: Especially with caramelized onions or mustard.

Sweet Pairings
- Apple pie or strudel: Cinnamon and fruit play off the malt.
- Carrot cake: Earthy sweetness and spice match beautifully.

Smoked Sirloin Steak

Sirloin is lean yet flavorful, especially when smoked—it develops a rich crust and deep umami. The smoke adds complexity without overwhelming the meat's natural character. The toasty malt backbone echoes the caramelized edges of the steak. Subtle sweetness balances the smoky bitterness. The beer's malt profile mirrors the Maillard reaction—those browned, savory notes from grilling and smoking. The low-to-moderate bitterness doesn't clash with smoke or seasoning, unlike hoppier beers. Add a side of roasted root vegetables or a smoky tomato chutney—Vienna lager will tie the whole plate together with its warm, amber charm.

Ingredients:
2 top sirloin steaks, about 1 pound each
2 Tbsp. Weber's "Cowboy Rub" or favorite dry rub

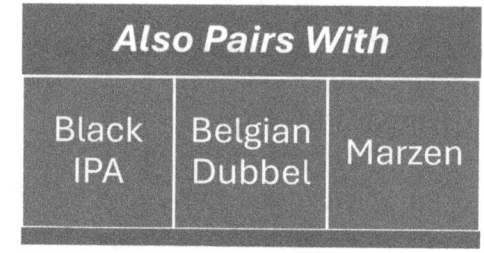

Instructions:
1. Pat the steaks dry with a paper towel.
2. Cover all sides with steak rub (dry brining). Dry brining steak brings out the natural flavors of meat and improves the texture. Salt draws moisture to the surface, which is then absorbed back into the meat, acting as a natural tenderizer.
3. Let it marinate for at least 30 minutes before cooking, and up to 24 hours.
4. Pre-heat the smoker to 225 °F.
5. Place on the grill and smoke until the internal temperature reaches 130-135 °F, about 45 minutes.
6. Remove from the smoker, cover with foil, and increase heat to 450 °F. or prepare gas grill to sear steaks alternatively.
7. Return the steaks to the smoker and sear for 3 to 3.5 minutes on each side until the internal temperature reaches about 145 °F (for medium) or your preferred level of doneness.
8. Remove the steaks from the grill and rest under foil at least 5 minutes before slicing.

Roasted Root Vegetables
2 Tbsp. avocado or olive oil
2 Tbsp. fresh oregano, chopped
2 medium sweet potatoes, chopped into chunks
1-pound carrots or parsnips, peeled and cut into ¾ inch thick rounds (about 4 cups)
1 medium red onion, peeled and cut into ½ inch thick wedges
1 tsp. sea salt
½ tsp. ground black pepper

Also Pairs With		
Black IPA	Belgian Dubbel	Marzen

1. Preheat oven to 425°F and line a baking sheet with parchment paper.
2. Add the oil and oregano to a large bowl and whisk to combine.
3. Add sweet potatoes, carrots (or parsnips), and onion to the bowl. Toss to coat veggies. Sprinkle the vegetables generously with sea salt and pepper.
4. Spread veggies onto the prepared baking sheet. Make sure they are in one layer, so they roast instead of steam. Roast vegetables until tender, about 50 minutes, tossing halfway.
5. This dish can be made up to 4 hours ahead. Let it stand at room temperature. If desired, rewarm in a 350°F oven for about 15 minutes, or serve at room temperature.

Bocks

Bock is a traditional German lager known for its rich malt character, smooth body, and higher alcohol content. Originally brewed in the town of Einbeck in the Middle Ages, the style was later adopted and popularized in Bavaria. The name "bock" comes from a Bavarian mispronunciation of "Einbeck," and means "goat" in German—hence the frequent goat imagery on bock labels.

Key Characteristics
Color: Deep amber to dark brown
Flavor: Toasted malt, caramel, toffee, sometimes nutty or chocolatey
Body: Medium to full, smooth, and creamy
Bitterness: Low to moderate (light hop presence)
ABV: Typically, 6% to 7.5%, but stronger versions can exceed 10%
Bock beers are bottom-fermented lagers that undergo extended cold storage (*lagering*), which helps develop their clean yet robust flavor profile.

Styles of Bock

Style	Description
Traditional Bock	Malty, smooth, and slightly sweet; classic springtime beer
Doppelbock	"Double bock"—stronger, richer, and more intense
Maibock / Helles Bock	Lighter in color, brewed for spring; more hop-forward
Eisbock	Concentrated by freezing and removing water; strong and rich
Weizenbock	Made with wheat and ale yeast; fruity and spicy notes

Food Pairings
Bock beers pair beautifully with hearty, roasted, and sweet-savory dishes:
- Roast pork or pork knuckle
- Aged Gouda or Emmental
- Duck breast with fruit glaze
- Chocolate desserts or nutty pastries

Awesome Food Pairings

Traditional Bock (Germany)	Roast pork with apples, Grilled bratwurst or kielbasa, Mushroom stroganoff, Aged Gouda, or Emmental
Doppelbock	Braised short ribs or beef stew, Duck confit or lamb shank, Blue cheese or aged cheddar, Chocolate cake, or bread pudding
Maibock (Helles Bock)	Grilled chicken or salmon, Spring vegetables (asparagus, peas), Soft cheeses like brie or Havarti, Lemon tart, or almond cake
Eisbock	Venison or wild game, Rich pâtés, or foie gras, Dark chocolate truffles, Stilton or Roquefort
Weizenbock	Roast turkey or ham, Sweet potato casserole, Camembert or triple cream brie, Banana bread, or spice cake

German Bock

A German-style Bock beer is a robust, malty beer with toasted or nut-like flavor notes. Bock is a strong beer, made with only barley malt. A bottom fermenting lager that takes extra months to smooth out. Rich sweetness balances strong spice components and intense flavors of Cajun, jerk, slow-roasted and seared foods. Drink with sausages, pork chops, or a nice cut of steak. They are great when paired with red meat, hearty soups, and potatoes.

German Bock: Key Characteristics		Notable German Bock
Attribute	**Description**	Spaten Optimator
ABV	6.3–7.2% — strong but smooth; warming without harshness	Weihenstephaner Korbinian
IBU (Bitterness)	20–30 — low to moderate; bitterness is clean and balanced	Einbecker Ur-Bock Dunkel
Color (SRM)	14–30 SRM — amber to dark brown; brilliant clarity with ruby highlights	Andechser Doppelbock Dunkel
Body	Medium to full — rich and rounded mouthfeel	Weltenburger Kloster Asam Bock
Carbonation	Moderate — supports drinkability and aroma	Einbecker Mai-Ur-Bock
Finish	Clean and malty — with lingering toast, caramel, and subtle dryness	

Taste: Malty | Rich | Toasty | Dark Fruit | High Alcohol
Food Pairings: Roast Pork or Duck | Smoked Meats | Carmel or Choc Desserts

Food Pairing Guide for German Bock

German Bock is a strong, malty lager known for its toasty malt complexity, higher alcohol content, and clean lager finish.

Hearty Meats & Roasts
- Roast pork or pork belly: Fatty richness balanced by smooth malt.
- Grilled bratwurst or kielbasa: Echoes the beer's toasty notes.
- Beef stew or pot roast: Deep flavors match the beer's intensity.
- Smoked meat: Especially with sweet glazes or spicy rubs.

Cheese Pairings
- Aged Gouda or Gruyère: Their caramel and nutty notes mirror Bock's malt.
- Blue cheese: Sharp contrast to the beer's sweetness.
- Beer cheese dip: Especially if made with Bock itself.

Rich Comfort Foods
- Shepherd's pie or meatloaf: Earthy and savory with a touch of sweetness.
- Mushroom stroganoff: Umami and malt are a natural match.

Breads & Sides
- Pretzels or rye bread: Toasty malt meets hearty grain.
- Spaetzle or dumplings: Soft textures and mild flavors complement the beer's body.

Sweet Pairings
- Bread pudding or sticky toffee pudding: Rich and indulgent.
- Chocolate cake or brownies: Cocoa and malt are a dream team.
- Apple strudel or caramel flan: Fruit and sugar meet smooth malt.

German Pot Roast in the Slow Cooker (Sauerbraten)

Marinated beef roast slow cooked with vinegar, spices, and aromatics develops deep, tangy, and savory flavors. The slow cooking process intensifies umami and creates a melt-in-your-mouth texture. Often served with gravy, red cabbage, and dumplings, it's a hearty, comforting meal. A German Bocks rich malt backbone and notes of caramel, toast, and subtle chocolate offer minimal bitterness, allowing the roast's spices and tang to shine. It's full-bodied and smooth; it complements the dish's weight without overwhelming it. The Bock's caramel malt sweetness balances the vinegar-based marinade and gravy. The beer's clean finish refreshes the palate between bites of rich meat and starchy sides.

Ingredients

For the marinade and beef:
- 2 cups water
- 1 cup dry red wine
- 1 cup red wine vinegar
- 2 medium carrots, peeled and chopped
- 2 medium celery stalks, chopped
- 1 medium onion, halved and sliced
- 2 cloves garlic, smashed
- 1 Tbsp. whole black peppercorns
- 1 Tbsp. juniper berries
- 1 Tbsp. mustard seeds
- 2 bay leaves
- 1 (3-to-4 pound) beef chuck roast or bottom round roast

For cooking and finishing the roast:
- 1 1/2 tsp. kosher salt
- 1/2 tsp. freshly ground black pepper
- 1 Tbsp. olive oil
- 2 Tbsp. unsalted butter
- 2 Tbsp. all-purpose flour

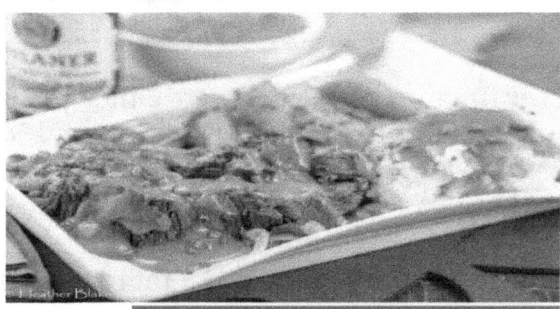

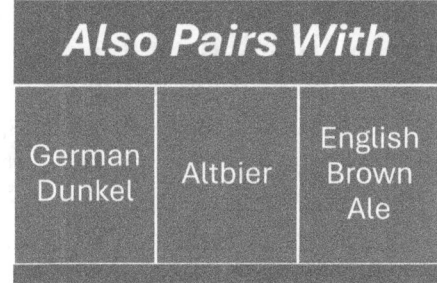

Also Pairs With: German Dunkel | Altbier | English Brown Ale

Instructions

Marinate the beef:
1. Stir all the ingredients except the beef together in a large saucepan. Bring to a boil over medium-high heat, then remove from the heat and cool completely.
2. Place the beef in a 6-quart or larger slow cooker and pour in the cooled marinade. (The meat will not be completely submerged.) Cover and place the bowl in the refrigerator to marinate for 2 days, flipping the meat once or twice per day.

Slow-cook the beef:
1. Remove the beef from the refrigerator about 30 minutes before cooking. Transfer the meat to a large plate and pat completely dry with paper towels. Do not discard the marinade. Generously season the meat all over with salt and pepper.
2. Heat the oil over high heat in a large cast iron or heavy-bottomed skillet until shimmering. Add the beef and sear each side until deeply browned, 4 to 5 minutes per side.
3. Return the beef to the marinade in the slow cooker. Cover with the lid. Cook until the beef is tender and cooked through, 8 to 9 hours on LOW, or 5 to 6 hours on HIGH. Transfer the beef to a cutting board and rest for about 5 minutes.
4. Meanwhile, strain the cooking liquid through a strainer or colander set over a bowl. Measure out 2 cups of the liquid and set aside (discard the remaining cooking liquid and solids).
5. Melt the butter in a medium saucepan over medium heat. Whisk in the flour and cook, whisking constantly, for 1 to 2 minutes. Gradually whisk in the 2 cups reserved cooking liquid. Cook, whisking frequently, until thickened, 3 to 4 minutes. Slice the meat and serve hot.

Maibock/Helles Bock

"Helles" in German translates to "light" in English. Maibock or Helles Bock is a pale version of a traditional bock. The style is usually enjoyed in warmer weather in the Spring or Summer. The color should be light yellow to light amber to gold, with notable clarity. The aroma should have a solid hint of malt sweetness, with notes of bready yeast or toasted grains. Hop aroma should be low or absent. The taste should have a notable malt sweetness, like the aroma. Also, there should be very mild hop bitterness, with mild flavors of pepper or spices. Good with BBQ chicken and sausages.

Maibock / Helles Bock:	Key Characteristics	Notable Maibock
Attribute	Description	Einbecker Mai-Ur-Bock
ABV	6.3–7.4% — strong but smooth; warming without harshness2	Ayinger Maibock
IBU (Bitterness)	23–38 — moderate; more hop bitterness than other Bocks	Hofbräu Maibock
Color (SRM)	6–11 SRM — deep gold to light amber; brilliant clarity	Paulaner Maibock
Body	Medium — rounded and smooth with a dry edge	Victory St. Boisterous
Carbonation	Moderate to high — enhances crispness and aroma	Capital Maibock
Finish	Moderately dry — with lingering malt and subtle hop spice	Rogue Dead Guy Ale

Taste: Bready | Lightly Sweet | Spicy | Herbal | Peppery
Food Pairings: Smoked Pork or Ham | Roasted Chicken | Grilled Sausages | Nutty Desserts

Food Pairing Guide for Maibock

Maibock is a springtime German lager that combines the strength and malt richness of traditional Bock with a lighter color and a more assertive hop profile.

Grilled & Roasted Meats
- Grilled bratwurst or pork chops: The beer's malt sweetness balances the smoky edges.
- Roast chicken or turkey: Especially with herbs or citrus glazes.
- Lamb skewers or gyros: Earthy meat meets crisp finish.

Cheese Pairings
- Havarti or Fontina: Mild and buttery, echoing the beer's smoothness.
- Aged Gouda or Gruyère: Nutty depth complements Maibock's malt.
- Goat cheese: Tangy contrast to the beer's richness.

Fresh Spring Fare
- Asparagus with lemon butter: The beer's clean finish balances vegetal bitterness.
- Spring salads with vinaigrette: Crisp greens meet malty depth.
- Deviled eggs or egg salad: Rich and creamy with a refreshing contrast.

Breads & Sides
- Soft pretzels with mustard: Classic Bavarian pairing.
- Potato salad (German-style): Vinegar and bacon play well with Maibock's malt.
- Spaetzle or buttered noodles: Mild starches let the beer shine.

Sweet Pairings
- Apple tart or strudel: Fruit and spice echo the malt.
- Lemon bars or citrus cake: Bright flavors contrast the beer's depth.
- Shortbread cookies: Buttery and simple, perfect with a crisp lager.

Sausage & Pepper Flatbread Pizza

Pairing sausage & pepper flatbread pizza with a Maibock beer is a delicious way to balance spice, richness, and malt sweetness. Sausage brings savory fat and spice. Peppers add sweetness and a touch of heat. Flatbread crust is crisp and light, letting the toppings shine. A toasty malt backbone complements the caramelized sausage and roasted peppers. Subtle sweetness balances the spice and salt. Medium to full body stands up to bold toppings without overwhelming. The Maibock's malt echoes the roasted notes in the pizza. Its crisp carbonation lifts the richness of the sausage.

Ingredients:
2 Stone-Ground Whole-Wheat Wraps
6 Tbsp. pizza sauce
1 cup sweet mini peppers, sliced
½ cup pre-cooked turkey sausage crumbles
½ cup shredded mozzarella cheese
2 Tbsp. shredded Parmesan cheese

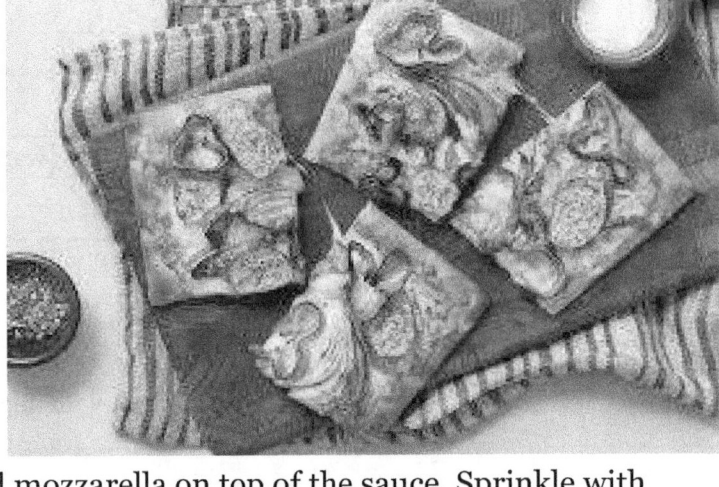

Instructions:
1. Preheat the oven to 350°F. Place Flat-out Flatbreads on a cookie sheet and bake for two minutes.
2. Remove from oven. Spread pizza sauce evenly over the flatbreads. Layer peppers, sausage, and mozzarella on top of the sauce. Sprinkle with Parmesan cheese. Return to the oven and bake for an additional 10-12 minutes.

Classic Tomato Bruschetta
1 baguette or rustic Italian bread, sliced into ½-inch thick pieces
4–5 ripe Roma tomatoes, finely diced
2–3 garlic cloves (1 for rubbing, the rest minced)
¼ cup fresh basil leaves, chopped
2 tbsp extra virgin olive oil
1 tbsp balsamic vinegar (optional)
Salt and freshly ground black pepper, to taste

For the bread:
Olive oil for brushing
Optional: pinch of sea salt or garlic powder

Also Pairs With		
Pale Ale	Pilsner	Christmas Ale

Preheat oven to 400°F. Brush bread slices lightly with olive oil. Toast on a baking sheet for 5–7 minutes until golden and crisp. Rub each slice with a cut garlic clove while warm for extra flavor. In a bowl, combine diced tomatoes, minced garlic, chopped basil, olive oil, and balsamic vinegar (if using). Season with salt and pepper. Let sit for 10–15 minutes to meld flavors. Spoon tomato mixture generously onto each toasted bread slice. Serve immediately so the bread stays crisp.

Doppelbock

"Doppel" meaning "double," this style is a bigger and stronger version of the lower-gravity German-style Bock beers. Originally made by monks in Munich, the Doppelbock beer style is very food-friendly and rich in melanoidins reminiscent of toasted bread. The color is copper to dark brown. Malty sweetness is dominant but should not be cloying. The malt character is more reminiscent of fresh and lightly toasted Munich-style malt than caramel or toffee malt. Doppelbocks are full-bodied, and alcoholic strength is on the higher end. Not only is this beer good with most barbecues, but it is great as an ingredient in popular barbecue sauces.

Doppelbock: Key Characteristics		Notable Doppelbock
Attribute	Description	Ayinger Celebrator Doppelbock
ABV	7.0–12.0% — high alcohol; warming and robust2	Paulaner Salvator
IBU (Bitterness)	16–26 — low to moderate; bitterness is clean and supportive	Weihenstephaner Korbinian
Color (SRM)	18–30 SRM — deep amber to dark brown; brilliant clarity with ruby highlights	Andechser Doppelbock Dunkel
Body	Full — velvety and rich with a smooth mouthfeel	Duck-Rabbator Doppelbock
Carbonation	Moderate — enhances drinkability without sharpness	Samuel Adams Double Bock
Finish	Malty and warming — with lingering notes of toast, caramel, and dark fruit	Double Vision Doppelbock

Taste: Carmel | Toffee | Bready | Malt-Forward | Dark Fruits
Food Pairings: Roast Pork or Game | Smoked Meats | Bread Pudding | Chocolate Cake

Food Pairing Guide for Doppelbock

Doppelbock is the malt-lover's powerhouse—a strong, full-bodied German lager originally brewed by monks as "liquid bread" to sustain them during fasting.

Hearty Meats & Roasts
- Braised short ribs: Fatty, tender meat meets malty sweetness.
- Roast duck or goose: Gamey flavors balanced by smooth malt.
- Beef stew or Sauerbraten: Tangy, savory, and perfect with a full-bodied beer.

Cheese Pairings
- Aged Gouda or Gruyère: Nutty and caramel-like, mirroring the beer's malt.
- Blue cheese: Sharp contrast to the beer's smooth richness.
- Triple cream Brie: Luxurious texture meets warming alcohol.

Comfort Foods
- Mushroom stroganoff: Umami and malt are a natural match.
- Shepherd's pie: Earthy and savory with a touch of sweetness.
- Spaetzle with gravy.

Breads & Sides
- Pretzels or rye bread: Toasty malt meets hearty grain.
- Red cabbage or sauerkraut: Tangy contrast to the malt.

Sweet Pairings
- Bread pudding with caramel sauce: Rich meets richer.
- Apple strudel or sticky toffee pudding: Fruit and sugar meet smooth malt.

Smoked Bologna and Pimiento Cheese Sandwich

This pairing is all about comfort meets complexity—a humble sandwich elevated by a regal beer. Smoked bologna brings salty, fatty richness with a hint of char. Pimiento cheese adds creamy texture, sharp cheddar bite, and a touch of peppery sweetness. A Doppelbock's rich caramel and toffee malt complements the smoky meat and sharp cheese. Full-bodied and low in bitterness, it won't clash with the sandwich's bold flavors. The beer's malt sweetness balances the salt and smoke of the bologna. Its depth mirrors the aged cheddar and pimiento tang, creating a flavor echo.

Ingredients:

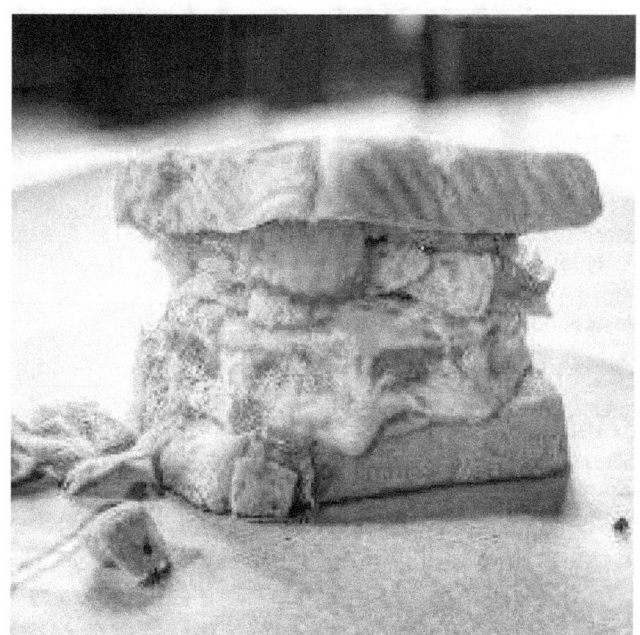

Pimiento Cheese:
16 ounces grated sharp Cheddar
8 ounces grated Monterey Jack or pepper jack cheese
3 ounces diced pimientos
1 1/4 cups mayonnaise, preferably Duke's
1/4 tsp. ground black pepper
1/8 tsp. cayenne pepper

Smoked Bologna Sandwich:
One 2-pound chub bologna
Butter, for buttering the bread
24 slices Texas toast
Barbecue sauce, yellow mustard, thin pickle slices, and corn chips, such as Fritos, for building sandwiches

Instructions:

For the pimiento cheese:
1. Add the cheese and pimientos to a mixing bowl, then add the mayo and mix. Add the seasoning and mix in. Cover and chill until it's cold, 1 hour.
2. Form the mixture into 12 pimiento cheese patties around the same diameter as the bologna and about 1/4-inch-thick. Set aside.

For the smoked bologna sandwich:
1. Slice the bologna chub into twenty-four 4-ounce, 1/2-inch-thick slabs.
2. Sear off the bologna on a hot flat top or in a hot cast-iron skillet, about 3 minutes. Alternatively, smoke for 30 minutes to 1 hour, flipping once.
3. Top the slice of bologna with a pimiento cheese slice. Cook until melted, then stack half the bologna slices with a second slice, with pimiento cheese slices on top. Butter the Texas toast and cook on a hot flat-top or in the hot cast-iron skillet until browned.
4. Spread liberal barbecue sauce and mustard on the Texas toast. Place pickles on the bottom toast. Place the bologna slices on top of the pickles. Add heaping handfuls of corn chips on top of the melted pimiento cheese and place toast on top to close the sandwiches.

Also Pairs With		
Cream Ale	American Wheat	Marzen

Eisbock

Eisbock is an extremely strong beer with a typical alcohol content well beyond 7% ABV. The brewing process involves freezing the beer to separate water from other components (alcohol and sugars). Because water freezes at a lower temperature than ethanol, the water ice is removed, leaving behind a more concentrated beer. Eisbock can range from near black to as light as tawny red. Hop bitterness takes a back seat, replaced by a big alcohol presence that can vary from sweet to spicy and fruity to fusel. Expect a heavy or almost syrupy body with tons of malty flavor.

Eisbock: Key Characteristics		Notable Eisbock
Attribute	Description	Schneider Aventinus Eisbock
ABV	7.0–14.0% — very high; warming and smooth despite strength	Ayinger St. Nikolaus Eisbock
IBU (Bitterness)	25–35 — low to moderate; bitterness is clean and subtle	Kulmbacher Eisbock
Color (SRM)	18–30 SRM — deep amber to near black; often with ruby highlights	Fassbender Eisbock
Body	Full to syrupy — velvety and rich with a luxurious mouthfeel	EKU 28
Carbonation	Low to moderate — supports smoothness and aroma	Alaskan Eisbock
Finish	Warming and lingering — with notes of dark fruit, toffee, and alcohol warmth	

Taste: Carmel | Toast | Port-Like | Spicy | Sweet | Malty
Food Pairing: Venison | Smoked Meats | Poultry | Short Ribs | Crème Brulee

Food Pairing Guide for Eisbock

Eisbock is a bold, rich, and warming beer created through a unique process called freeze distillation, where water is partially frozen and removed to concentrate the remaining liquid.

Rich & Roasted Meats
- Roast duck or goose: Gamey richness balanced by malt and alcohol warmth.
- Braised short ribs: Fatty, tender meat meets caramel and dried fruit notes.
- Smoked pork belly: Sweet glaze and char echo the beer's intensity.
- Venison or wild boar: Earthy and bold, perfect with Eisbock depth.

Bold Cheese Pairings
- Aged Gouda or Comté: Nutty and caramel-like, mirroring the beer's malt.
- Blue cheese or Roquefort: Sharp contrast to Eisbock sweetness.
- Triple cream Brie: Rich and buttery, softened by the beer's warmth.

Hearty Comfort Foods
- Beef Wellington: Pastry, mushroom duxelles, and tender beef match the beer's elegance.
- Mushroom stroganoff: Umami and cream meet malt and fruit.

Decadent Desserts
- Sticky toffee pudding: Rich meets richer.
- Chocolate lava cake or flourless torte: Cocoa and malt are a dream team.
- Bread pudding with bourbon sauce: Boozy, sweet, and indulgent.
- Caramel flan or crème Brulee: Silky textures and burnt sugar echo the beer's profile.

Stout Beer Chili Recipe

Stout beer in the chili adds roasted malt, coffee, and chocolate notes. Beans, beef, and spices create a rich, hearty base with layers of umami and heat. Eisbock sweetness balances the chili's spice, creating a smooth, rounded flavor experience. Concentrated caramel and dried fruit flavors soften the chili's spice and bitterness. Full-bodied and syrupy, it stands up to the chili's richness. Warming alcohol enhances the comfort factor without clashing with heat. Low bitterness ensures it doesn't compete with the stout's roasted edge.

Ingredients:
For The Chili:
2 Tbsp. olive oil
2 cups yellow onions, chopped (2 medium onions)
1½ tsp. salt and pepper
4 cloves garlic, minced
2 Tbsp. fresh oregano (or 1 tsp. dried)
⅓ cup chili powder
2 Tbsp. ground cumin
1 Tbsp. coriander
¾ tsp. cayenne
2 pounds lean ground beef (or ground turkey)
2 15-ounce cans kidney beans, drained & rinsed
1 28-ounce can fire roasted diced tomatoes
4 Tbsp. tomato paste
18 ounces stout beer (about 1 ½ bottles)
1-2 Tbsp. molasses (depending on your preferred sweetness)

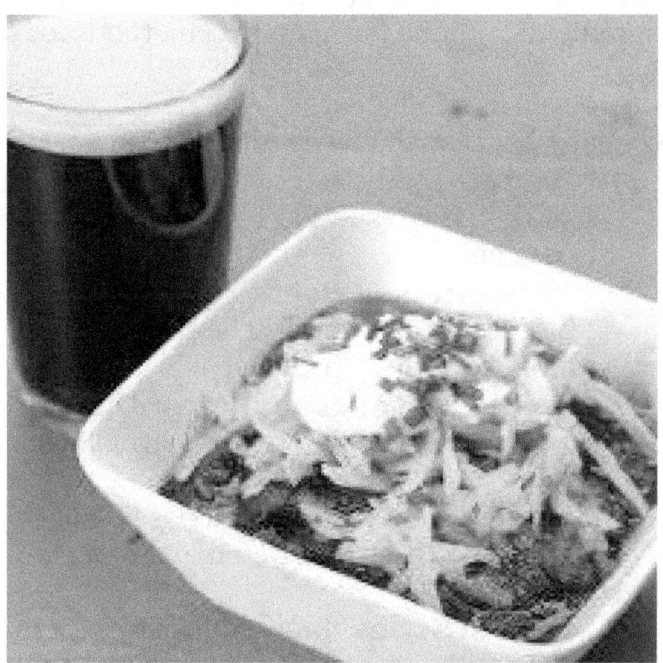

For Serving:
Shredded cheddar cheese
Sliced scallions
Sour cream
Cilantro
Fresh or jarred jalapenos

Also Pairs With

Dry Irish Stout	American Citrus IPA	Vienna Lager

Instructions:
1. Heat the oil in a large pot. Add the onions and season with ½ tsp. salt and pepper. Cook on medium high heat, stirring occasionally, until softened, about 6 minutes.
2. Stir in the garlic and oregano and cook for 1 more minute.
3. Add chili powder, cumin, coriander, and cayenne, and stir for about 1 minute.
4. Add the ground beef and another ½ tsp. salt & pepper. Break the meat into small pieces with a spatula and cook for 8 minutes or until the meat is no longer pink.
5. Stir in the kidney beans, diced tomatoes and the tomato paste, and bring to a simmer. Mix in the stout beer, molasses, and final ½ tsp. salt and pepper and return to a simmer.
6. Serve with shredded cheddar cheese, chopped green onions, cilantro, sour cream, and jalapenos.

Specialty Beers

Specialty beers are the adventurous heart of the brewing world—crafted with intention, creativity, and often a touch of rebellion. Unlike mass-produced lagers or standard ales, specialty beers push boundaries in flavor, style, and technique. They're brewed to stand out, whether through rare ingredients, unique fermentation methods, or seasonal inspiration.

A Spectrum of Styles
Specialty beers span a wide range of categories, each offering its own story and sensory experience:
- **Barrel-Aged Beers**: These are matured in oak barrels that once held bourbon, wine, or other spirits. The result is a complex blend of wood, vanilla, and alcohol warmth layered over the base beer.
- **Fruit-Infused Beers**: From tart cherry lambics to juicy mango lagers, fruit additions bring brightness and depth. They're especially popular in summer and among those seeking a lighter, more refreshing profile.
- **Spiced and Seasonal Ales**: Think cinnamon-laced Christmas ales, pumpkin-spiced fall brews, or coriander-kissed spring Saisons. These beers evoke the flavors and moods of the calendar.
- **High-Gravity Brews**: Styles like barleywine, wheat wine, and doppelbock boast elevated alcohol content and rich malt character. They're ideal for slow sipping and often improve with age.
- **Hybrid Styles**: Brewers love to experiment—blending sour techniques with stouts, crossing IPAs with lagers, or fermenting with wild yeasts for funky, unpredictable results.

The Art of Innovation
Specialty beers are often brewed in small batches, allowing for experimentation and refinement. Brewers might use heirloom grains, local honey, smoked malts, or even botanicals like lavender and spruce tips. Some are collaborations between breweries; others are one-off releases tied to festivals or anniversaries.

Pairing Possibilities
These beers shine at the dinner table. A barrel-aged stout complements chocolate cake; a Saison with citrus zest elevates grilled seafood; a spiced winter ale warms up roast pork and root vegetables. Specialty beers invite thoughtful pairing and elevate casual meals into culinary experiences.

Where to Begin?
For newcomers, start with a seasonal release from a local brewery or a well-known specialty like Sierra Nevada Bigfoot Barleywine, The Bruery's White Chocolate Wheatwine, or Great Lakes Christmas Ale. Visit taprooms, attend beer festivals, and don't be afraid to ask for tasting flights—exploration is part of the fun.

SPECIALTY & FOOD PAIRINGS

Beer	Food
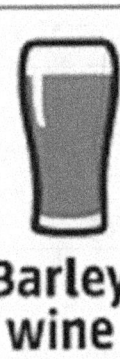 Barley wine	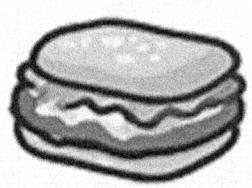 Cheesesteak
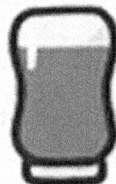 Scotch Ale	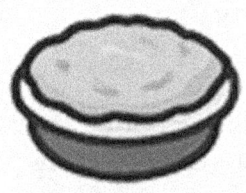 Shepherd's pie
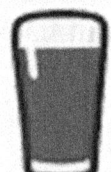 Altbier	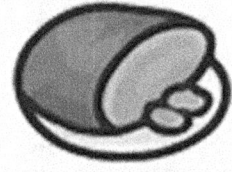 Roast beef
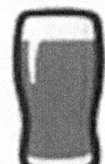 Wheat wine	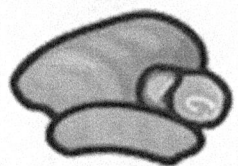 Smoked salmon
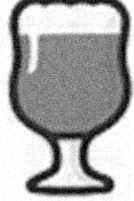 Strong Ale	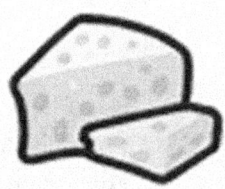 Blue cheese
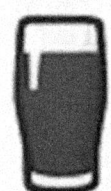 Christmas Ale	 Gingerbread
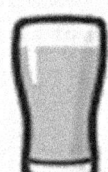 Kölsch	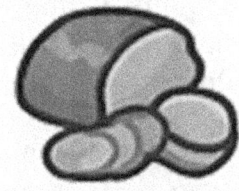 Roast beef
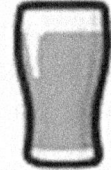 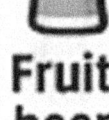 Fruit beer	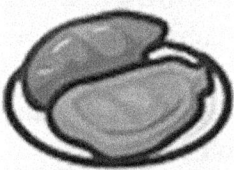 Chocolate cake

Barleywines Ales

The riches and strongest of British ales. Typically enjoyed in a snifter for its warming qualities. High Alcohol content. Strength of flavor often overpowers main dishes; better suited as a complement with strong cheeses or rich, sweet chocolate and caramel desserts. This goes great with, and things slowly roasted.

English Barleywine: Key Characteristics		Notable Barleywines
Attribute	**Description**	Revolution Straight Jacket
ABV	8–12%	Sierra Nevada Bigfoot
IBU (Bitterness)	35–70	Anchor Old Foghorn
Color (SRM)	8–22 (light copper to dark brown)	Bourbon County Barleywine
Body	Full and chewy	Old Backus Barleywine
Carbonation	Low to moderate	
Finish	Malty and warming	

Taste: Caramel | Toffee | Molasses | Bread Crust | Dried Fruit | Sherry-like
Food Pairings: Roast Beef | Lamb | Chocolate | Hearty Stews

Food Pairing Guide for Barleywine Ales
Barleywine Ales are bold, boozy, and packed with complex malt character. Despite the name, they're very much beer, not wine, but they share wine-like strength and aging potential.

Bold & Rich Meats
- Braised short ribs or oxtail: Fatty, slow-cooked meats match the beer's intensity.
- Roast duck or lamb: Gamey flavors complement the ale's dried fruit and caramel notes.
- Smoked brisket or pork belly: Sweet glaze and char echo the beer's malt backbone.
- Steak with blue cheese butter: Sharp, funky contrast to the beer's warmth.

Cheese Pairings
- Aged cheddar or Stilton: Sharpness cuts through the sweetness.
- Gorgonzola or Roquefort: Funky and rich, perfect with American-style Barleywine.
- Parmesan or aged Gouda: Nutty and crystalline, echoing the beer's depth.

Hearty Comfort Foods
- Beef stew or chili: Especially with smoky or spicy notes.
- Mushroom risotto: Earthy umami meets malt complexity.
- Shepherd's pie or meatloaf: Classic comfort with bold flavor.

Decadent Desserts
- Sticky toffee pudding: Rich meets richer.
- Carrot cake with cream cheese frosting: Spice and sweetness play off the malt.
- Chocolate torte or flourless cake: Cocoa and alcohol are a dream team.
- Bread pudding with bourbon sauce.

Rancher's Texas Chili Recipe (Chili con Carne)

Texas-style chili is all about beef, spice, and depth—no beans, just slow-simmered meat with bold chili peppers and smoky seasoning. It's rich, hearty, and often fiery, with layers of umami and a touch of bitterness from tomato and spice. Barleywine's high ABV (8–12%+) gives it warming power to match the chili's heat. Its rich malt backbone with notes of caramel, toffee, and dried fruit balances the spice and salt. The beer's sweetness tames the chili's heat, creating a smoother flavor experience. Its intensity matches the dish's richness, so neither gets lost. If the chili includes smoked or grilled meat, the beer's toasty malt echoes those flavors beautifully.

Ingredients:

Chili Paste Starter:
3 Tbsp each: ancho chili powder AND cornmeal
1 Tbsp each: chipotle chili powder, ground cumin, cocoa powder, smoked paprika
2 tsp each: ground coriander, Mexican oregano

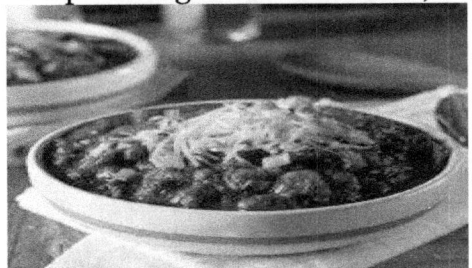

Texas Chili:
3 ½ -4 pounds stew meat (or chuck roast cut into 1 - 1¼ inch chunks)
2 Tbsp. each: oil & Worcestershire sauce
1 large onion, diced
2 poblano peppers, diced (or bell peppers)
1-5 jalapeno, minced
8-12 cloves garlic, minced
1 Tbsp. brown sugar
4 cups beef broth*
1 (14-ounce can) tomato sauce
2 (14-ounce) cans rinsed/drained pinto beans

Instructions:

1. **PASTE:** Combine the ingredients for the paste in a small bowl and slowly stir in 1/2 cup of hot water. Mix and set this aside for now.
2. **SEAR THE MEAT:** Season the meat with a generous pinch of salt and pepper. Heat a large chili pot over medium-high heat. Add 1 Tbsp. of oil to the pot and add a few pieces of meat at a time. Sear the meat on all sides, about 2-3 minutes and remove it to a plate. Repeat the process until all the meat is seared. You may need a little more oil than what's listed just depending on how well marbled the meat is.
3. **CHILI:** If you need it, add another drizzle of oil to the pan along with the chopped onions and the poblanos. Use a wooden spoon to help scrape any brown bits left behind by the meat and cook for 5 minutes. Then, add the garlic and jalapeno and continue to cook for another 1-2 minutes or until fragrant. Add the prepared chili paste to the pot and stir it in so that it coats everything nicely. Allow the paste to cook for 1 minute before adding the brown sugar, Worcestershire, beef broth, tomato sauce, 1 cup water and ½ tsp. salt. Use the wooden spoon to scrape the bottom so that none of the chili paste sticks.
4. **COOK:** Add the seared meat and allow the chili to come to a boil before lowering the heat to low and allowing it to cook for 2 ½ - 3 ½ hours. Set aside 1 cup of water and add in a ¼ cup every time you stir the chili if it's thickened. Stir the chili every 30-45 minutes to make sure it's not stick. You may not need all the water if you're going bean-free; with beans you need a little more. I like to add beans around the 2-hour mark so that they cook for at least half an hour before serving. Serve topped with all your favorite chili toppings.

Also Pairs With		
Smoked Porter	Robust Porter	Mexican-Style Dark Lager

English Ale

English Pale Ale originated when breweries started using pale barley malt, resulting in lighter brews. This style balances hop bitterness and malty sweetness. They're brewed to be sessionable, flavorful, and deeply tied to British pub culture.

English Barleywine: Key Characteristics		Notable English Ale
Attribute	Description	Newcastle Brown Ale
ABV	4.5–5.5%	Fuller's ESB
IBU (Bitterness)	20–40	Timothy Taylor's Landlord
Color (SRM)	5-12 (light copper to dark brown)	Samuel Smith's Old Brewery Pale Ale
Body	Full and chewy, with a velvety texture	Adnams Southwold Bitter
Carbonation	Low to moderate	Theakston Old Peculier
Finish	Caramel undertones, floral hops	Wychwood Hobgoblin

Taste: Malty | Nutty | Caramel | Bready | Fruity || Earthy
Food Pairings: Fish & Chips | Roast Beef | Banger & Mash | Steak & Ale Pie

Food Pairing Guide for English Ale

English Ales are the soul of British brewing—rich in tradition, layered in flavor, and brewed for balance and drinkability.

Classic British Dishes
- Fish and Chips. The ale's light carbonation and earthy bitterness cut through the crispy batter and complement the salt and vinegar.
- Steak and Ale Pie. Deep roasted malt flavors mirror caramelized beef and rich gravy, creating a seamless experience.
- Roast Beef & Yorkshire Pudding. The beer's malty base supports the savory roast while its dry finish balances the fluffy pudding and gravy.
- Bangers & Mash. Malty sweetness enhances the savory sausage and cuts through onion gravy.

Cheese Pairings
- Ploughman's Lunch. Ale won't overpower cheddar, pickles, or chutney. For stronger cheeses, switch to a porter or stout.
- English Cheddar or Stilton. The malt sweetness complements aged cheese, while bitterness balances richness.

Hearty Comfort Foods
- Shepherd's Pie. The ale's light body and subtle hops match the dish's earthy meat and potato layers.
- Chicken & Mushroom Pie. Caramel malt and floral hops enhance the umami of mushrooms and the richness of pastry.
- Roast Lamb. Herbal hop notes and a robust malt base pair beautifully with rosemary-seasoned lamb.

Breads & Sides
- Crusty Bread & Pickles. Earthy malt tones balance tangy pickles and hearty bread.
- Savory Pastries (Pork Pies, Sausage Rolls) The ale's bitterness cuts through fat while malt complements the filling.

London Broil

London Broil is typically made with marinated flank or top round steak, grilled, or broiled and sliced thin. The marinade often includes soy sauce, garlic, vinegar, and herbs, adding tang and umami. The meat is lean but flavorful, with a charred exterior and juicy interior. Moderate bitterness from earthy hops balances the meat's richness. Toasty, caramel-like malts complement the charred edges and marinade sweetness. Low carbonation and smooth body make it easy to sip alongside grilled meats. Styles like English Bitter, Pale Ale, or ESB offer just enough backbone without overpowering.

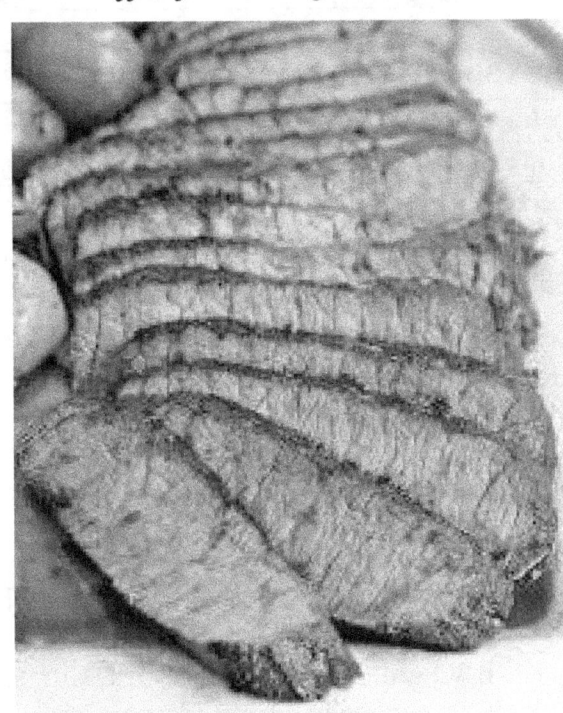

Ingredients:
1 (3 lb.) top round roast
1 Tbsp. salt
1/2 tsp. ground black pepper
2 tsp. granulated garlic
2 tsp. onion powder
8 Tbsp. salted butter (1 stick), room temperature
1 tsp. soy sauce
3 Tbsp. olive oil

Instructions:
1. Using a sharp knife, on both the top and bottom, make shallow diagonal slices across the roast, about ⅛-inch deep. Repeat in the opposite direction to create hash marks.
2. In a small bowl, combine salt, pepper, garlic powder, and onion powder. Divide the mixture evenly between top and bottom and rub into hash marks.
3. Transfer the roast to a wire rack fitted onto a sheet pan. Refrigerate roast at least 30 minutes or for up to three days, uncovered.
4. Meanwhile, in a small bowl, combine butter and soy sauce. Refrigerate until ready to use.
5. Remove the roast from the refrigerator. Let's stand while the oven is preheated.
6. Preheat the oven to 420°F.
7. In a large, oven-proof skillet, heat olive oil over medium-high heat until it shimmers. Place the roast in the pan. Sear on one side, for about 3 minutes.
8. Flip the roast over and place the pan in the oven.
9. Roast 10-12 minutes or until an instant-read thermometer inserted into the thickest part of the roast registers 130°F for medium-rare, or until the desired temperature is reached based on the chart below.
10. Remove the pan from the oven. Let it stand for 10 minutes. Transfer the roast to a cutting board. Top roast with pan drippings and the soy sauce butter. Slice thinly against the grain and serve.

Also Pairs With		
Golden Stron Ale	Czech Amber Lager	Honey Blonde Ale

American Ale

American ale beers are medium-bodied beers with a focus on hop flavor and aroma. They display floral, fruity, citrus-like, piney, and resinous American hops. The malt profile includes low to medium caramel, providing a balanced backdrop. APAs are often clean-fermented with ale yeast.

American Ale: Key Characteristics		Notable American Ale
Attribute	**Description**	Sierra Nevada Pale Ale
ABV	4.3–6.2%	Dale's Pale Ale
IBU (Bitterness)	20–40	Sierra Nevada Pale Ale
Color (SRM)	18–35	Stone Pale Ale 2.0
Body	Full and chewy, with a velvety texture	Fat Tire Amber Ale
Carbonation	Low to moderate	Dale's Pale Ale
Finish	Caramel undertones, floral hops	Deschutes Mirror Pond

Taste: Citrus | Pine Hops | Light Caramel Malt High Carbonation
Food Pairings: Grilled Chicken | Roast Vegetables | Fish Tacos | Smoked Brisket | Pecan Pie

Food Pairing Guide for American Ales
American Ales are the flag bearers of U.S. craft brewing—bold, hop-forward, and endlessly adaptable.

Savory & Grilled Dishes
- Grilled burgers with cheddar: The beer's hops cut through the fat and enhance the cheese's sharpness.
- BBQ chicken or pulled pork: Citrusy hops brighten smoky sweetness.
- Fish tacos with lime crema: Crisp bitterness balances citrus and spice.
- Grilled bratwurst or sausages: Toasty malt complements savory links.

Spicy & Zesty Fare
- Buffalo wings: Hops cool the spice, while malt echoes the sauce's sweetness.
- Spicy Thai noodles: Refreshing contrast to chili and peanut sauce.
- Jambalaya or Cajun shrimp: Earthy spice meets citrusy hops.
- Street tacos with salsa Verde: Bright, herbal flavors match the beer's profile.

Cheese Pairings
- Sharp cheddar: Classic match for APA's malt and hops.
- Goat cheese: Tangy contrast to citrusy bitterness.
- Pepper jack: Spice and creaminess balance the beer's edge.

Fresh & Light Dishes
- Grilled vegetable skewers: Charred edges meet crisp hops.
- Cobb salad with vinaigrette: Bitterness balances tangy dressing and bacon.
- Avocado toast with chili flakes: Creamy and spicy, perfect with a pale ale.

Sweet Pairings
- Lemon bars or citrus tarts: Echo the beer's bright notes.
- Shortbread cookies: Buttery simplicity meets crisp finish.
- Apple crisp: Toasty malt complements baked fruit.

Oven Fried Nashville Hot Chicken

Nashville Hot Chicken is spicy, cayenne-heavy coating delivers serious heat. Oven-fried method keeps it crispy without deep-frying, but still rich and savory. Often served with pickles and white bread, adding tang and softness. Bright citrus and piney hops cut through the heat and fat. Moderate bitterness balances the cayenne's burn without overwhelming. The light malt backbone complements the chicken's crust and seasoning. Carbonation and a dry finish refresh the palate after each fiery bite.

Ingredients:

Marinade
2 cups of buttermilk
1/4 cup pickle brine
2 tsp. Cajun seasoning salt
1/3 cup of hot sauce

Oven Fried Chicken
3 large chicken breasts . cut lengthwise and then widthwise
4 cups of cornflakes
1/4 cup of all-purpose flour
2 tsp. salt
1 tsp. cayenne
olive oil for brushing

Hot Chicken Cayenne Glaze
4 Tbsp. cayenne
2 Tbsp. brown sugar
1 Tbsp. smoked paprika
1 tsp. garlic powder
1 tsp. chili powder
1 tsp. onion powder
1 tsp. Cajun seasoning salt
pickles and white bread ... optional but highly suggested
3/4 cup vegetable oil
4 Tbsp. of butter

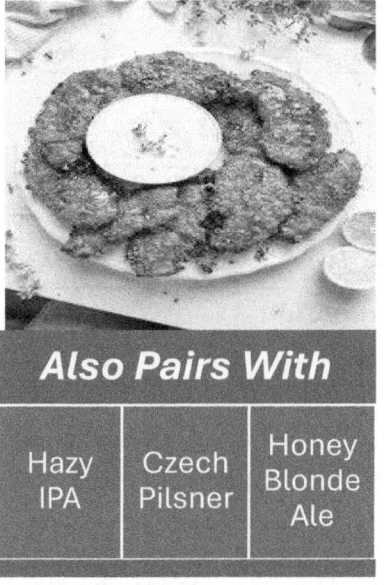

Also Pairs With

| Hazy IPA | Czech Pilsner | Honey Blonde Ale |

Instructions:

Marinade
To make your Oven Fried Nashville Hot Chicken, start with the marinade. Whisk together buttermilk, pickle brine, your favorite hot sauce and two tsp. of Cajun seasoning salt and then pour it into a large zip-top bag. Cut your chicken breasts lengthwise and then in half (across) and add them to the buttermilk marinade. Push out the excess air, seal the bag, and move your chicken to the refrigerator to marinate for at least six hours, but overnight is best.

Oven Fried Chicken
Once your chicken is marinated, remove your chicken breasts from the buttermilk and move to a baking rack to drain. Add cornflakes to a food processor and pulse to create cornflake crumbs. Move your cornflake crumbs to a large bowl and stir in the all-purpose flour along with cayenne and salt. Preheat your oven to 450 degrees and line a baking pan with parchment paper or tinfoil. Dredge the chicken pieces in the cornflake crumbs, pressing firmly to adhere the crumbs to all sides of the chicken. Move the coated chicken to the baking pan and repeat until all chicken pieces are coated in cornflakes. Lightly brush each of the chicken pieces with olive oil and bake for 20-25 minutes, turning your chicken over halfway through the cooking time and continuing cooking.

Hot Chicken Cayenne Glaze
As your oven fried chicken is baking, make your hot chicken cayenne glaze. In a small saucepan, add vegetable oil and butter, and heat over medium heat. Increase its temperature slightly until you just see little bubbles form. Whisk together your spices in a separate bowl and then slowly start whisking

into your heated oil. Once your oven fried chicken is done, remove from the oven and, using a basting brush, coat both sides of your chicken in the cayenne glaze. Serve with pickles.

Strong Ales

Strong ale is a type of ale, usually above 5% ABV and often higher, between 7% to 11% ABV, which spans several beer styles, including old ale, barley wine, and Burton ale. Strong Ales are brewed throughout Europe and beyond, including in England, Belgium, and the United States. Pair the Ale, with slow cooked meats, pit beef, lamb, game grilled or smoked.

Strong Ales: Key Characteristics		Notable Strong Ales
Attribute	Description	Kentucky Bourbon Barrel Ale
ABV	7.0–11.3% (can reach 20% in American styles)	Arrogant Bastard Ale
IBU (Bitterness)	30–65 (British); 40–100 (American)	Old Ruffian
Color (SRM)	8–21 (Amber to dark brown)	Old Stock Ale
Body	Medium to full	Double Bastard Ale
Carbonation	Moderate to low	Wicked Weed Oblivion
Finish	Warming, often sweet or vinous	

Taste: Carmel | Toffee | Molasses | Bready | Earthy
Food Pairings: Chinese Food | Hearty Stews | Prime Rib | Lamb | Duck | Barbecue

Food Pairing Guide for Strong Ales

Strong Ales are not for the faint of palate—they're contemplative, complex, and often best enjoyed slowly.

Hearty & Bold Meats
- Roast beef or prime rib: The beer's malt sweetness complements the meat's caramelized crust.
- Smoked brisket or pork shoulder: Bold flavors meet the ale's warming depth.
- Duck or venison: Gamey meats match the beer's earthy complexity.
- Lamb chops with rosemary: Herbal notes play off the ale's spice and malt.

Cheese Pairings
- Aged cheddar or Stilton: Sharp and salty contrast to the beer's sweetness.
- Gorgonzola or Roquefort: Funky and bold, ideal for American or Belgian strong ales.
- Triple cream Brie: Rich and buttery, softened by the beer's warmth.

Comfort Foods & Rich Dishes
- Beef stew or pot roast: Deep flavors echo the ale's malt and spice.
- Mushroom risotto: Earthy umami meets warming alcohol.
- Shepherd's pie or meatloaf: Classic comfort with bold flavor.
- Barbecue ribs with a sweet glaze: Caramelized edges match the beer's body.

Decadent Desserts
- Sticky toffee pudding: Rich meets richer.
- Chocolate lava cake or flourless torte: Cocoa and alcohol are a dream team.
- Bread pudding with bourbon sauce: Boozy, sweet, and luxurious.
- Caramel flan or crème Brulee: Silky textures and burnt sugar echo the beer's profile.

Chicken in Ale Sauce

Chicken in Ale Sauce is typically made with tender chicken simmered in a rich, malty ale-based gravy, often with onions, herbs, and a touch of sweetness. The sauce is deep and savory, with caramelized notes from the ale and pan drippings. Strong Ale with High ABV (usually 7–11%) adds warming depth and richness. Its robust malt character (caramel, toffee, dried fruit) mirrors the sauce's sweetness and browning. The beer's malt sweetness echoes the sauce's caramelized flavors, creating a seamless match. The ale's depth and body stand up to the richness of the gravy, without overwhelming the chicken's delicate texture. If the dish is made with the same beer style, the pairing becomes even more cohesive and layered. making each bite feel fresh.

Ingredients:
4 tsp. cooking oil
6 skinless and boneless chicken breast halves
1/3 cup chopped yellow onion
2 ½ cups chopped mushrooms
1 ¼ cups chicken broth
1/3 cup brown ale
4 tsp. white wine Worcestershire sauce
1 Tbsp. snipped fresh thyme
1/4 tsp. salt
1/4 tsp. freshly ground black pepper
3 Tbsp. all-purpose flour

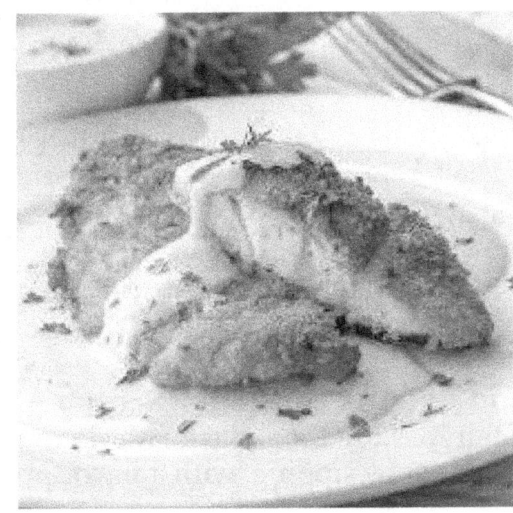

Instructions:
1. In a large nonstick skillet, heat the cooking oil. Add chicken and brown in hot oil over medium-high heat, turning the chicken once, to brown on all sides. Stir in mushrooms, 3/4 cup chicken broth, beer, Worcestershire sauce, and thyme. Season with salt and black pepper.
2. Remove the cooked chicken and transfer it to a serving platter. Cover with aluminum foil to keep warm.
3. In a mixing bowl, combine the remaining chicken broth and all-purpose flour. Stir well. Add to skillet. Cook, stirring, until thickened and bubbly. Pour ale sauce over the chicken and serve.

Honey Glazed Parsnips
1 ½ lbs. parsnips, peeled and cut into batons (like thick fries)
2 tbsp butter (or olive oil for a lighter version)
2 tbsp honey
1 tbsp brown sugar
Salt and freshly ground black pepper, to taste
1 tsp fresh thyme leaves (or ½ tsp dried thyme)

Also Pairs With		
English Bitter	Helles Lager	English Porter

Prep the Parsnips. Preheat the oven to 400°F. Peel the parsnips and trim the ends. If they're large, cut them in half lengthwise and then into evenly sized sticks. In a bowl, toss the parsnips with butter (or oil), honey, and brown sugar. Season with salt, pepper, and thyme. Spread evenly on a parchment-lined baking sheet — don't overcrowd. Roast for 25–30 minutes, turning once halfway through, until golden, caramelized, and slightly crisp on the edges. Drizzle lightly with more honey.

Scotch Ale

Scotch ale is a style of beer originating in Scotland that is fermented with ale yeast. Low in bitterness with rich malt sweetness, the caramel-colored beer often uses a pale malt base backed by darker malts. Though it can vary, many are comparable to English barley wine. Some American interpretations of Scotch ales are paired and smoky brisket.

Scotch Ales: Key Characteristics		Notable Scotch Ale
Attribute	Description	Founders Backwoods Bastard
ABV	6.0–10.0%	Belhaven Scottish Ale
IBU (Bitterness)	15–30 (low to moderate)	Founders Dirty Bastard
Color (SRM)	13–22 (deep amber to dark brown)	Traquair House Ale
Body	Medium to full	Orkney Skull Splitter
Carbonation	Low to moderate	Oskar Blues Old Chub
Finish	Malty, warm, often slightly sweet	Odell 90 Shilling Ale

Taste: Carmel | Toffee | Brown Sugar | Toasty | Smokey | Dark Fruit
Food Pairings: Roast Lamb | Duck | Smoked Brisket

Food Pairing Guide for Scotch Ales

Scotch Ales are the malt-forward monarchs of Scottish brewing tradition. They're rich, warm, and built for slow sipping, with a flavor profile that's all about depth and caramelized complexity.

Hearty & Savory Meats
- Roast lamb or beef: The beer's caramel notes complement the meat's char and richness.
- Smoked sausage or kielbasa: Smoky fat meets malty sweetness.
- Grilled pork chops with apple glaze: Sweet and savory harmony.
- Venison or duck: Gamey meat matches the ale's earthy depth.

Cheese Pairings
- Aged cheddar or Gouda: Sharp and caramel-like, echoing the malt.
- Smoked cheese: Enhances the beer's roasted character.
- Brie or Camembert: Creamy contrast to the beer's warmth.

Comfort Foods & Pub Fare
- Shepherd's pie or meatloaf: Classic comfort with malty depth.
- Beef stew or pot roast: Slow-cooked richness meets smooth sweetness.
- Scotch eggs: Savory and crispy, perfect with a Wee Heavy.
- Mushroom risotto: Earthy umami pairs beautifully with roasted malt.

Breads & Sides
- Rye or brown bread: Toasty grains echo the beer's malt.
- Roasted root vegetables: Caramelized edges match the ale's sweetness.
- Mashed potatoes with gravy: Creamy and hearty, ideal with a full-bodied beer.

Sweet Pairings
- Sticky toffee pudding: Rich meets richer.
- Pecan pie or bread pudding: Nutty and sweet, perfect with malt.
- Chocolate cake or brownies: Cocoa and caramel are a dream team.

Brown Sugar Glazed Pork Chops

Brown sugar glaze adds caramelized sweetness and a sticky, rich coating. Pork chops bring savory, slightly fatty meat with a mild flavor that absorbs glaze beautifully. Often grilled or pan-seared, adding charred edges and depth. Rich malt profile with notes of caramel, toffee, and roasted grain mirrors the glaze's sweetness. Low bitterness ensures it doesn't clash with the sugary crust. Full body and warm alcohol stand up to the pork's richness and enhance its flavor. Subtle smoky undertones in some Scotch Ales echo the seared or grilled meat.

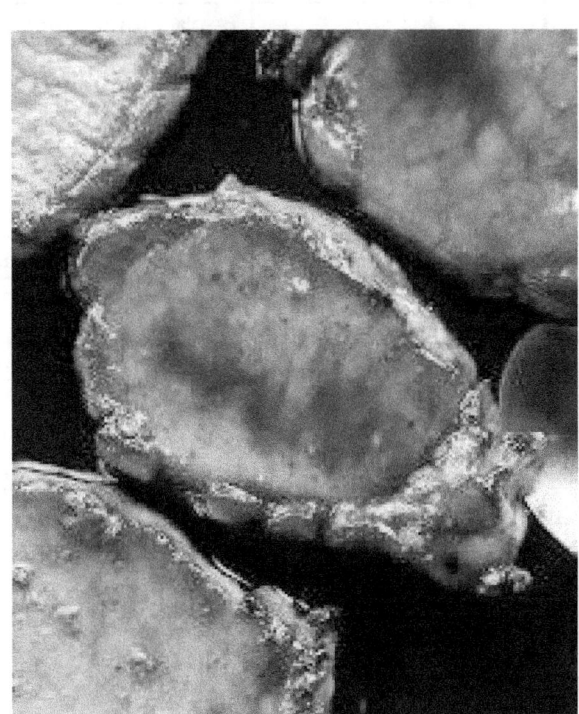

Ingredients:
4 bone-in thick cut pork chops
2 Tbsp. flour
2 tsp. smoked paprika
1 ½ tsp. salt
½ tsp. ground black pepper
Olive oil
3 Tbsp. white wine vinegar
3 tsp. soy sauce
3 Tbsp. brown sugar
3 tsp. Dijon mustard

Instructions:
1. Pat the pork chops dry with a clean kitchen towel. Combine the flour, smoked paprika, salt and freshly ground black pepper in a shallow dish. Dredge all sides of the pork chops with the seasoned flour.
2. Heat a large skillet over medium-high heat. Add enough olive oil to coat the pan and sear the pork chops until evenly browned, about 2 minutes per side. Sear the edges of the pork chops as well.
3. Reduce the heat to medium-low and cover the pan with a lid. Cook the pork chops over low heat for 6 to 10 minutes until they reach an internal temperature of 145°F with an instant-read thermometer inserted into the center of the chops. (Timing will depend on the thickness of the pork chops.) Transfer the chops to a plate and cover them loosely with aluminum foil.
4. Turn the heat under the pan up to medium and add the white wine vinegar, soy sauce, brown sugar, and Dijon mustard. Whisk the ingredients together and bring the mixture to a boil. Lower the heat and return the pork chops to the pan. Coat both sides of the pork chops with the glaze and cook for another minute. Season with freshly ground black pepper.

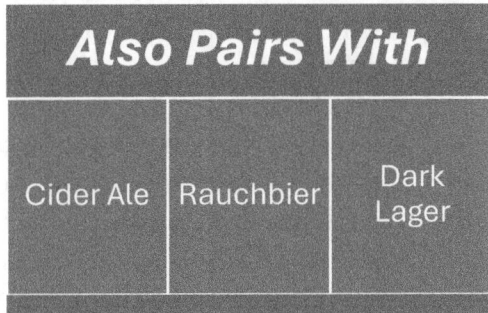

Also Pairs With

Cider Ale	Rauchbier	Dark Lager

Christmas Ale

A stronger, darker spiced beer that often has a rich body and warming finish suggesting a pleasant accompaniment for the wintry weather season. Pair with heavy smoked meat, brisket, pit beef, and beef ribs.

Christmas Ales: Key Characteristics		Notable Christmas Ales
Attribute	**Description**	Great Lakes Christmas Ale
ABV	6–9% (some go higher for extra warmth)	Anchor Christmas Ale
IBU (Bitterness)	15–35 (low to moderate)	Delirium Noël
Color (SRM)	10–30 (amber to deep brown)	Sierra Nevada Celebration Ale
Body	Medium to full	Bell's Christmas Ale
Carbonation	Moderate	St. Bernardus Christmas Ale
Finish	Malty, sweet, often spiced, or vinous	

Taste: Complex | Honey | Ginger | Cinnamon | Carmel | Orange Peel
Food Pairings: Roast Turkey or Ham | Stuffing | Fruitcake | Christmas Cookies

Food Pairing Guide for Christmas Ales
Christmas Ales are the liquid embodiment of holiday cheer—rich, spiced, and brewed to warm you from the inside out.

Hearty & Festive Mains
- Roast beef or prime rib: The beer's sweetness and spice echo the meat's caramelized crust.
- Glazed ham with cloves or brown sugar: the sweet and spiced glaze matches the ale's festive notes.
- Roast turkey with stuffing: Earthy herbs and savory meat pair beautifully with warming spices.
- Duck or goose: Gamey richness meets the beer's depth and warmth.

Cheese Pairings
- Aged cheddar or Stilton: Sharp and salty contrast to the ale's sweetness.
- Brie with cranberry compote: Creamy and tangy, perfect with spiced malt.
- Smoked Gouda or blue cheese: Adds depth and funk to match the beer's complexity.

Seasonal Sides & Breads
- Stuffing with herbs and sausage: Savory and aromatic, ideal with spiced ale.
- Sweet potato casserole: Caramelized sweetness complements the malt.
- Cranberry sauce: Tart contrasts with the beer's richness.
- Gingerbread or molasses bread: Echoes the ale's spice and body.

Holiday Desserts
- Fruitcake or plum pudding: Dried fruit and spice mirror the beer's profile.
- Gingerbread cookies: Spiced and sweet, a perfect match.
- Pecan pie or apple crisp: Nutty and caramelized flavors pair beautifully.
- Chocolate yule log: Rich cocoa meets warming malt.

Baked Ham with Pineapple and Brown Sugar Glaze

Baked Ham with Pineapple & Brown Sugar Glaze creates a caramelized crust. Salty, smoky ham provides a rich, savory base. Pineapple's acidity adds brightness and contrast. The dish is bold, sweet-savory, and holiday-ready. Christmas Ale is typically brewed with warming spices like cinnamon, clove, nutmeg, and orange peel. Rich malt backbone offers caramel, toffee, and toasted bread notes. Medium to full body stands up to the ham's richness. Low to moderate bitterness keeps the pairing smooth and festive.

Ingredients:

For the Ham:
8-10 lb. smoked ham, fully cooked
20 oz. can pineapple rings, save juice
6 oz. jar maraschino cherries, save juice

Pineapple Brown Sugar Glaze:
juice from canned pineapple rings
juice from maraschino cherries
1/3 cup pure honey
1/4 cup yellow mustard
1/4 cup brown sugar, dark or light
1/4 tsp ground nutmeg
1 tsp ground cinnamon
1/4 tsp ground ginger
1/4 tsp ground clove
1/4 cup cornstarch

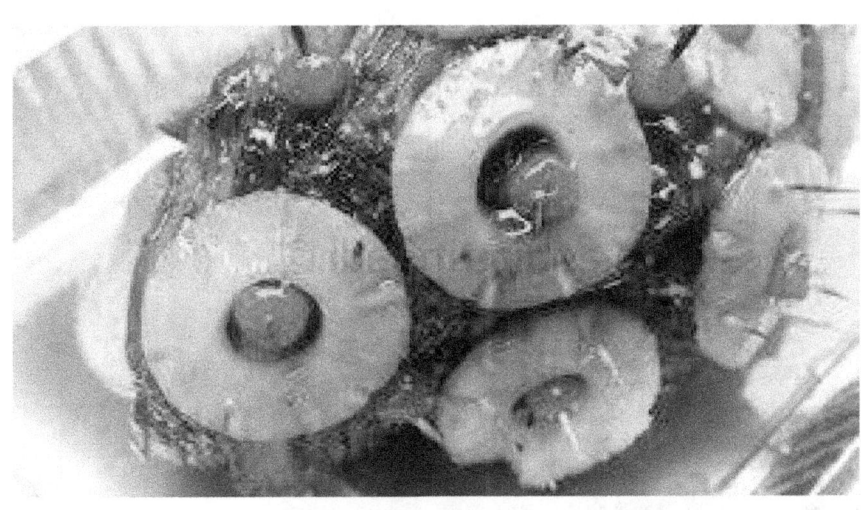

Also Pairs With		
Vienna Lager	Golden Strong Ale	Fruited Sour Lambric

Instructions:
1. Preheat oven to 325 F. Make sure that the ham is completely thawed.
2. Decorate the ham with pineapples and cherries, using the toothpicks to hold everything in place.
3. In a large measuring cup or bowl, combine the pineapple juice, cherry juice, brown sugar, mustard, honey, ginger, clove, nutmeg, and cinnamon. Stir everything, then sprinkle in the cornstarch. Whisk everything until lump free, then transfer the sauce/glaze to a saucepan.
4. Bring the sauce to a boil over medium-high heat and whisk constantly. Let boil for about 3-5 minutes, then turn the heat off. Pour the glaze all over the ham.
5. Bake the ham, uncovered, for 30 minutes.
6. Remove the ham from the oven and baste and extra glaze and pan juices.
7. Place it back in the oven for 20-30 minutes (still uncovered).
8. Remove from the oven and let the ham sit for about 15 minutes.

Weizen

Weizenbier, also known as Hefeweizen, is a traditional German beer style that originates from Bavaria. Weizenbier (German for "white beer") is a beer in which a significant proportion of malted barley is replaced with malted wheat. By law, Weissbier brewed in Germany must use a "top-fermenting" yeast, which produces fruity overtones of banana and clove during fermentation. It is often unfiltered, resulting in a cloudy appearance because of suspended yeast and wheat proteins. It has low hop bitterness (about 15 IBUs) and high carbonation.

Christmas Ales: Key Characteristics		Notable Weizen
Attribute	Range / Description	Schneider Weisse
ABV	4.3–5.6%	Franziskaner
IBU (Bitterness)	8–15 (very low)	Live Oak Hefeweizen
Color (SRM)	2–9 (pale straw to deep gold)	Altstadt Hefeweizen
Body	Medium-light to medium	Shotgun Betty
Carbonation	High	Brooklyner Weisse
Clarity	Cloudy (unfiltered); clear in Krystalweizen	

Taste: Banana | Clove | Vanilla | Spice | Bready | Slightly Sweet
Food Pairing: Sausages | Banana Bread |

Food Pairing Guide for Weizen
Weizen beers are summer staples and aromatic showstoppers, perfect for pairing with grilled fare or sipping solo on a warm afternoon.

Light & Savory Proteins
- Grilled chicken with lemon or herbs: Citrus notes in the beer echo the seasoning.
- Weisswurst: A traditional pairing—mild sausage meets clove and banana.
- Roast turkey or pork loin: Light meats match the beer's body and spice.
- Seafood (shrimp, scallops, white fish): Delicate flavors lifted by the beer's effervescence.

Fresh & Tangy Dishes
- Goat cheese citrus vinaigrette salad: Cheese and bright dressing mirror the beer's fruitiness.
- Ceviche or sushi: Clean, citrusy flavors pair beautifully with wheat beer.
- Grilled vegetable skewers: Smoky char meets banana and clove notes.

Cheese Pairings
- Goat cheese or feta: Bright and acidic, perfect with Weizen's fruit.
- Brie or Camembert: Creamy texture complements the beer's smooth body.
- Mild cheddar or Havarti: Balanced and approachable.

Breads & Sides
- Pretzels with mustard: Classic Bavarian pairing—salt and spice meet malt and clove.
- Potato salad with vinegar dressing: Tangy and hearty, ideal with wheat beer.
- Soft rolls or rye bread: Toasty grains match the malt base.

Sweet Pairings
- Banana bread or spicy cake: Echoes the beer's natural flavors.
- Apple strudel or fruit tart: Fruity and flaky, perfect with wheat beer.
- Lemon bars or citrus sorbet: Bright acidity complements the beer's zest.

Garlic Grilled Shrimp Skewers

Shrimp is light, slightly sweet, and delicate in texture. Garlic marinade adds savory depth and aromatic punch. Grilling introduces smoky char and caramelization. Often served with lemon or herbs, adding brightness and zest. Banana and clove notes from yeast add subtle sweetness and spice. High carbonation scrubs the palate, refreshing after each bite. Low bitterness ensures it doesn't overpower the shrimp. Citrusy undertones echo lemon or herb accents in the dish. The beer's fruity esters complement the shrimp's natural sweetness.

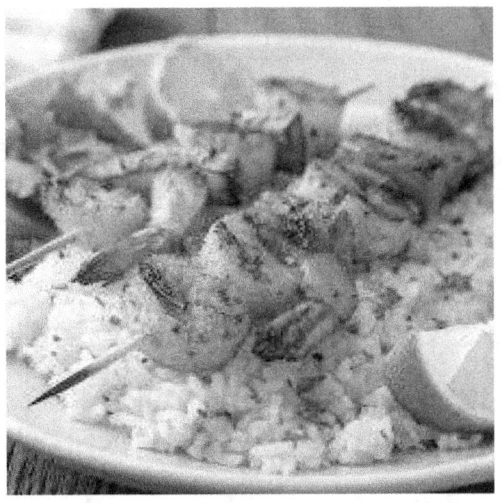

Ingredients:
1-pound large shrimp
¼ cup olive oil
¼ cup fresh cilantro, finely chopped
¼ cup fresh parsley, finely chopped
4 cloves garlic, minced
1 Tbsp. lemon juice
Season with salt, black pepper & cayenne pepper, to spice preference

Instructions:
1. Mix the marinade. Add the olive oil, lemon juice, herbs, garlic, and spices to a small mixing bowl and whisk together.
2. Marinate the shrimp. Place the shrimp in a bowl and pour ¾ of the marinade on top of the shrimp. Mix gently until the shrimp are well coated. Cover the bowl and marinate the shrimp for 30 minutes to an hour.
3. Prep the shrimp for grilling. Thread the shrimp onto the skewers. Get all the good garlic and herbs from the bowl and spread on to the shrimp.
4. Grill the shrimp. Heat a grill or grill pan on medium high heat. Once the grill is hot, place the shrimp skewers on the grill and cook for 2 to 3 minutes each side, or until they turn pink and opaque.
5. Serve. Remove the shrimp to a plate and spoon the remaining marinade on top before serving.

Coconut Lime Rice
1 cup jasmine or long-grain white rice
1 cup canned coconut milk (full-fat for richness)
1 cup water
½ tsp. salt
Zest of 1 lime
2 Tbsp. fresh lime juice
Optional: 1 Tbsp. chopped cilantro or mint for garnish

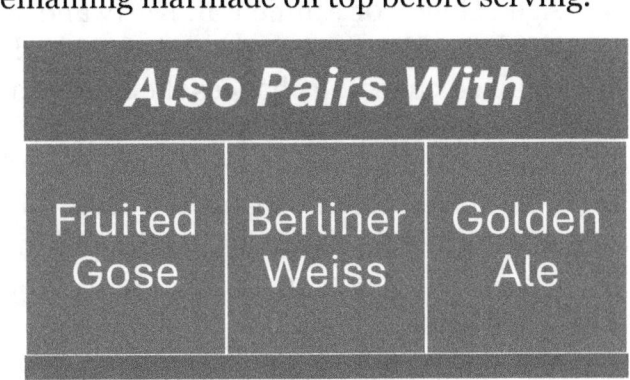

Also Pairs With		
Fruited Gose	Berliner Weiss	Golden Ale

Rinse the rice under cold water until the water runs clear. This helps prevent stickiness. In a saucepan, combine the rice, coconut milk, water, and salt. Bring to boil over medium heat. Reduce heat to low, cover, and simmer for 15–18 minutes until rice is tender and liquid is absorbed. Remove from the heat and let sit covered for 5 minutes. Fluff with a fork. Stir in lime zest and juice. Taste and adjust salt or lime as needed. Sprinkle with chopped herbs and serve warm.

Altbier

Altbier, which translates to "Old Beer" in German, is a distinctive German beer style primarily brewed in the Rhineland region, especially around the city of Düsseldorf. Altbier is top-fermented, which means it ferments at a moderate temperature using ale yeast. After fermentation, Altbier is matured at a cooler temperature, resulting in a flavor profile more akin to lager beer styles than typical top-fermented ales. Altbier typically has a dark, copper color. Its flavor exhibits a subtle fruitiness because of the top-fermenting yeast.

Altbier: Key Characteristics		Notable Altbier
Attribute	**Range / Description**	Utepils Alt 1848
ABV	4.3–5.5%	Uerige Alt
IBU (Bitterness)	25–40 (moderate)	Zum Schlüssel Original Alt
Color (SRM)	11–20 (copper to deep amber)	Füchschen Alt
Body	Medium	Schumacher Alt
Carbonation	Moderate	Diebels Alt
Finish	Clean, dry, slightly bitter	Alaskan Amber

Taste: Malt-Forward | Toasty | Carmel | Earthy | Floral | Fruity
Food Pairings: Grilled Pork | Beef | Apple Strudel

Food Pairing Guide for Altbier
Altbier is a distinctive German beer style that bridges the gap between ales and lagers—top-fermented like an ale, but cold-conditioned like a lager.

Savory & Grilled Meats
- Roast pork or pork schnitzel: Crisp bitterness cuts through fat and breading.
- Grilled steak or burgers: Caramelized crust echoes the beer's malt backbone.
- Smoked ham or bacon: Smoky richness pairs with Altbier's subtle roast.

Cheese Pairings
- Aged Gouda or Emmental: Nutty and sweet, perfect with malt.
- Mild cheddar or Havarti: Balanced and approachable.
- Smoked cheese: Enhances the beer's earthy depth.

Comfort Foods & German Classics
- Sauerbraten (German pot roast): Sweet-sour marinade meets smooth malt.
- Potato pancakes or spaetzle: Toasty edges and buttery richness match the beer's body.
- Roasted chicken with herbs: Crisp skin and savory meat pair beautifully.
- Mushroom gravy or ragout: Earthy umami complements Altbier's subtle bitterness.

Breads & Sides
- Pretzels with mustard: Salt and spice meet malt and hops.
- Rye or pumpernickel bread: Deep grain flavors echo the beer's toastiness.
- German potato salad (vinegar-based): Tangy contrast to smooth malt.

Sweet Pairings
- Apple strudel or baked apples: Fruit and spice match the beer's warmth.
- Carrot cake or a spicey cake: Earthy sweetness and soft texture pair well.
- Nut-based desserts (pecan tart, walnut cake): Toasty and rich, ideal with Altbier.

Hot Smoked Salmon

Salmon is rich, flaky texture with a deep, smoky flavor from the hot smoking process. Often seasoned with herbs, pepper, or a touch of sweetness. The smoke adds earthy depth, while the salmon's natural oils create a luxurious mouthfeel. The toasty malt backbone of Altbier with notes of caramel and bread crust complements the salmon's smoky richness. Clean fermentation and cold conditioning give Altbier a crisp finish that refreshes the palate. Moderate bitterness balances the salmon's fat and seasoning without overpowering. Subtle fruitiness from ale yeast adds a gentle contrast to the savory fish.

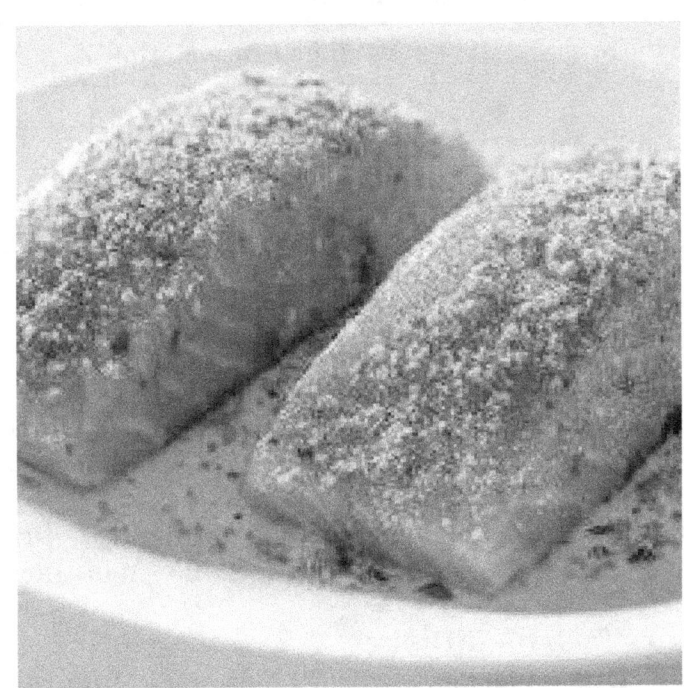

Ingredients:
4 lb. sockeye salmon, 2 pieces, 2 lb. each

For the brine:
1-quart cold water
1/3 cup kosher salt

For the brown sugar rub:
2 tbsp brown sugar
1 tsp salt
1/4 tsp black pepper
1 tsp paprika

For the garlic dill rub:
2 tbsp chopped fresh dill
1 tsp garlic powder
1/2 tsp salt
1 tbsp olive oil

Instructions:
1. In a large plastic container with a lid, combine the water and salt. Add fish skin-side up. Brine for 4-8 hours in the fridge.
2. Remove from the brine, rinse well with cold water and pat dry.
3. Set a drying rack on top of a large baking sheet and place the fish, skin side down, on it.
4. Let the fish dry for 8-12 hours in the fridge to form a pellicle.
5. Preheat your pellet grill. Set the temperature to 180 F. You can start smoking the fish at 150 F and gradually increase the temperature to 180 F.
6. Remove the fish from the fridge.
7. In two small bowls, combine the ingredients for the sweet and savory rubs.
8. Rub one piece with the sweet rub and the other with the garlic dill rub.
9. Place the salmon on the smoker, skin side down, and smoke for 3-5 hours, until the internal temperature reaches 135-140 F.
10. You can baste the fish (the sweet, rubbed piece) while it is smoking with maple syrup or orange juice.

Also Pairs With

Tripel	Baltic Porter	Golden Ale

Cream Ale

Cream ale is an American beer style; it doesn't contain any dairy or lactose. The term "cream" is marketing jargon, referring to the beer's silky taste or richness. It's a light, refreshing ale (though sometimes made with lager yeast) that typically falls around 5% ABV. Cream ales often include adjuncts like rice and corn, which contribute to their smooth mouthfeel. They have a crisp finish, making them highly drinkable. While they're not exceptionally creamy, they offer a medium body and a refreshing mouthfeel.

Cream Ale: Key Characteristics		Notable Cream Ales
Attribute	Range / Description	Urban Growler Cowbell Cream Ale
ABV	4.2–5.6%	Genesee Cream Ale
IBU (Bitterness)	8–20 (low to moderate)	Little Kings Cream Ale
Color (SRM)	2.5–5 (pale straw to light gold)	Sunshine City Cream Ale
Body	Light to medium-light	Cream Ale
Carbonation	Moderate to high	Spotted Cow
Finish	Clean, dry, slightly sweet	Caldera Ashland Amber

Taste: Grainy | Biscuity | Honey | Floral | Herbal
Food Pairings: Hot Dogs | Grilled Chicken | Cornbread | Fruit Salad

Food Pairing Guide for Cream Ale

Cream Ale is one of America's most charming hybrid beer styles—light, crisp, and quietly complex, blending ale fermentation with lager-like smoothness.

Savory & Grilled Dishes
- Grilled chicken or turkey burgers: Light proteins match the beer's body.
- Hot honey butter chicken: Cream Ale's smoothness tames the heat and echoes the honey glaze.
- BBQ pork sliders: Sweet and smoky meat meets crisp refreshment.
- Grilled corn or veggie skewers: Toasty malt complements charred edges.

Cheese Pairings
- Mozzarella or Havarti: Soft and buttery, perfect with Cream Ale's smooth texture.
- Goat cheese: Tangy contrast to the beer's subtle sweetness.

Comfort Foods & Pub Fare
- Mac & cheese: Creamy richness meets crisp carbonation.
- Fried chicken or fish: Light bitterness cuts through the crust.
- Soft pretzels with mustard: Salt and spice meet malt and fizz.
- BLT or club sandwich: Crisp veggies and savory bacon pair beautifully.

Fresh & Light Dishes
- Caesar or garden salad: Crisp greens match the beer's refreshing finish.
- Avocado toast with chili flakes: Cream Ale softens heat and complements richness.
- Shrimp tacos or grilled fish: Bright flavors lifted by the beer's clean profile.

Sweet Pairings
- Lemon bars or citrus sorbet: Zesty and refreshing.
- Shortbread cookies or pound cake: Buttery and simple, ideal with smooth beer.
- Apple crisp or peach cobbler.

Hot Honey Butter Grilled Chicken

Hot Honey Butter Grilled Chicken is made with a sweet and spicy glaze made from honey, butter, and chili or cayenne, delivering sticky heat and richness. Grilling adds smoky char and caramelization. The chicken is juicy and savory, with layers of flavor from the glaze and grill. Cream Ale is light-bodied and smooth, with subtle malt sweetness and a crisp finish. Low bitterness keeps the pairing gentle and refreshing. Often has a slightly creamy mouthfeel, which softens spicy edges. Mild corn or grain notes complement grilled flavors without overpowering.

Ingredients:

Chicken and Marinade
1 cup Hot Sauce
1/4 cup honey
3 lb. chicken breasts cut into 1-inch cubes
Avocado oil for brushing before grilling

Hot Honey Butter
1/2 cup Hot Sauce
1/2 cup salted butter, melted
1/2 cup honey
1/2 tsp fine sea salt

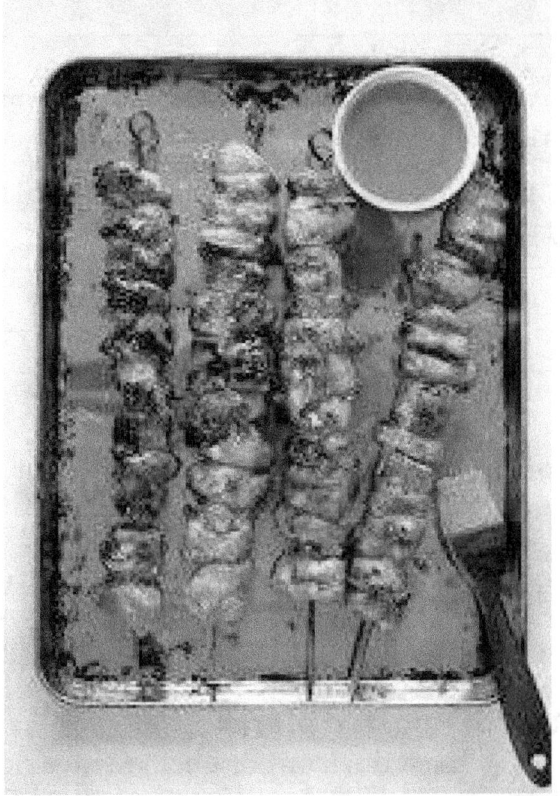

Instructions:
1. Make the marinade by whisking together 1 cup Hot Sauce and 1/4 cup honey in a large mixing bowl. Place cubed chicken in marinade, toss to coat, and allow you to sit for 1 hour at room temperature (Preheat grill to medium-high heat 425°F.
2. Skewer chicken to make kabobs.
3. Make hot honey butter by whisking together all ingredients in a medium mixing bowl. Reserve half of the mixture for serving and use the other half for basting while grilling.
4. Grill chicken. Once the grill is hot, brush chicken kabobs and grill grates with avocado oil (approx. 1/4 cup). Grill chicken for 5 minutes (with the lid closed), brush with hot honey butter, then flip the kabobs. Grill for 5 more minutes, then baste and flip again. Grill for about 2-5 more minutes. Total grilling time will be 12-15 minutes or until the internal temperature reaches 165°F. Brush the kabobs one more time with hot honey butter before removing them from the grill.
5. Serve with reserved hot honey butter for dipping or drizzling!

Also Pairs With

American Wheat Ale	American Brown Ale	Gose

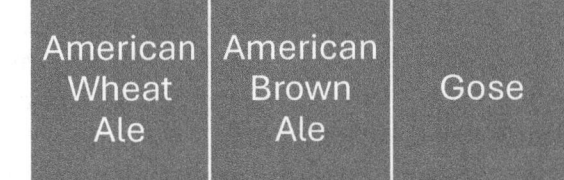

Wheat Wine

Wheat wine is a strong ale that includes a portion of wheat in its grain bill. Like barleywine, it is characterized by being sweet, malty, and high in alcohol (typically between 8% and 12% ABV). The amount of wheat can vary, but it typically comprises about half of the grain bill, 40% to 60%. The rest is barley malt1. Wheat wines are lighter and body compared to traditional barleywines. They are less aggressively hopped, resulting in a less bitter flavor. Because of wheat's higher protein content, wheat wine has a thicker texture than a typical brew. Brewers often use lighter malts in wheat wines, making them softer and fruitier.

Wheat wine: Key Characteristics		Notable Wheat Wine
Attribute	Range / Description	Cascade Brewing Pear Therapy
ABV	8–12% (sometimes higher)	The Bruery White Chocolate
IBU (Bitterness)	30–60 (balanced to moderately bitter)	Perennial Barrel-Aged Wheat Wine
Color (SRM)	6–14 (light amber to golden brown)	Wren House
Body	Full and creamy	Lewis & Clark Halo Huckleberry Wheatwine
Carbonation	Moderate	
Finish	Warming, smooth, often slightly sweet	

Taste: Bready | Honey | Carmel | Light Spice | Fruity | Citrus
Food Pairings: Grilled Pork | Smoked Brisket | Rost Duck or Pork Belly

Food Pairing Guide for Wheat Wines

Wheat wine is the silky, high-octane cousin of barleywine, blending the strength of a strong ale with the smooth, bready character of wheat malt.

Rich & Roasted Meats
- Roast duck or pork belly: Fatty richness balanced by fruity esters and warming alcohol.
- Beef Wellington or prime rib: Malty depth complements the crust and savory filling.
- Lamb chops with rosemary: Herbal notes play off the beer's spice and wheat character.
- Smoked turkey or ham: Sweet glaze and smoke echo the beer's caramel and citrus tones.

Cheese Pairings
- Triple cream Brie or Camembert: Rich and buttery, softened by wheat wine's smooth texture.
- Aged Gouda or cheddar: Sharp and nutty, perfect with malt sweetness.
- Blue cheese or Gorgonzola: Funky contrast to fruity esters and alcohol warmth.

Hearty Sides & Breads
- Buttery mashed potatoes or gratin: Creamy richness meets silky wheat body.
- Stuffing with herbs and dried fruit: Echoes the beer's spice and sweetness.
- Rye or whole grain bread: Toasty grains match the malt profile.

Decadent Desserts
- Bread pudding with bourbon sauce: Boozy, sweet, and luxurious.
- Spice cake or carrot cake: Earthy sweetness and warm spices match the beer's profile.
- Peach cobbler or apple crisp: Fruit and caramel pair beautifully with wheat esters.
- White chocolate cheesecake: Creamy and sweet, ideal with wheat wine's soft citrus notes.

Penne Arrabiata with Smoked Sausage

Arrabiata sauce is fiery and tangy, made with garlic, chili flakes, and tomatoes. Smoked sausage adds savory depth, fat, and a touch of sweetness. The dish is robust and layered, with heat, acidity, and umami. Wheat wine with a high ABV (8–12%) brings warmth and body to match the dish's intensity. Wheat malt adds a smooth, creamy texture that softens the spice. Fruity esters (like apricot, pear, or citrus) contrast the tomato's acidity and chili heat. Caramel and honey-like malt sweetness complement the sausage's smoky richness.

Ingredients:
2 1/2 tbsp good quality Olive Oil
7 oz Smoked Sausage, sliced
3 fat cloves of Garlic, thinly sliced
1 tsp Chilli Flakes, or to taste
3 tbsp Tomato Puree
2x 14oz good quality Chopped Tomatoes
pinch of Sugar
Salt & Black Pepper, to taste
12 oz Penne
1 oz freshly grated Parmesan, plus more to serve
2 tbsp finely diced Fresh Parsley, plus extra to serve

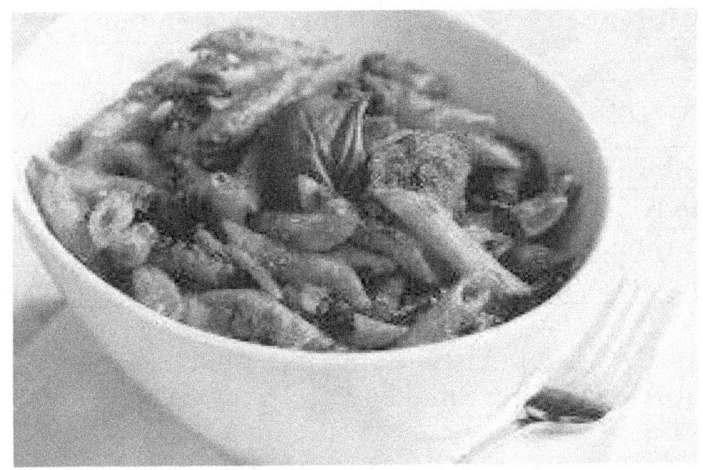

Instructions:
1. Drizzle the olive oil into a large deep pan over medium heat. Once hot, add the sausage & fry for a few minutes each side until browned.
2. Push to the edges of the pan, then add the garlic & chili flakes into the center. Fry for a minute until the garlic begins to lightly color (careful it doesn't burn).
3. Stir in the tomato puree and fry for 1-2mins, then add in the chopped tomatoes. Season to taste with salt, pepper and sugar, then simmer for 10mins, or until the sauce thickens.
4. Meanwhile, pop your pasta in salted boiling water and cook until al dente, reserving 1 cup starchy pasta water just before draining.
5. Stir the drained pasta through the sauce with a splash of the pasta water, then stir in the Parmesan and parsley until the Parmesan melts. If the sauce looks a little dry, stir through some more pasta water, a splash at a time. The pasta water will also help emulsify the oils (discard any water you don't use). The final texture should be saucy but not watery and should cling to the pasta. Continue tossing/stirring until it does.
6. Serve with extra parmesan/parsley.

Also Pairs With

Eisbock	American Stout	Wild

Kolsch

Kölsch is a subtle beer, with a light, grainy Pilsner malt aroma and flavor. It is subtle and soft with some grainy malt sweetness up front but with a crisp enough finish that the beer. It is gently bittered with Noble hops and, overall, well balanced. Its simultaneous softness and snap deliver a refreshing and utterly enjoyable drinking experience. It typically has a low alcohol content. Fruit, bread and citrus, sausages, grilled chicken, burgers, pizza, and anything off the grill that becomes a sandwich.

Kolsch: Key Characteristics		Notable Kolsch
Attribute	Range / Description	Leinenkugel's Canoe Paddler
ABV	Typically, 4.4–5.2%	Reissdorf Kölsch
IBU (Bitterness)	20–30 (balanced, not assertive)	Früh Kölsch
Color (SRM)	Pale straw to light gold; brilliantly clear	Gaffel Kölsch
Body	Full and creamy	Sünner Kölsch
Carbonation	Moderate	
Finish	Light body, moderate carbonation, smooth texture	

Taste: Clean | Crisp | Complex | Acidic | Earthy
Food Pairings: Smoked Poultry | Grilled Seafood | Brats | Tangy Coleslaw and Pickles

Food Pairing Guide for Kolsch
Kölsch is a masterclass in subtlety—clean, crisp, and quietly complex. It's the beer that doesn't shout, but whispers with elegance.

Light Proteins & Seafood
- Grilled white fish (cod, halibut): Clean malt and soft hops enhance the fish's freshness.
- Shrimp cocktail or ceviche: Bright acidity and seafood meet Kölsch's crisp finish.
- Chicken with lemon and herbs: Herbal notes pair beautifully with the beer's soft fruitiness.
- Sushi or sashimi: Light and clean, ideal with Kölsch's gentle profile.

Fresh & Herbaceous Dishes
- Caprese salad or tomato bruschetta: Sweet tomato and basil match the beer's subtle fruit.
- Spring greens with vinaigrette: Crisp bitterness balances tangy dressing.
- Grilled asparagus or zucchini: Earthy char meets clean malt.

Cheese Pairings
- Fresh mozzarella or burrata: Soft and milky, perfect with Kölsch's light body.
- Goat cheese: Tangy contrast to the beer's subtle sweetness.
- Mild cheddar or Swiss: Balanced and approachable.

Pub Fare & Comfort Foods
- Soft pretzels with mustard: Classic German pairing—salt and spice meet crisp refreshment.
- Turkey sandwich or grilled cheese: Simple and satisfying with Kölsch's clean finish.
- Bratwurst with sauerkraut: Mild sausage and tangy kraut pair beautifully.

Light Desserts
- Lemon bars or citrus sorbet: Bright and refreshing.
- Shortbread cookies or sponge cake: Buttery and light, ideal with Kölsch's crispness.
- Fresh berries with whipped cream: Fruity and delicate.

Reuben Sandwich

A Reuben Sandwich is made with corned beef, Swiss cheese, sauerkraut, and Russian or Thousand Islands dressing, all grilled between slices of rye bread. It's salty, fatty, tangy, and creamy, with bold flavors and a toasted crunch. The sauerkraut adds acidity, while the dressing brings sweetness and spice. Kölsch is light-bodied and crisp, with subtle fruitiness and gentle hop bitterness. A clean finish refreshes the palate between bites. Low alcohol and carbonation make it easy-drinking and food-friendly. Slight grainy malt sweetness complements the rye bread and dressing.

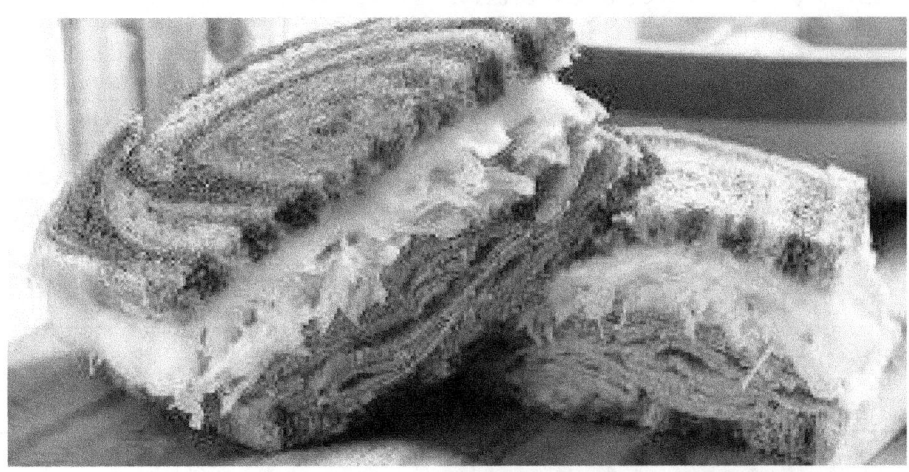

Ingredients:
2 lb. pastrami, sliced thin
10 slices light rye bread
10 slices Swiss cheese
Butter, *for spreading*
1 can sauerkraut
1 tsp caraway seeds

Russian Dressing:
1 tbsp onion, *finely minced*
1 tbsp dill pickle/gherkin, *finely minced*
3/4 cup mayonnaise
1/4 cup sour cream
2.5 tbsp sriracha, spicy ketchup or Chili Sauce *(or 1/4 cup ketchup + 2 tsp Tabasco)*
3 tsp horseradish, *to taste*
1 tsp Worcestershire sauce
1/4 tsp sweet paprika

Also Pairs With		
Irish Red Ale	Barrek Aged Stout	Dortmunder

Instructions:
Russian Dressing:
1. Mix ingredients, refrigerate 20 minutes+ (keeps 2 weeks).

Prepare Pastrami:
1. Thinly slice still cold pastrami. Place in a container with a couple of Tbsp. of pastrami liquid and Russian dressing.
2. Microwave to warm through.

Assemble Reuben:
1. Preheat grill/broiler to medium high with shelf about 10" from heat source.
2. Toast bread. Spread with butter, then 1 tbsp Russian Dressing on each piece.
3. Pick up the pastrami and let excess juices drip away, then place on bread.
4. Do the same for sauerkraut, pile onto pastrami, then top with cheese.
5. Also, place cheese on the other slice of bread (i.e., with just Russian Dressing).
6. Place it under the grill until the cheese is just melted. Sandwich together and devour while hot!

Fruit/Herb/Spice Lagers

Any time a fruit, vegetable or spice is added to a beer, it is classified as a fruit/vegetable beer. Fruit and vegetables can be added to your typical beer styles such as pilsner, a wheat beer, a sour or a lager to make them possess a sweeter and fruit taste or profile. You should be keen to complement the barbeque and the beer. If you feel the need to be more industrious is stronger than becoming normal, try not to contrast the beer and meal sharply. Pairs well with barbeque meals used as appetizers.

Fruit-Style Beer: Key Characteristics		Notable Fruit Lagers
Attribute	Range / Description	REDD's Apple Ale
Base Style	Can be any style—wheat, IPA, stout, sour, lager, etc.	Hell or High Watermelon
Fruit Additions	Fresh fruit, puree, juice, peel, zest, or extract	Bud Light Chelada Mango
Aroma	Prominent fruit notes (e.g., berries, citrus, stone fruit, tropical)	Wild Berry Lager
Flavor Profile	Ranges from sweet and juicy to tart and tangy, depending on fruit and base	Peach Lager
Appearance	May take on fruit hues—pink, orange, purple—with hazy or clear body	Strawberry Blonde Lager
ABV Range	Wide spectrum: 2.5% (e.g., Lambics) to 8%+ (e.g., fruit IPAs or stouts)	Pineapple Mana Wheat Lager
Finish	Often light to medium body; carbonation varies by style	

Taste: Vary from Fruity | Grainy | Berry Based | Citrus | Fruity | Tropical
Food Pairings: Barbecue | Brisket Tacos | Mango Coleslaw | Pulled Pork | Smoked Turkey

Food Pairing Guide for Fruit Beers

Fruit-style beers are a vibrant, expressive category that blends traditional brewing with the natural sweetness, tartness, or aroma of real fruit.

Savory & Spicy Dishes
- Spicy Thai or Indian curries: Mango, passionfruit, or apricot beers cool the heat complement bold spices.
- Grilled chicken with fruit glaze: Cherry or peach beer echo the glaze and add depth.
- Pulled pork BBQ sauce: Berry-forward beers cut through richness & enhance smoky sweetness.
- Duck with cherry or plum sauce: Dark fruit beer mirrors the sauce and elevate the dish.

Cheese Pairings
- Goat cheese or Brie: Soft and tangy cheeses match well with raspberry or strawberry beers.
- Blue cheese: Bold funk balanced by sweet fruit beers like fig or pear.
- Aged cheddar or Gouda: Nutty and sharp, ideal with apple or cranberry beers.

Fresh & Fruity Dishes
- Arugula salad with berries and vinaigrette: Berry beers amplify the fruit and balance the greens.
- Prosciutto-wrapped melon: A peach or apricot beer enhances the sweet-salty contrast.
- Citrus-marinated shrimp or scallops: Lemon or lime-infused beer echo the zest.

Desserts & Sweet Pairings
- Cheesecake with fruit topping: Match the topping—raspberry beer with raspberry swirl.
- Chocolate cake with cherry beer: Think Black Forest vibes.
- Lemon tart or berry cobbler: Tart beers like sour cherry or blackberry add brightness.
- Vanilla ice cream float: Try strawberry or peach beer for a grown-up twist.

Slow-Cooker Carnitas Tacos

Slow-cooked pork is tender, fatty, and deeply flavorful. Often topped with onions, cilantro, lime, and salsa, adding brightness and acidity. The dish is rich and layered, with crispy edges and juicy meat. Fruit Beer offers bright fruit flavors like cherry, raspberry, mango, or citrus. Tartness and sweetness cut through the pork's richness. Effervescence and acidity refresh the palate after each bite. Adds a playful contrast to the savory depth of Caritas. Its sweet-tart profile complements lime and salsa, enhancing the taco's toppings. Together, they offer a street-food-meets-craft-beer vibe—perfect for casual gatherings or sunny afternoons.

Ingredients:
3 pounds boneless pork shoulder
3/4 cup lower-sodium chicken broth
1/4 cup fresh orange juice (from 1 orange)
4 garlic cloves, smashed
1 tsp. black pepper
1 Tbsp. plus 1 tsp. kosher salt, divided
Warm corn tortillas, shredded cabbage, diced avocado, queso fresco (fresh Mexican cheese), lime wedges, for serving

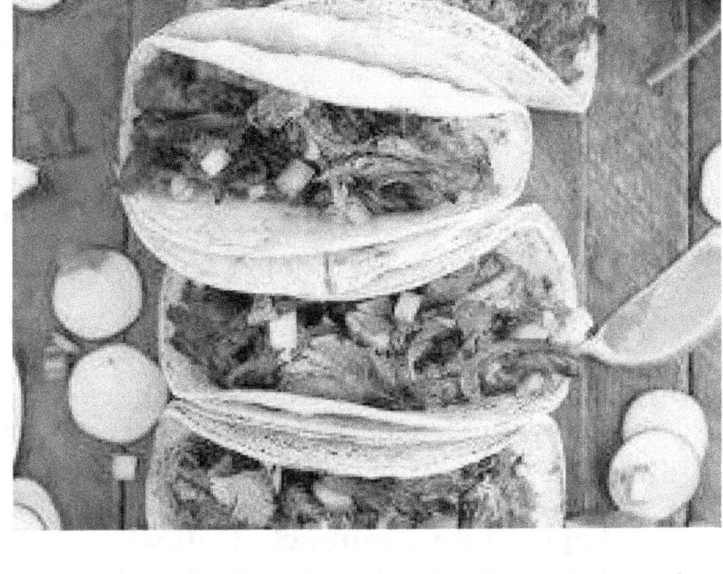

Instructions:
1. Combine pork, chicken broth, orange juice, garlic, pepper, and 1 Tbsp. of salt in a 6-to 7-quart slow cooker. Cover and cook on LOW until pork is fork-tender, about 8 hours.
2. Preheat broiler to high with oven rack 6 inches from heat. Shred pork in slow cooker. Remove the pork from the liquid, and transfer it to a large, rimmed baking sheet. Spread into an even layer. Broil until the pork is brown and crisp, about 8 minutes. Stir and broil 2 more minutes. Sprinkle with the remaining 1 tsp. salt and toss well. Transfer to a serving platter.
3. Serve pork with tortillas, shredded cabbage, diced avocado, queso fresco, and lime wedges.

Salsa Verde (Tomatillo Green Sauce)
1 lb. fresh tomatillos (husks removed, rinsed)
1–2 jalapeno or serrano peppers (stemmed; adjust for heat)
1 small white onion, quartered
2 cloves garlic, peeled
½ cup fresh cilantro
Juice of 1 lime
Salt to taste
Optional: 1 Tbsp. olive oil for richness

Also Pairs With		
Mexican-Style Lager	Cream Ale	Czech Pilsner

Place the tomatillos, peppers, onion, and garlic on a baking sheet. Broil until charred (about 5–7 minutes). Transfer the cooked ingredients to a blender. Add cilantro, lime juice, and salt. Blend until smooth. Add more lime, salt, or cilantro to balance the flavor. For a thinner sauce, add a splash of water or cooking liquid.

Seasonal Lagers

Pumpkin beer, Octoberfest, March beer originally brewed in the spring and stored in icy caves in the summer for fall celebrations. Strong with malty sweetness and low hop flavor. Caramelization of malts complements that of char-grilled and seared meats or hearty, spicy Mexican dishes. Seasonal brews go best when paired with dishes meant for their season.

Fruit-Style Beer: Key Characteristics		Notable Seasonal Lagers
Attribute	Range / Description	
Base Style	Seasonal Variations Mader in Lager Style	Lakefront Pumpkin Lager
ABV	4.5 – 7.5%	Jack's Abby Copper Legend
IBU (Bitterness)	Various by style 15-30	Einbecker Mai-Ur-Bock
Color (SRM)	Light to Dark	Victory Winter Cheers
Body	Medium body and creamy	
Finish	Clean, crisp, refreshingly smooth	

Taste: Malty | Spicy | Smooth | Toasty | Floral | Rich | Crisp Carbonation
Food Pairings: Roasted Chicken | Grilled Asparagus | Fish Tacos | Fried Foods | Choc Cake

Food Pairing Guide for Seasonal Lagers

Seasonal lagers are like nature's way of brewing—each one tuned to the mood, weather, and flavors of its times, especially if you're exploring barbecue fusion.

Spring Lagers (e.g., Maibock, Helles)
Bright, bready, and slightly stronger than typical lagers:
- Grilled asparagus or spring vegetables: Earthy and fresh, perfect with malt sweetness.
- Roast chicken with herbs: Clean flavors match the beer's smooth body.
- Soft cheeses (Brie, Camembert): Creamy textures meet gentle bitterness.
- Lamb chops or schnitzel: Rich meats balanced by crisp finish.

Summer Lagers (e.g., Pilsner, Mexican Lager, Kölsch-style lagers)
Light, crisp, and thirst-quenching:
- Fish tacos or ceviche: Bright citrus and spice lifted by carbonation.
- Caprese salad or watermelon feta: Fresh and juicy, ideal with subtle hops.
- Grilled corn or veggie skewers: Charred sweetness meets clean malt.
- Bratwurst or hot dogs: Classic summer fare with a refreshing contrast.

Fall Lagers (e.g., Märzen, Festbier, Vienna Lager)
Toasty, amber-hued, and malt-forward:
- Roast pork or sausages with mustard: Rich meat echoes the beer's caramel notes.
- Pretzels with cheese dip: Salt and malt in perfect harmony.
- Stuffed mushrooms or root vegetables: Earthy flavors match toasted malt.
- Aged cheddar or Gruyère: Nutty and sharp, ideal with amber lagers.

Winter Lagers (e.g., Dunkel, Baltic Porter, Winter Bock)
Dark, warm, and full-bodied:
- Beef stew or pot roast: Deep umami meets roasted malt.
- Smoked meat or brisket: Smoke and caramelized crust pair beautifully.
- Spice cake or gingerbread: Sweet and spiced, perfect with dark lagers.
- Blue cheese or aged Gouda: Bold flavors balanced by malt richness.

Honey Dijon Mustard Pork Loin

Savory pork loin is lean yet flavorful, often roasted to develop a caramelized crust. Honey adds sweetness, while Dijon mustard brings tang and spice. The glaze creates a sweet-savory balance with a touch of heat and depth. Typically, Fall Lagers are amber-hued and malt-forward, with notes of caramel, toasted bread, and subtle spice. Smooth body and moderate carbonation make it ideal for rich, roasted dishes. Low to moderate bitterness keeps the pairing warm and balanced. Together, they evoke the comfort and warmth of fall, perfect for harvest dinners or festive gatherings.

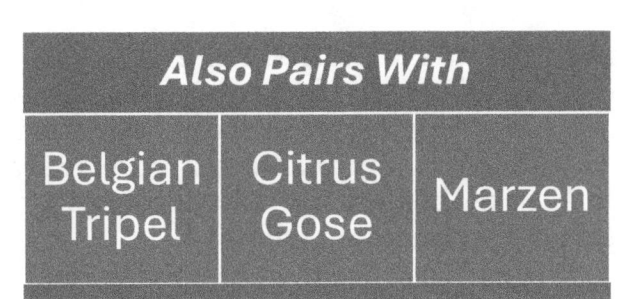

Ingredients:
1 (3 to 4-pound) boneless pork loin
Salt and freshly cracked black pepper
2 Tbsp. white wine vinegar
3/4 cup Dijon mustard
1 Tbsp. freshly chopped parsley leaves
1 Tbsp. freshly chopped chives
1 Tbsp. freshly chopped tarragon leaves
3 Tbsp. vegetable oil

Instructions:
1. Preheat oven to 350 degrees F.
2. Season the pork loin with salt and pepper.
3. In a small bowl, mix the vinegar, mustard, and herbs together. Reserve mustard sauce for pork.
4. In a large oven-proof sauté pan over medium-high heat, warm the vegetable oil. Sear pork loin on all sides. Brush with mustard sauce and roast in the preheated oven until the internal temperature reaches 145 degrees F on an instant-read thermometer, about 20 minutes. Remove from the oven and rest for 15 minutes before slicing and serving.

Blackberry Honey Mustard Sauce
1 cup fresh or frozen blackberries
2 tbsp honey
2 tbsp Dijon mustard (or whole grain for texture)
1 tbsp apple cider vinegar
1 tsp lemon juice
Pinch of salt
1/2 tsp cracked black pepper or cayenne for heat

Also Pairs With		
Belgian Tripel	Citrus Gose	Marzen

In a small saucepan over medium heat, add blackberries and a splash of water. Simmer for 5–7 minutes until berries burst and soften. Use a fork or potato masher to crush the berries. Strain through a fine-mesh sieve to remove seeds (optional for a smoother texture). Return the strained juice to the pan. Stir in honey, mustard, vinegar, lemon juice, and salt. Cook for another 3–5 minutes until slightly thickened. Taste and adjust sweetness or tang.

Weiss Lagers

This beer is one of the oldest beers you can find on the market today. It was first brewed in Bohemia and belonged to Bavaria's 500-year long tradition. Initially, it was referred to as "Weiss's beer," meaning white beer, and the only beer made from wheat during summer. Reflect for Texas style BBQ brisket and sausage.

Weiss Lager Beer: Key Characteristics		Notable Weiss Lagers
Attribute	**Range / Description**	Leinenkugel's Berry Weiss
Base Style	Lager (bottom-fermented), brewed with a high percentage of wheat	Franziskaner Weissbier
Appearance	Pale straw to golden; often hazy because of wheat and yeast	Ayinger Bräuweisse
Aroma	Light banana, clove, subtle citrus, mild malt	Live Oak Hefeweizen
Flavor Profile	Clean lager finish with soft wheat sweetness and gentle spice	Altstadt Hefeweizen
ABV Range	Typically, 4.5–5.5%	
Bitterness (IBU)	Low (10–20), allowing fruit and yeast notes to shine	
Finish	Medium-light body, smooth texture, moderate to high carbonation	

Taste: Fruity | Grainy | Banana | Spice | Fruit
Food Pairings: Grilled Foods | Salads with fruit | Barbecue | Pulled Pork | Smoked Chicken

Food Pairing Guide for Weiss Lagers

Weiss lager is a bit of a unicorn—the refreshing smoothness of a lager with the fruity, spicy character of wheat beer.

Light Proteins & Grilled Fare
- Grilled Lemon chicken: Bright and savory, perfect with wheat malt and subtle hops.
- Pork tenderloin or schnitzel: Mild richness balanced by the beer's crisp finish.
- Grilled shrimp or scallops: Delicate seafood lifted by fruity esters and carbonation.
- Turkey burgers with avocado: Creamy and clean, ideal with the beer's smooth body.

Fresh & Herbaceous Dishes
- Arugula salad with citrus vinaigrette: Peppery greens and bright dressing match the beer's zest.
- Caprese salad or tomato bruschetta: Sweet tomato and basil echo the malt's softness.
- Grilled vegetable skewers: Earthy char meets clean malt and gentle hops.

Cheese Pairings
- Goat cheese or feta: Tangy contrast to the beer's fruitiness.
- Brie or Camembert: Soft and buttery, perfect with wheat malt.
- Mild cheddar or Swiss: Balanced and approachable.

Pub Fare & Comfort Foods
- Grilled cheese or turkey sandwich: Simple and satisfying with a clean finish.
- Fish and chips: Crisp batter and flaky fish match the beer's refreshing character.

Light Desserts
- Lemon bars or citrus sorbet: Zesty and bright, ideal with wheat malt.
- Fruit tarts or berry shortcake: Juicy and sweet, echoing the beer's subtle esters.
- Vanilla sponge cake or shortbread: Buttery and light, perfect with a crisp lager.

Dry Rub Smoked Chicken Wings

Smoked wings offer a deep, savory flavor with crispy skin and juicy meat. A dry rub adds layers of spice, herbs, and subtle sweetness. The dish is bold but not saucy, letting the smoke and seasoning shine. A Weiss Lager combines the clean finish of a lager with the soft fruitiness and bready character of wheat malt. Light to medium body keeps the pairing refreshing. Subtle esters (like citrus or pear) complement spice and smoke. Smooth carbonation lifts the palate between bites. Weiss Lager's crispness cuts through the richness of the chicken skin and smoky meat.

Ingredients:
1 tsp. each paprika, granulated garlic, onion powder
½ tsp. cayenne pepper
2 tsp. chili powder
½ tsp. cumin
1 tsp. kosher salt
1 tsp. ground black pepper
2 pounds chicken wings
2 Tbsp. vegetable oil

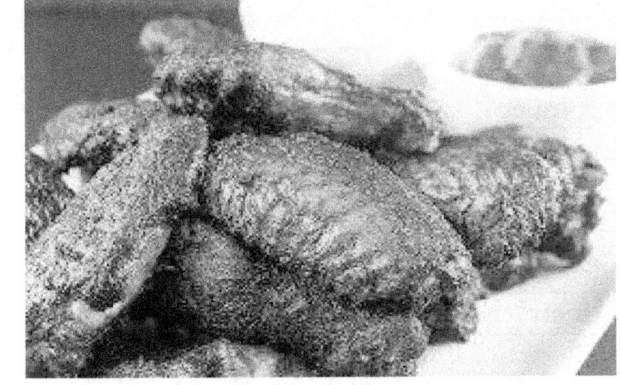

Instructions:
1. Preheat the smoker to 225°F. In a small bowl, combine the paprika, granulated garlic, onion powder, cayenne pepper, chili powder, cumin, kosher salt, and ground black pepper. Mix well.
2. Cut the chicken wings at the joints, separating them into drumettes, wingettes, and wing tips. Discard the wing tips or save them to make stock.
3. Pat dry the wingettes. Place half of them into a large plastic zip-top bag along with half of the dry rub and half of the oil. Massage the seasoning onto the chicken. Then, remove the chicken from the bag and place it onto a wire rack. Repeat with the remaining chicken, spices, and oil.
4. Smoke the wings for 1 to 1 ½ hours until the chicken reaches an internal temperature of 160°F. Remove the wings from the smoker.
5. Increase the temperature of the smoker to 450°F. When the proper temperature has been reached, return the wings to the smoker for 3 to 5 minutes per side. Remove the chicken wings from the smoker and serve immediately.

Sweet Chili Lime Sauce
½ cup Thai sweet chili sauce
1½ Tbsp. fresh lime juice
1 tsp. lime zest
1 tsp. rice vinegar
½ tsp. soy sauce or fish sauce
pinch of red pepper flakes or minced chili for heat
1 Tbsp. chopped cilantro for garnish

Also Pairs With

Smoked Helles	Dry Irish Stout	Flanders Red Ale

In a small bowl, whisk together sweet chili sauce, lime juice, zest, vinegar, and soy or fish sauce. Add red pepper flakes for heat or more lime juice for brightness.

Cider Beers

This is an alcoholic cider that is typically made from apple cider and wheat beer. It has a higher alcohol content (4.5~5.0%) than other types of cider and is often served cold. Pair with pulled pork, chopped pork, sausages and even a cheeseburger.

Fruit-Style Beer: Key Characteristics		Notable Ciders
Attribute	**Range / Description**	Stella Artois Cidre Hard Cider
Base Ingredient	Fermented apple juice (sometimes pear or other fruits)	Wölffer No. 139 Dry Rosé Cider
Appearance	Pale gold to amber; clear or slightly hazy	Virtue Cider Michigan Brut
Aroma	Fresh apple, pear, citrus, sometimes floral or spice notes	Angry Orchard Stone Dry
Flavor Profile	Ranges from dry and tart to sweet and juicy; acidity is often prominent	Eden Imperial 11° Rosé
ABV Range	Typically, 4–8%	Seattle Cider Dry
Carbonation	Can be still or sparkling; most commercial ciders are lightly carbonated	Reverend Nat's Revival
Finish	Light to medium body; crisp and refreshing	

Taste: Fruit Forward | Apple | Acidic | Sweet Rich
Food Pairings: Thai Food | Fried Fish | Indian Food | Sushi | Roast Pork and Chicken

Food Pairing Guide for Cider Beers

Cider's acidity and fruit-forward profile make it a brilliant match for a wide range of foods. Here's how to pair it like a chef:

Cheese Pairings
- Sharp cheddar: Classic pairing—apple notes complement the cheese's bite.
- Brie or Camembert: Creamy richness balanced by cider's acidity.
- Goat cheese: Tangy and earthy, perfect with fruit-forward ciders.
- Blue cheese: Funky softened by cider's sweetness.

Pork & Poultry Dishes
- Roast pork loin with apples: Echoes the cider's core flavors.
- Pulled pork sandwiches: Sweet and smoky meat meets crisp refreshment.
- Chicken with rosemary or thyme: Herbal notes pair beautifully with cider's fruit.
- Turkey burgers or sausages: Mild meats lifted by bright acidity.

Fresh & Herbaceous Dishes
- Arugula salad with apple slices and vinaigrette: Crisp and tangy harmony.
- Grilled vegetables: Earthy char meets clean fruit.
- Beet and goat cheese salad: Sweet, earthy, and tangy all in one.

Spicy & Global Fare
- Carnitas tacos or BBQ chicken: Sweet-savory meat balanced with tart cider.
- Thai curry or Indian biryani: Fruitiness softens spice and adds contrast.
- Korean fried chicken: Crispy, spicy, and perfect with cider's zing.

Desserts & Sweet Pairings
- Apple pie or crumble: Classic pairing—echoes and enhances the flavors.
- Carrot cake or spice cake: Warm spices meet crisp fruit.
- Vanilla ice cream or Panna cotta: Creamy textures lifted by acidity.

Crisp Cider-Braised Pork Belly

Pork belly is rich, fatty, and tender, often finished with a crispy crust. Braised in cider, it absorbs fruity acidity and subtle sweetness. The result is a dish that's savory, slightly sweet, and deeply flavorful, with hints of apple and spice. Cider Beer offers a crisp apple character, ranging from dry and tart to semi-sweet and juicy. Bright acidity and carbonation cut through the pork's fat and refresh the palate. Fruit-forward notes echo the braising liquid, enhancing flavor continuity. Some cider beers include spices or hops, adding complexity that complements the dish.

Ingredients:
1 large carrot, chopped
1 onion, chopped
few celery sticks, chopped
2 garlic cloves, smashed
sprig Fresh Thyme
2 bay leaves
16 oz good-quality cider
Small splash cider vinegar, plus extra to season
32 ounces fresh chicken stock
2 ½ pound piece, unscored boneless pork belly
2 tbsp sunflower oil
apple mash and Mustard cabbage, to serve

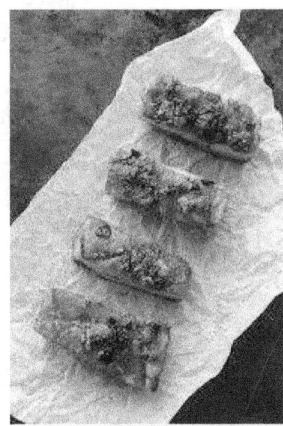

Also Pairs With

Belgian Saison	Cider Gose	Belgian White

Instructions Day 1:

1. Heat oven to 350°F. Place all the ingredients except the pork and sunflower oil in a flameproof pan that will fit the pork snugly – a casserole dish is ideal. Season, bring everything to the boil, then turn down the heat and slide the pork into the pan. The pork should be totally submerged – if it is not, top up with water. Cover the dish with a lid or tight tent of foil and place it in the oven for 3 hrs. undisturbed.
2. When the pork is cooked, leave it to cool slightly in the stock. Line a flat baking tray with cling film. Carefully lift the pork into the tray and make sure you get rid of any bits of vegetables or herbs as they will end up pressed into the pork. Cover the pork with another sheet of cling film and cover with a flat tray or dish – the tray must be completely flat as any indentations will be pressed into the pork. Weigh the pork down with another dish or some cans and leave to cool in the fridge overnight. Strain the juice into a jug or small saucepan, cover and chill.

Instructions Day 2:

1. Unwrap the pork and place it on a board. Trim the uneven edges so that you have a neat sheet of meat. Cut the meat into 4 equal pieces and set aside until ready to cook. Lift off any bits of fat from the braising juices and tip what will now be jelly into a saucepan, then bubble down by about two-thirds until it becomes slightly syrupy. Add a few more drops of vinegar to taste.
2. Heat the oil in a large frying pan until hot, then turn the heat down. Add the pork to the pan, skin-side down – be careful as it spits. Sizzle the pork as you would bacon for 5 mins until the skin is crisp. Flip it over and cook for 3-4 mins until browned. Place a small pile of cabbage on the side of each plate and sit a piece of pork on top. Place a spoonful of mash on the other side of the plate, drizzle over the sauce and serve.

Beer Style Comparison Chart

Style	ABV	IBU	Malt/Grain Character	Hop Aroma	Balance	Esters
Blonde Ale	4.0–5.5%	15–28	Light malt, biscuit, honey	Mild floral or citrus	Balanced	Low
Amber Ale	4.5–6.2%	25–40	Toasted caramel, medium body	Earthy, piney	Malt-forward	Low to moderate
Brown Ale	4.5–6.0%	20–30	Nutty, chocolate and caramel	Mild floral or earthy	Malt-heavy	Low
Pale Ale	4.5–6.0%	30–50	Biscuit, light caramel	Citrus, pine	Balanced	Low to moderate
India Pale Ale (IPA)	5.5–7.5%	40–70+	Subtle malt, dry finish	Bold citrus, resinous	Hop-forward	Moderate (can be fruity)
Amber Lager	4.5–5.5%	18–30	Toasted malt, smooth body	Mild floral or herbal	Malt-forward	Low
Pilsner (Lager)	4.5–5.2%	25–45	Crisp, grainy, light malt	Herbal, spicy	Hop-forward	Very low
Helles Lager	4.7–5.4%	16–22	Soft malt, bready, clean	Mild floral or spicy	Malt-balanced	Very low
Bock (Lager)	6.3–7.5%	20–30	Rich malt, caramel, toast	Minimal	Malt-dominant	Low
Wheat Beer (Ale)	4.0–5.5%	10–20	Bready, wheat-forward	Low, sometimes spicy	Malt-forward	High (banana, clove, citrus)
Saison (Specialty Ale)	5.0–7.0%	20–35	Peppery, dry, grainy	Herbal, earthy	Dry and spicy	High (fruity, spicy)
Sour Ale	3.0–6.0%	5–15	Minimal malt, wheat, or pilsner	Low to none	Acidic/tart	High (wild yeast, fruit)
Belgian Dubbel	6.0–7.6%	20–30	Rich malt, dark fruit, caramel	Low to moderate	Malt-forward	High (plum, raisin, spice)
Stout (Ale)	5.0–8.0%	30–60	Deep roast, espresso, dark malt	Low to moderate	Malt-heavy	Low to moderate
Porter (Ale)	5.0–6.5%	25–50	Roasty, chocolate, coffee	Subtle, earthy or floral	Malt-dominant	

BBQ Style and Beer Varietal Recommendations

BBQ Style	Flavor Profile and Notes	Recommendations
Kansas City	Sweet & Tangy, Molasses based Sauces The stars here are pork and ribs, but you will also find brisket. This is the saucy, finger-licking barbecue that requires a wine equally over the top, and intense, showing spicy, juicy, and ripe characteristics. Sweet sauces need something assertive. **Featured Cuts:** Burnt ends, Kansas City bacon, ribs, brisket, pulled pork, chicken, sausage, "all-purpose sauce"	Amber Ale Pale Ale Wheat Stouts IPA Belgian Ale Irish Red Ale Porter Brown Ale Pilsner American Porter
Memphis	Dry Rubs, Tangy & Tomatoey & Sweet Sauces Known for pulled pork & ribs. Memphis ribs are heavily seasoned with a dry rub made of brown sugar, chili powder, pepper, and cumin, and they are slowly cooked. **Featured Cuts:** Wet ribs, dry ribs, pulled pork, chicken, beef shoulder, brisket	Brown Ale Smoked Porter Irish Red Ale Porters Belgian Saison American IPA Bock Amber Lager
Texas	Dry Rubs, Spicy & Drippings & Worcestershire & thin sauces here we are talking beef (brisket is the key). We focus on dry rubs and smoke, not sauces. Focus on wines with earthy and complex characteristics. **Featured Cuts:** Brisket, beef ribs, pork ribs, and sausages are the foundation of Texas BBQ, but you will find pulled pork, turkey, and chicken, too.	Bold Stout Hoppy Pale Ale Pilsner Czech Pilsner Mexican Lagers Brown Ales Berliner Weisse
South Carolina "Gold Sauce"	Tangy & Mustard Based Sauces Whole hog or sometimes just the shoulders. Though the sauce may also contain ketchup and either honey or brown sugar, we focus here on the spice from the mustard. **Featured Cuts:** Pulled Pork, chicken, pork ribs	Blonde Ale Hefeweizen Monk Beers Pale Ales American IPAs Rye Beers Kolsch
East North Carolina	Tangy & Vinegar & Hot & Pepper Based Sauce Featured Cuts: whole hog	IPA American Brown Ale Scotch Ale Various Pilsners American Barley
West North Carolina "Lexington"	Ketchup & Vinegar & Pepper Sauce & Sweet & Thick Western North Carolina sauce is like the E. North version but thickens it up a bit using ketchup and adds some brown sugar to reduce the effect of the vinegar. **Featured Cuts:** Chopped or sliced pork, pulled pork, quartered chicken, "Mop Sauce"	IPA Pilsner Blonde Ale Pale Ales Ambers Dubbel Brown Ales
St. Louis	Sweet & Vinegar & Spicy & Thin **Featured Cuts:** St Louis Ribs, Pork Steaks	IPA German Styled Beers American Brown Ales Brown Lagers Porters Nut Brown

Region	Sauce / Style	Beer Pairings
Nashville	Tangy & Vinegar & Smokey **Featured Cuts:** Brisket, pork tacos, dry ribs, yardbird, sausage, pulled pork, whole hog.	Lagers Bonde Ales Hefeweizen Witbiers Light Beers
Alabama	White & Mayo, Cider Vinegar, Brown Mustard & Horseradish **Featured Cuts:** Chicken and other poultry, pork & coleslaw.	Sour Rauchbier IPA Pilsner Belgian Witbiers
Oklahoma	Ketchup & Worcestershire & Sweet & Tangy. **Featured Cuts:** Brisket, beef, beef ribs, sausage.	Sour Rauchbier India Pale Ale Brown Ale
Florida	Caribbean Spicy & Vinegar. **Featured Cuts:** Mullet, grilled fish.	Kolsch Pilsner India Pale Ale Citrus
Baltimore	Horseradish & Spicy. **Featured Cuts:** Grilled Pit Beef Sandwich.	Light Lager Blonde Pilsner Stout Brown Ale American Wheat IPA Porter
Kentucky	Worcestershire & Gamey. **Featured Cuts:** Mutton, Burgoo, other roasted meats.	Stouts American IPA Coder Amber Bock
Santa Maria	Spicy dry rub, with salsa, not sauced, on oak fire pit. **Featured Cuts:** Tri-tips, top sirloin, ribeye.	Dubbel American Ale Belgian Ales Imperial Stout
Southern	Tangy & Lemon Juice & Tabasco. **Featured Cuts:** Pork, beef & chicken.	Blonde Ale Pilsner Saisons Witbiers

Plan a Party

Cheese	Salad	Soup	Entree	Vegetables	Dessert
Pale Ale + Mild Cheddar	Pale Ale + Grilled Chicken Caesar Salad	Dunkelweizen/Oatmeal Stout & Bean Chili	Pale Ale + Grilled Chicken Thighs	Pale Ale + Grilled Asparagus with Lemon Zest	Pale Ale + Lemon Bars
IPA + Blue Cheese	IPA + Thai Peanut Salad	Pale Ale + Chicken Noodle Soup	IPA + Spicy Pulled Pork	IPA + Spicy Roasted Cauliflower	IPA + Carrot Cake with Cream Cheese Frosting
Amber Ale + Gruyère	Amber Ale + Roasted Beet & Goat Cheese Salad	IPA + Spicy Thai Coconut Soup (Tom Kha)	Amber Ale + BBQ Ribs	Amber Ale + Glazed Carrots with Thyme	Amber Ale + Apple Crisp
Brown Ale + Smoked Gouda	Brown Ale + Warm Spinach & Bacon Salad	Amber Ale + Butternut Squash Soup	Brown Ale + Smoked Sausage	Brown Ale + Mushroom Stroganoff	Brown Ale + Bread Pudding
Porter + Stilton	Porter + Steak & Blue Cheese Salad	Brown Ale + French Onion Soup	Porter + Braised Short Ribs	Porter + Roasted Brussels Sprouts with Balsamic	Porter + Chocolate Lava Cake
Stout + Brie	Stout + Roasted Root Vegetable Salad	Porter + Black Bean Soup	Stout + Smoked Brisket	Stout + Charred Eggplant with Garlic Yogurt	Stout + Espresso Tiramisu
Wheat Beer + Feta	Wheat Beer + Citrus Arugula Salad	Stout + Beef Stew	Wheat Beer + Lemon-Herb Chicken	Wheat Beer + Zucchini Fritters	Wheat Beer + Orange Sorbet
Sour Ale + Chèvre	Sour Ale + Strawberry Spinach Salad	Wheat Beer + Gazpacho	Sour Ale + Duck Confit	Sour Ale + Pickled Vegetable Medley	Sour Ale + Raspberry Cheesecake
Pilsner + Swiss	Pilsner + Greek Salad	Sour Ale + Chilled Cucumber Yogurt Soup	Pilsner + Pork Schnitzel	Pilsner + Corn and Tomato Salad	Pilsner + Vanilla Bean Ice Cream
Amber Lager + Monterey Jack	Amber Lager + Cobb Salad	Pilsner + Miso Soup	Amber Lager + Bacon-Wrapped Meatloaf	Amber Lager + Stuffed Bell Peppers	Amber Lager + Peach Cobbler
Bock + Aged Manchego	Bock + Apple & Walnut Salad	Amber Lager + Corn Chowder	Amber Lager + Bacon-Wrapped Meatloaf	Bock + Sweet Potato Mash	Bock + Chocolate-Dipped Pretzels
Saison + Camembert	Saison + Herbed Quinoa Salad	Bock + Lentil Soup	Bock + Roasted Lamb Shank	Saison + Ratatouille	Saison + Honey Almond Tart
Belgian Dubbel + Morbier		Saison + Rustic Vegetable Soup	Saison + Herb-Crusted Pork Tenderloin	Belgian Dubbel + Roasted Beets with Goat Cheese	Belgian Dubbel + Fig and Walnut Cake
Tripel + Triple Cream Brie			Belgian Dubbel + Glazed Ham		Tripel + Crème Brûlée
Barleywine + Aged Parmesan			Tripel + Moroccan-Spiced Chicken		Barleywine + Dark Chocolate Truffles
			American IPA & Cheeseburger		
			Hoppy Lager & banh mi		
			Pale Ale & Fried Chicken		
			Stout & Salmon with lemon butter		
			Black IPA Brisket		
			Weizenbock & Pulled Pork		

Recipe Index

Beer Can Chicken	28
Pan Fried Pork Chops	30
Chicken Fried Chicken Recipe	32
Bacon Smash Burger	34
Spiced Pork Chops with Apple Chutney	36
BBQ Brisket Nachos	38
Cedar Planked Salmon	40
Braised Beef Short Ribs	42
Crock-Pot Dr. Pepper Shredded Beef	44
Shrimp Tacos with Mango Salsa	46
Santa Fe Pork Medallions with Peach Salsa	48
Grilled Leg of Lamb With Garlic and Lemon	50
Fish Tacos	54
The Best Ever Cheeseburger	56
Cioppino (Fisherman's Stew)	58
Crispy Smoked Pork Belly Recipe	60
Slow Cooker Short Ribs	62
Roast Chicken with Rosemary and Lemon	64
Grilled Chicken Thighs	66
Grilled Ham and Cheese Sandwich	68
Ceviche	71
Smoked Chicken Wrap	73
Bratwurst Stewed with Sauerkraut	75
Smoked Ribeye	77
Shrimp Po' Boy	80
Chicken Satay with Peanut Sauce	82
Smoked Skirt Steak	84
Beef Rouladen	86
Vietnamese Pork Banh Mi Sandwiches	88
Smoked Brisket	91
Pulled Pork Sandwich with Apple Slaw	93
Smoked Ham and Grilled Cheese	96
Cowboy Sliders	98
Pepper Stout Beef	101

Pulled Pork Mac and Cheese	103
Sticky Ribs	105
KC Burnt Ends	107
Crockpot Bourbon BBQ Meatballs	109
Jamaican Jerk Chicken	111
Smoked Baby Back Ribs	113
Chicken in White Wine Sauce	118
Green Chile Stew	120
Carolina Pulled-Pork Sandwiches	122
Crispy Beer Batter Fish	124
Pork Cabbage Rolls	126
Carne Asada Street Tacos	128
Grilled Chicken Caesar Salad	130
Smoked Pork Tenderloin	132
Santa Maria Grilled Tri-Tip Beef	134
Savory Smoked Sausage and Potatoes	137
Chicken Sausage and Vegetable Foil Packet Dinner	139
Flat Iron Steak	141
Caramelized Pork Ribs	143
Taco Chicken Enchiladas	145
Blackened Salmon	150
Sausage Mushroom Pizza	152
Beer Braised Chicken with Carrots and Red Potatoes	154
BBQ Dry Rub Ribs	156
Bourbon Brown Sugar Smoked Pork Loin	158
Smoked Sirloin Steak	160
German Pot Roast in the Slow Cooker (Sauerbraten)	163
Sausage & Pepper Flatbread Pizza	165
Smoked Bologna and Pimiento Cheese Sandwich	167
Stout Beer Chili Recipe	169
Rancher's Texas Chili Recipe (Chili con Carne)	173
London Broil	175
Oven Fried Nashville Hot Chicken	177
Chicken in Ale Sauce	179
Brown Sugar Glazed Pork Chops	181
Baked Ham with Pineapple and Brown Sugar Glaze	183
Garlic Grilled Shrimp Skewers	185

Hot Smoked Salmon	187
Hot Honey Butter Grilled Chicken	189
Penne Arrabiata with Smoked Sausage	191
Reuben Sandwich	193
Slow-Cooker Carnitas Tacos	195
Honey Dijon Mustard Pork Loin	197
Dry Rub Smoked Chicken Wings	199
Crisp Cider-Braised Pork Belly	201

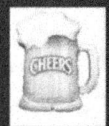

Brewery Spotlight

South Shore Brewery – Bayfield, Wisconsin

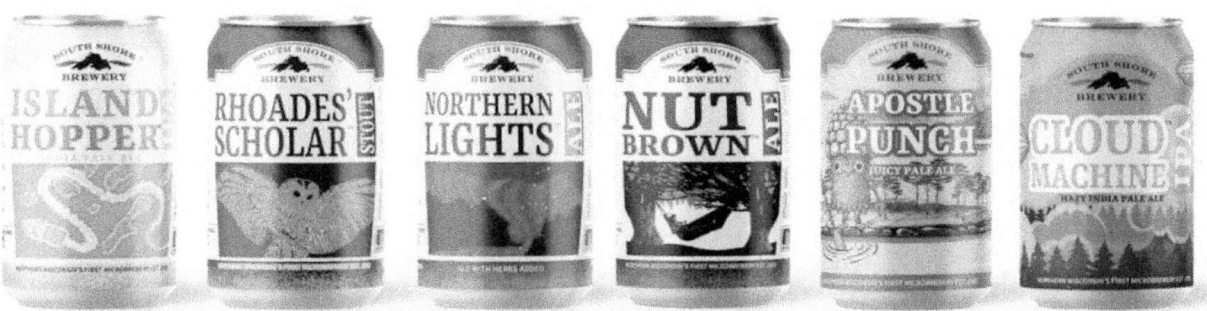

ABOUT THE BREWERY

Founded in 1995, South Shore Brewery is one of Wisconsin's pioneering craft breweries in Bayfield. With a commitment to local ingredients and sustainable brewing, the brewery captures the spirit of Lake Superior in every pint.

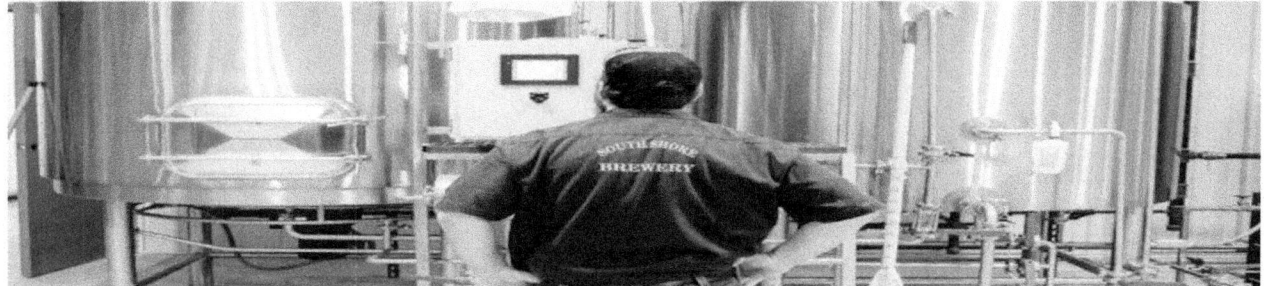

BEER & RECIPE PAIRINGS

Beer	Style	Recipe
Nut Brown Ale	English Brown	Smoked Bologna
Rhoades' Scholar Stout	Oatmeal Stout	Stout Chili
South Shore IPA	American IPA	Hot Honey Chicken
Red Lager	Vienna Lager	Brisket Nachos
Wheat Ale	American Wheat	Grilled Shrimp
Blueberry Ale	Fruit Ale	Baked Ham

CONTACT INFORMATION

Production:
532 W Bayfield St
Washburn, WI 54891

Taproom:
117 Rittenhouse Ave
Bayfield, WI 54814

Phone: (715) 682-9199
Web: southshorebrewery.com

IG: @southshorebrewery
FB: /southshorebrewery
Untappd: South Shore Brewery

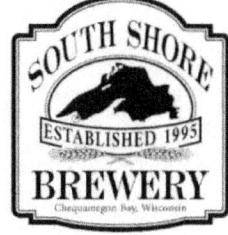

Wisconsin Brewery Directory

Brewery	**Address**	**City**	**Website**

Wisconsin Microbrewery Directory

Microbrewery	Address	City	Website

Wisconsin Taphouse Directory

Taphouse	**Address**	**City**	**Website**

Wisconsin Brewpub Directory

Brewpub	Address	City	Website